CARCINOGENESIS

Edited by **Kathryn Tonissen**

Carcinogenesis
http://dx.doi.org/10.5772/2982
Edited by Kathryn Tonissen

Contributors

Francesca Duraturo, Raffaella Liccardo, Angela Cavallo, Marina De Rosa, Paola Izzo, Maria Auxiliadora Vieira do Carmo, Patrícia Carlos Caldeira, Andrés Castillo, Anna Ptak, Ewa Lucja Gregoraszczuk, Ming-Chei Maa, Tzeng-Horng Leu, Ewa Balcerczak, Aleksandra Sałagacka, Malwina Bartczak-Tomczyk, Marek Mirowski, Maneet Bhatia, Therese C. Karlenius, Giovanna Di Trapani, Kathryn F. Tonissen, Hiroko Kuwabara, Masahiko Yoneda, Zenzo Isogai, M.E. Hernández-Caballero, Jinhui Zhang, Lei Wang, Yong Zhang, Junxuan Lü, Naoki Ashizawa, Takeo Shimo, Magdy Sayed Aly, Amani Abd ElHamid Mahmoud, Pornngarm Limtrakul, Pornsiri Pitchakarn, Shugo Suzuki, Mohamed F. El-Refaei, Essam A. Mady

Published by InTech

Janeza Trdine 9, 51000 Rijeka, Croatia

Publishing Process Manager Oliver Kurelic
Technical Editor InTech Prepress, Novi Sad
Cover InTech Design team

Additional hard copies can be obtained from orders@intechopen.com

Carcinogenesis, Edited by Kathryn Tonissen
p. cm.
ISBN 978-953-51-0945-7

For EU product safety concerns:
IN TECH d.o.o., Prolaz Marije Krucifikse Kozulić 3, 51000 Rijeka, Croatia,
info@intechopen.com or visit our website at intechopen.com.

Meet the editor

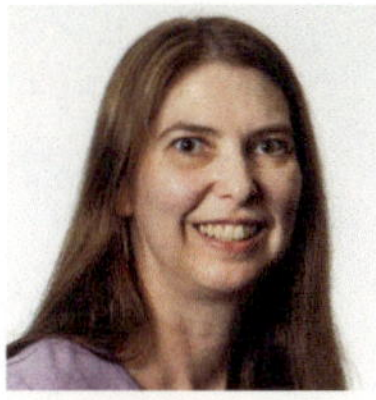

Associate Professor Kathryn Tonissen received her Bachelor of Science with Honours (B.Sc. Hons) degree in 1986 from the University of Adelaide, South Australia. She completed her PhD in biochemistry and molecular biology at the University of Adelaide in 1991, followed by postdoctoral training at the University of Texas at Austin, USA. She is currently an Associate Professor in the School of Biomolecular and Physical Sciences at Griffith University in Brisbane, Australia and a member of the Eskitis Institute for Cell and Molecular Therapies, also based at Griffith University. Her research is focussed on the cellular and molecular aspects of redox control, with a particular emphasis on cancer research and she has published more than 30 papers in international journals.

Contents

Preface

An increased understanding of the molecular, biochemical and cellular processes governing carcinogenesis can only be of benefit in improving the effectiveness of strategies used to prevent and treat cancer. Since cancer is a multifaceted and complex disease a number of factors can contribute to its development and progression. A broad knowledge of these factors may aid in understanding how they interact and influence the processes of initiating and promoting cancer. This in turn enables more effective preventative and therapeutic strategies to be devised and more relevant prognostic tools to be developed. This book includes comprehensive reviews and some specialized experimental findings that cover diverse processes that contribute to carcinogenesis, its diagnosis and treatment. The goal is for these examples to inform and influence a reader's own specialty by stimulating thinking across a diverse range of topics. A cross fertilization of ideas arising from understanding the various preventative, diagnostic and therapeutic approaches together with a broad knowledge of factors that affect cancer progression could be the impetus for further progress in tackling a disease that still exerts a heavy human toll worldwide.

Section 1 includes genetic, molecular and morphological approaches to assessing cancer susceptibility and classifying the risk of developing a cancer. While individual mutations are known to influence cancer formation a knowledge of the synergistic effects of low-risk variant alleles are also important when assessing predisposition to cancer. This section also describes a binary system using morphology and molecular analysis for classifying pre-cancerous lesions into either high or low-risk potential to subsequently develop into oral carcinoma.

Section 2 contains chapters that discuss the various mechanisms and stimuli that may contribute to the initiation of cancer or influence progression of the disease into a metastatic state. These stimuli include infection by the human papillomavirus and hormonal stimuli such as oestrogens. Specific proteins may also play a role in carcinogenesis and therefore have prognostic or therapeutic value. Examples of oncogenes and tumor markers, along with their characterisation in cancer cells, are described in this book. The oxygen environment of a cancer cell is an important determinant of carcinogenesis and a description of the redox and hypoxic signaling pathways and how they influence cancer development and metastasis is provided. The cancer microenvironment also plays a role in cancer progression and is the focus of a chapter that assesses the expression of specific stromal proteins in cancer tissues. Metastasis involves the movement of tumor cells to a distant tissue and the process of epithelial-mesenchymal transition (EMT) is described in detail in the final chapter of this section.

The study of cancer and how it develops, progresses and responds to treatments or chemopreventive agents is often conducted in animal models. Section 3 contains chapters that describe specialized models for studying cancers and offer key insights into interpreting and adapting animal studies into human consequences.

Natural products are increasingly becoming recognised as an important tool for both preventing and treating cancer. Section 4 contains chapters describing naturally sourced compounds, including dietary polyphenols, and their characterisation as chemopreventive or therapeutic agents.

This book is aimed towards researchers, students and medical practitioners wishing to obtain knowledge of the processes that underpin the broader carcinogenesis field. The goal is to inspire new ideas and innovative research directions, so that ultimately cancer will be defeated. The contributions by each of the specialist authors for their chapters and by Professor Krystyna Frenkel for the initial concept and reviews, together with the assistance from the extremely professional staff at InTech is greatly valued and appreciated in preparing this book.

Associate Professor Kathryn Tonissen
School of Biomolecular and Physical Sciences and
Eskitis Institute for Cell and Molecular Therapies
Griffith University
Nathan, Qld
Brisbane
Australia

Section 1

Cancer Pre-Disposition and Pre-Cancerous Risk Classification

Chapter 1

Synergistic Effects of Low-Risk Variant Alleles in Cancer Predisposition

Francesca Duraturo, Raffaella Liccardo,
Angela Cavallo, Marina De Rosa and Paola Izzo

Additional information is available at the end of the chapter

http://dx.doi.org/10.5772/55417

1. Introduction

It has long been known that cancer can be the result of a genetic predisposition. About 5% of total cancers are associated with known Mendelian susceptibility; in these cancer types the clinical manifestations of disease are due to mutations in high-risk alleles, with a penetrance usually at least of 70%. However, there are many tumors in which the cause of hereditary predisposition can not be explained as the Mendelian syndromes. For colorectal cancer (CRC), for example, about 30% of cases are thought to be due to inherited susceptibility, which only in part can be explained by the known Mendelian inheritance, as FAP, MAP and Lynch syndrome [1]. Breast cancer has a similar gap between Mendelian and overall genetic risk. For prostate cancer, the risk is even higher, as very few cases are attributable to high-risk alleles. This gap needs to be filled by studies to identify predisposition alleles that explain the cases of hereditary tumors for which no association with gene variants has been found, so far [2].

With the advent of high-throughput technology it is now possible to analyze a great number of polymorphic variants in large cohorts of cases and controls. These studies have been used successfully by many groups leading to the identification of a large number of rare variant alleles in patients with an inherited risk of cancer [3, 4]. The simultaneous presence of rare genetic variants in the same patient might contribute in a cooperative manner to increase the risk of tumor development. Another problem is represented by variants of unknown significance (VUSs) within the cancer predisposition highly penetrant genes. These variants are usually missense or silent changes which are generally rather uncommon or rare and thus of doubtful clinical relevance, that make troublesome the genetic counseling for these cancer families. The interpretation of these variations is not easy and requires the combination of different analytical strategies to get a proper assessment of their pathogenicity [5]. In some cases, VUSs make a more substantial overall contribution to cancer risk than the well-assessed severe Mendelian variants. It is also possible that the simultaneous presence of some polymorphisms and VUSs in cancer predisposition genes that behave as low-risk alleles, might contribute in a cooperative manner to increase the risk of hereditary cancer [6]. Therefore, current literature data suggest that a significant proportion of the inherited susceptibility to relatively common human diseases may be due to the addition of the effects of a series of low frequency variants of different genes, probably acting in a dominant and independent manner, with each of them conferring a moderate but even detectable increase in the relative cancer-risk.

Our studies are concerned with the molecular basis of the Lynch syndrome, which is commonly associated with mutations in mismatch repair (MMR) genes, MLH1 and MSH2. However, mutations in these genes do not account for all Lynch syndrome families. In our experience we have also identified germ-line genetic variants in the other MMR genes, called minor MMR genes: MSH6, PMS2, MLH3 and MSH3. We have shown that several patients were carriers of at least two genomic variants within the "minor" genes or a VUS in a major gene associated to a genetic variant in minor genes. We therefore speculate that the association between weak alleles in the MMR genes could determine the onset of the tumor.

2. Hereditary cancer syndromes

Over 200 hereditary cancer susceptibility syndromes have been described, the majority of which are inherited in an autosomal dominant manner. Although many of these are rare syndromes, they are thought to account for at least 5–10% of all cancer, amounting to a substantial burden of morbidity and mortality in the human population (Figure 1).

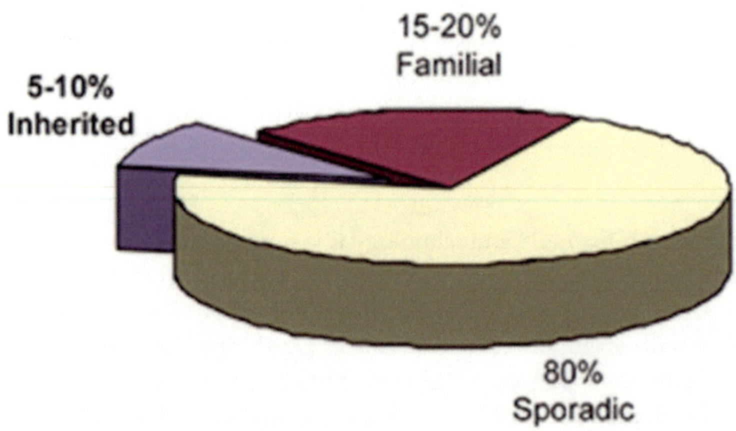

Figure 1. The majority of most common cancers are sporadic, 5–10% are inherited and arise due to highly penetrant germ-line mutations. An additional 10–15% are referred to as 'familial' and may be caused by the interaction of low-penetrance genes, gene–environment interactions, or both.

While characterized by their markedly increased risk of malignancy, these syndromes often predispose to benign tumors and generalized disease, as in Cowden syndrome (CS) and the multiple endocrine neoplasias [7]. When the benign and malignant manifestations are considered together, many of these syndromes show almost complete penetrance by age 70. An inherited cancer susceptibility is suspected in families with the following characteristics: two or more relatives with the same type of cancer on the same side of the family; several generations affected; earlier ages of cancer diagnosis than what is typically seen for that cancer type; individuals with multiple primary cancers; the occurrence of cancers in one family, which are known to be genetically related (such as breast and ovarian cancer, or colon and uterine cancer); and the occurrence of nonmalignant conditions and cancer in the same person and/or family [8]. In table 1 are reported the more frequent hereditary cancer

Syndrome	*MIM#[a]*	*Gene(s)*	*Population incidence*	*Penetrance[b]*
Cowden syndrome	158350	*PTEN*	1/200 000	90–95%
Familial adenomatous polyposis (FAP or MAP)	175100 608456	*APC* *MYH*	1/8000	<100%
Hereditary breast–ovarian cancer syndrome	113705, 600185	*BRCA1 and BRCA2*	1/500 to 1/1000	Up to 85%
Hereditary diffuse gastric cancer	137215	*CDH1*	Unknown, rare	90%
Hereditary nonpolyposis colon cancer	114500	*MLH1, MSH2, MSH6, MLH3, PMS2*	1 in 400	90%
Juvenile polyposis syndrome	174900	*MADH4 (SMAD4), BMPR1A*	1/100 000	90–100%
Li–Fraumeni syndrome	151623	*TP53*	Rare	90–95%
Multiple endocrine neoplasia type 1	131100	*MEN1*	1/100 000	95%
Multiple endocrine neoplasia type 2	171400, 162300	*RET*	1/30 000	70–100%c
Peutz–Jeghers syndrome (PJS)	175200	*LKB1 (STK11)*	1/200 000	95–100%
Retinoblastoma, hereditary (RB)	180200	*RB*	1/13 500 to 1/25 000	90%
von Hippel–Lindau (VHL)	193300	*VHL*	1/36 000	90–95%

[a] MIM numbers beginning with 1 indicate autosomal dominant inheritance; those beginning with 6 are autosomal loci or phenotypes entered into the catalogue after May 1994. [b] Penetrance estimates are up until age 70 years, include both malignant and benign features and with the exception of MEN2, describe clinical penetrance. [c] By biochemical testing (pentagastrin-stimulated calcitonin levels) is 95–100% by age 70.

Table 1. Highly penetrant cancer syndromes

syndromes that are associated with mutations in high penetrance alleles. Because of phenotypic variability, age-related penetrance, and gender-specific cancer risks, however, many families with an inherited cancer syndrome will not meet these criteria. Furthermore, because cancer is relatively common in the general population, it is possible to have a chance clusterings of the same or related cancers within a family. These familial clusterings are most likely due to low-penetrance alleles that are more common than mutations in high penetrant alleles. Thus, they will potentially account for a larger proportion of cancer in the general population than the mendelian classic syndromes. For colorectal cancer (CRC), for example, Mendelian syndrome includes FAP, MAP and Lynch syndrome.

However, about 30% of the variation in CRC risk is thought to be due to inherited susceptibility, which only in part can be explained by the known Mendelian inheritance [2]. Breast cancer has a similar gap between Mendelian and overall genetic risk and for prostate cancer the risk is even higher, as very few cases are attributable to high-risk alleles. It is that gap which must be filled by studies to identify cancer predisposition alleles in the general population [9]. Localization and characterization of low-penetrance alleles are the focus of much research, but the challenges are great due to the multi-factorial nature of cancer and the underlying genetic heterogeneity.

2.1. High-throughput technology for detection of the multiple alleles associated to cancer predisposition

The history of human genetics has focused on mapping regions of the genome that can explain part or all of a disease or human trait.

The 'rare variant hypothesis' proposes that a significant proportion of the inherited susceptibility to relatively common human diseases may be due to the sum of the effects of a series of low frequency variants of a variety of different genes, perhaps dominantly and/or independently acting, each conferring a moderate but detectable increase in relative risk [2]. Regardless, there is good supporting evidence that rare variants will often have stronger effects on cancer risk than common variants. This evidence is based on several works whose purpose was to determine whether evaluating rare single-nucleotide polymorphism (SNPs) in case-control association studies could help to identify causal SNPs for common diseases. The sources of data of these works were generally the International HapMap Project and the SeattleSNPs project and they suggest that slightly deleterious SNPs subjected to weak purifying selection are major players in genetic control of susceptibility to common diseases, including cancer. These results suggests that studies with large sample sizes (5000 and higher) targeting SNPs will be a better strategy to identify causal disease SNPs [10]. Instead, genome wide association studies (GWAS) have emerged as an important tool for discovering regions of the genome that harbor uncommon genetic variants that confer risk for complex tumors, whose nature is probably polygenic [11]. These variants include single nucleotide variants (SNVs) or single nucleotide polymorphisms (SNPs), small insertions and deletions and structural genomic variants.

One of the fundamental elements for the success of GWAS is represented by a large collection of biospecimens in case-control and cohort studies so as to have a high degree of reliability of results. The first approaches in this regard were based on technologies such as the Denaturing High Performance Liquid Chromatography (DHPLC) and classical sequencing analysis, that provide a high degree of analytical sensitivity and specificity. However, the new challenge in the field of biotechnology has surely been to make the techniques increasingly automated in order to process multiple samples simultaneously and especially more quickly.

The method becoming more widely used is high-throughput sequencing, which allows a massive study of DNA. This is a system able to obtain more than 400,000 different readings in a single stroke of about 8 hours. The operating principle is based on clonal amplification of DNA *in vitro* by emulsion PCR and on a protocol of pyrosequencing that, unlike the classic method of Sanger, is based on the detection of pyrophosphate released by the incorporation of a nucleotide during DNA synthesis. In high-throughput sequencing 454 instrumentation, the sample may be any DNA larger than 1500 base pairs (genomic DNA or portions, cDNAs and large amplicons). The sequences obtained are analysed, properly aligned and oriented in contigs from the sequencer software, according to the shotgun and paired-end strategy. The accuracy of the data obtained is measured in terms of "coverage", that is based on the average number of times that each is accessed (read). This technology, therefore, is able to ensure high accuracy of the results (> 99.5%), thanks also to the careful management of the enormous amount of bioinformatics sequences obtained, which minimizes the production of raw redundant data. This feature, coupled with the extraordinary speed of processing, which makes the method also more economical than the classic automated sequencer, allows the user to analyze and quantify at the same time a large amount of samples. Therefore, the sequencer ultra-massive is an extremely versatile technique for a large number of applications such as resequencing and de novo assembly of entire genomes, and the massive sequencing of amplicons.

This latter approach is now widely applied, for example, for the identification of rare variants that presumably contribute in a synergistic way and in association with other factors predisposing to the development of complex genetic diseases characterized by genetic heterogeneity. This technology therefore offers a great contribution to the studies of Genome Wide Association, because it allows quick identification of the allele frequencies of SNPs in population studies, and to analyze a given target gene in multiple genomes, or a panel of target genes in a single patient, even at the level of gene expression (transcriptome analysis) [4]. However, the high number of next generation sequencing information requires accurate statistically studies. The threshold value for discovery has been established at a high level, known as genome-wide significance, which serves two dual purposes [12]. First, it needs careful consideration of the power to detect the effect sizes expected to be observed in the study. Second, the high bar of genome wide significance protects against the probability of a false-positive finding. The latter is critical because GWAS are discovery tools that point investigators toward long arduous follow-up studies for unraveling the underlying biology and the pursuit of markers for risk assessment [11, 13]. However, the common cancer alleles detected by GWAS account for only 10% of the familial relative risk of disease.

2.2. Variants of unknown significance in hereditary cancer predisposition genes

Variants of unknown significance (VUS) within the cancer predisposition genes could be responsible for cancer development, in particular when associated with another VUS or SNPs. The influence of these variants on the development of cancer is often difficult to predict [5, 14]. Several criteria have been established for the characterization of these phenotypic variants, particularly for the missense variants [15, 16]; these criteria included the co-segregation of the variant with the disease and the presence/absence of variation in the healthy population. However, these criteria are not always pursued to establish the pathogenetic significance of these variants [17, 18].

Segregation analysis is not always practicable, since, often the families are small or part of family members is reluctant to participate to molecular investigation. Population studies to exclude the polymorphic nature of the variant is often laborious. Recent studies have revealed new strategies to classify the VUS as pathogenic. These strategies include "in silico" analysis, using computational programs such as PolyPhen (Polymorphism Phenotiping) and SIFT (Sorting Intolerant From Tolerant) to assess whether the VUS missense type falls into a phylogenetically conserved domain and / or makes changes to the physical-chemical properties of proteins [19 -21].

The program Human Splicing Finder (HSF) [22, 23], which simultaneously uses a set of matrices already available on the network is useful to predict the effects of missense, silent and intronic variants on the signals of splicing and to identify regulators motifs associated with the processing of the mRNA. However, the results of the computational accuracy have a predictive value of about 80% and, therefore, do not always reflect the functional consequences of the variant *in vivo*. Several papers suggest to combine the results from several bioinformatics approaches especially those based on amino acid conservation status, to increase the predictive value of about 10% [19, 24].

Other studies complemented "in silico" analysis to a direct study of the mRNA, to confirm or rule out the effects of splicing variants [25, 26]. In addition, many recent literature data emphasize the importance of developing functional assays *in vitro* and *in vivo* to assess the effects of VUS on specific biological functions [18]. All studies conducted so far show that none of the above criteria, including functional assays, is an indicator of pathogenicity, if considered individually; it is necessary that most of these strategies are used in combination with each other so that they can lead to a correct evaluation pathogenicity of numerous variant data.

2.3. The simultaneous presence of low-risk alleles increases the risk of hereditary cancer: review of literature data

Genome–wide association studies in cancer based on high-throughput sequencing approaches have already identified over 150 regions associated with two dozen specific cancers, such as breast, prostate and colorectal cancer, providing new insights into common mechanisms of carcinogenesis. Since each region confers a small contribution to the cancer risk, it is daunting to consider any single nucleotide polymorphism as a clinical test, rather one should think about the synergistic action of different SNP as well as the environmental factor [11, 27]. These studies allowed researchers to identify large susceptibility chromosomal regions for many unrelated cancers. For example, the 8q24 region harbor multiple cancer susceptibility SNP loci associated with prostate cancer, colorectal cancer and precancerous colorectal adenomas, and bladder cancer risk; these loci affect genes such as MYC oncogene and the prostate stem cell antigen gene (PSCA) [11, 28].

Another common cancer susceptibility chromosomal region is the 5p15.33; in this region common variants in the TERT-CLPTM1L have been identified by GWAS in association with the prostate, uterine cervix and skin cancers [11]. TERT is an attractive candidate gene, because it encodes the reverse transcriptase component of the telomerase, a gene that is critical for telomere replication and stabilization by controlling telomere length. TERT promotes epithelial proliferation and telomere maintenance has been implicated in the progression from KRAS-activated adenoma to adenocarcinoma in a murine model. There is additional evidence for its association with bladder, prostate, uterine cervix and skin cancers [11]. Moreover, phenotypic heterogeneity in the breast cancer, such as merging estrogen receptor negative and positive cases, has been need to identify other loci that might contribute to different phenotypes. Preliminary GW analysis has shown that a subset of the discovered loci may be specific to ER-pos breast cancer while select loci could be more important for ER-neg breast cancer [29]. Similar studies have identified an association between coding variants in CASP8 gene and breast cancer [30]. CASP8 belongs to many key pathways, including p53 signaling, apoptosis, and cancer [31]. The decreased risk for breast cancer with CASP8 Asp302His was revealed in an another recent association study [32]. Others proposed that rare variants within the double strand break repair genes CHEK2, BRIP1 and PALB2 predispose to breast cancer [33].

Other large studies have identified 31.7% of the novel gene-variant breast cancer significant associations between 145 variants analyzed. A large GWAS conducted with East Asian women provided convincing evidence for an association with a novel independent susceptibility locus located at 6q25.1, near the TAB2 gene (TGF-beta activated kinase 1). Furthermore this study shows that genetic variants in the ESR1 gene (estrogen receptor 1) may be related to breast cancer risk [34]. A recent study of populations conducted by Smith et al. [35] has pointed out that the simultaneous presence of mutations in the TP53 gene and single nucleotide polymorphisms (SNPs) in genes belonging to different repair systems such as complex BER, NER, MMR and DSBR (Double-Strand Break Repair) is associated with earlier age of onset of breast cancer (<50 years), thus suggesting the idea of an additive or multiplicative effect.

In prostate cancer, there are at least 35 distinct loci harboring common susceptibility alleles identified by GWAS that could distinguish between aggressive and non-aggressive disease, but other studies are required [36]. These analyses were conducted in both European and Asian populations [37]. Moreover, a fine mapping of a region of chromosome 11q13 showed a complex genomic architecture characterized by multiple independent signals contributing to prostate cancer risk. This study further annotates common and uncommon variants across this region. In particular, a variant in the promoter of the MSMB gene on chromosome 10q13, is known to have influence in the gene expression, and in the protein PSP94 (prostate secretory protein 94) levels, showing significant association with prostate cancer. This chromosomal region was extensively resequenced and it is possible that a neighboring gene, the androgen receptor coactivator (NCOA4), could also be a candidate gene for analysis [38]. Moreover, GWAS for chromosomal 19q13.33 region, that harbors the gene responsible for the prostate serum antigene (PSA), suggested that variants in this gene, including a nonsynonymous SNP, could contribute to both prostate carcinogenesis and PSA levels [39].

A large GWAS conducted in several populations (European Americans and African Americans) showed that genetic associations by race are modified by interactions between individual SNPs and prostate cancer and that significance of particular GWAS "hits" is not the same between racial groups. This study highlights the need to conduct GWAS and GWAS replication studies in a variety of racial groups in order to gain a more complete understanding of differences in risk alleles by race and in order to study gene-gene and gene-environment interactions [40]. A similar study conducted in two European populations suggested a list of SNP–SNP interactions that can be followed in other confirmation studies. to explore the etiology of prostate cancer [41].

Finally several papers report numerous GWAS for colorectal cancer, identifying a total of 16 new susceptibility loci for colorectal cancer. SNPs both in common genes as MMR genes and in other novel loci as SMAD7 and MYC seem to associate with different clinical outcomes [42], or different pharmacological responses [43]. Moreover, GWAS for chromosomal 20p12.3 region, a site bereft of genes or predicted protein-encoding transcripts, suggested that particular SNP in this region could contribute to colorectal cancer progression. Interestingly, the bone morphogenetic protein 2 (BMP2) maps 342 kb telomeric to this locus, which is an initiator of BMP signaling by binding to its corresponding receptors. BMP signaling can suppress the Wnt pathway to ensure a balanced control of intestinal stem cell self-renewal. As reflected by earlier studies, mutations of BMP pathway have been described in juvenile polyposis, an inherited syndrome that predisposes to CRC. Considering all this information, it has been speculated that this locus might alter the BMP signaling transduction by the effect on BMP2 and thus affect CRC incidence [44].

A different GWAS study assessed a set of single-nucleotide polymorphisms (SNPs) near 157 DNA repair genes in three studies on colorectal cancer (CRC). Although no individual SNP showed evidence of association, the set of SNPs as a whole was associated with colorectal cancer risk, in particular the MLH1 promoter SNP -93G>A (rs1800734) and rare variants in

CHEK2 (I157T and possibly del1100C) [45]. Numerous GWAS data for susceptibility cancer specially for colorectal cancer have been the subject of several functional studies to demonstrate the effective association and to test the hypothesis of a synergistic effect between low risk allelic variants.

In a recent study on the genome of yeast, it has been shown that the weak alleles of MMR complex cause a weak mutator phenotype, but when these interact with each other cause a strong mutator phenotype. In this work, 11 SNPs and 14 missense variants of doubt pathogenetic meaning, previously identified in these genes, have been studied. The mutator effect of these variants both individually and in combination with each other was assayed by testing complementation, in selective media for the amino acids lysine and tyrosine, and for resistance to canavanine [46]. Finally, Demogines et al. [47] have used yeast strains, that differed in terms of geographic and environmental factors, to demonstrate that the association of polymorphic variants, identified in the MMR genes MLH1 and PMS1, affecting the same or different genetic loci, may act as modifiers intra - or inter-gene and this phenomenon may play a role in both the penetrance of the colorectal disease (mutator phenotype) and in the process of evolutionary adaptation (genomic compatibility).

3. The Lynch syndrome

In this chapter we report the results of our studies on detection of mutations in MisMatch Repair (MMR) genes as responsible for Lynch syndrome. Because many patients with hereditary cancer syndrome did not show mutations in high penetrance genes, we speculate that association of several low penetrance alleles could determine a genetic predisposition to cancer development.

Colon cancer is a multifactorial disease. It's caused by enviromental factors, nutritional factors and genetic predisposition. Our studies are related to the genetic susceptibility of colon cancer, in particular the molecular basis of Lynch syndrome (Hereditary Non Polyposis colorectal cancer, HNPCC). The Lynch Syndrome is one of the syndromes of hereditary cancer with higher incidence in the population [48]. It has an autosomal dominant transmission and occurs in two forms: as Lynch I with an early age of occurrence (25% at 50 years and 70–80% within 70 years), predilection for the proximal colon (60–80%), and high rates of metachronous colorectal cancer (30% at 10 years and 50% at 15 years from the first tumor); and Lynch II, has the same characteristics but also extracolonic tumors involving the uterus (25–60%), ovaries (8–14%), stomach (13%), and urinary tract (4%) (Figure 2).

This syndrome accounts for 5–15% of all colorectal cancers, although the true incidence is unknown, confounded by incomplete penetrance (<80%), rapid progression of adenoma to carcinoma (<5 years), development of extracolonic neoplasms, and the inter- and, occasionally, intra-familiar heterogeneity of the lesions [49]. In Lynch syndrome, the adenomas have the same frequency as in sporadic cases, but a more rapid progression to carcinoma. Due to the deficiency in DNA-repair genes, adenomas accumulate mutations about three times faster than in sporadic disease. These mutations occur predominantly in microsatellite DNA sequences, a condition defined as microsatellite instability (MSI), which are more susceptible to errors in these genes replication because of their repetitive nature. The microsatellite sequences are also present in very important colorectal cancer tumorigenesis genes, thus the accumulation of errors in these genes determine rapid cellular proliferation. MSI is present in over 90% Lynch cases [50]. The clinical diagnosis of Lynch syndrome is performed upon the Amsterdam Criteria (Tab. 2). However, the Amsterdam Criteria do not identify up to 30% of potential Lynch syndrome carriers [51].

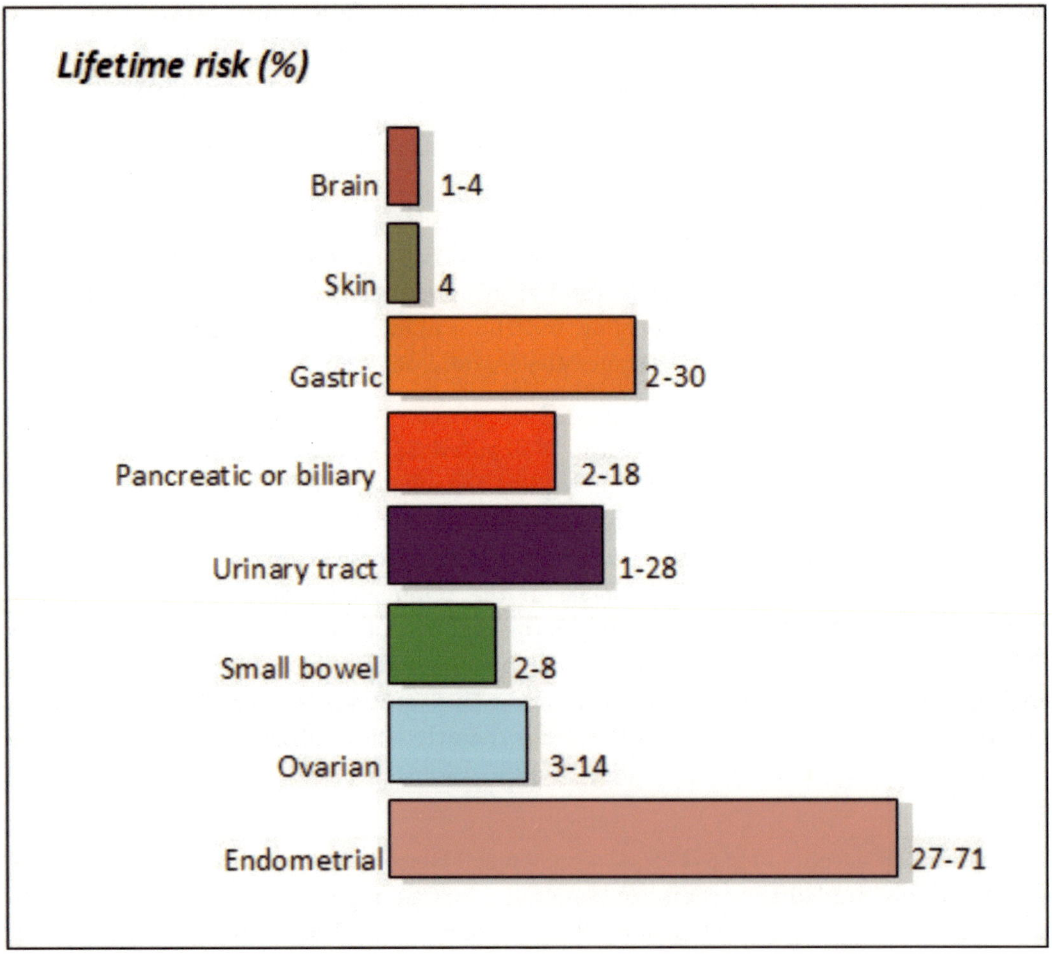

Figure 2. Lifetime Risk of development of cancer associated with Lynch Syndrome.

All of the following must apply for a putative diagnosis of HNPCC to be made in a family
There are at least three relatives with an HNPCC-associated cancer (large bowel, endometrium, small bowel, ureter, or renal pelvis, although not including stomach, ovary, brain, bladder, or skin)
One affected person is a first-degree relative of the other two
At least two successive generations are affected
At least one person was diagnosed before the age of 50 years
Familial adenomatous polyposis has been excluded
Tumors have been verified by pathologic examination

Table 2. Amsterdam Criteria I and II

For this reason, in some patients with colon cancer, as suggested by the Bethesda guidelines (Table 3) [52], it is possible to analyse microsatellite instability in colon tumor specimens, to identify the inefficiency of DNA mismatch repair complex. If there is microsatellite instability, there is a higher likelihood for a Lynch syndrome diagnosis.

Tumors from any of the following should be tested for MSI and then positive patients should continue for MMR testing
Individuals with cancer in families that meet the Amsterdam Criteria
Individuals with two HNPCC-associated cancers, including synchronous and metachronous CRC or associated extracolonic cancers
Individuals with CRC and a first-degree relative with CRC and/or HNPCC-related extracolonic cancer and/or a colorectal adenoma diagnosed at age < 40 years
Individuals with CRC or endometrial cancer diagnosed at age < 45 years
Individuals with right-sided CRC with an undifferentiated pattern (solid or cribriform) on histopathology diagnosed at age < 45 years
Individuals with signet-ring–cell-type CRC diagnosed at age < 45 years
Individuals with adenomas diagnosed at age < 40 years

Table 3. Bethesda Guidelines for MSI Testing

Germ-line mutations in the MLH1 and MSH2 genes account for a majority of families with Lynch Syndrome. The majority of research into mutations has focused on MLH1 and MSH2, however mutations in these two gene are not present in many patients. So far, 10% of mutations in MMR genes have been identified in the MSH6 gene and a total of 5% in MLH3 and PMS2 and very recently germ-line mutations in the MSH3 gene [53]. These genes are defined as "minor MMR genes" because they have redundant functions in mismatch repair in replication. It is known that as well as being involved in mismatch repair in replication, the MMR system also has other functions [54], such as: DNA damage response, diversification of antibody, promotion of meiotic crossover. In these functions the "minor" MMR genes play an important role.

3.1. Results of mutation detection analysis in MMR genes

Recently, several studies have shown that association of low penetrance alleles could determine a genetic predisposition to cancer development [46,47]. For this reason, we studied 63 Lynch families recruited from various health centres in Campania (Southern Italy). Of these, forty families met the Amsterdam criteria and twenty-three patients with high microsatellite instability (MSI-H) met the Bethesda guidelines, in which no pathogenetic germline mutations were identified in MLH1 and MSH2 genes. We performed detection mutation analysis in each minor MMR gene (MSH6, MLH3, PMS2 and MSH3) by DHPLC. All samples exbiting abnormal DHPLC profiles were analyzed by directed sequencing (Figure 3). In our studies we have identified overall 65 genetic variants in these "minor" MMR genes.

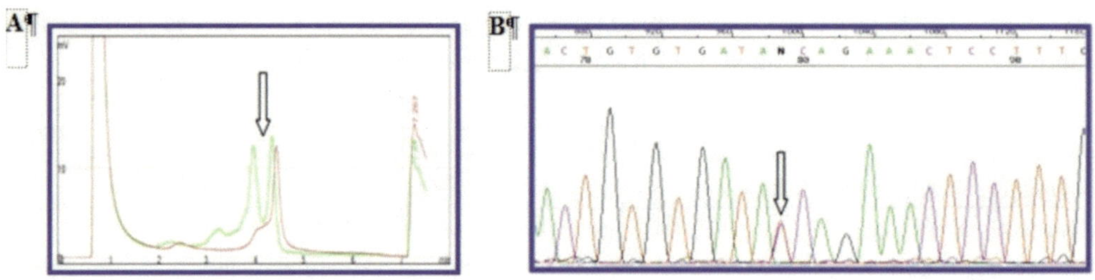

Figure 3. A) Chromatogram and B) electropherogram of the missense mutation c.2732 T>G (Leu>Trp) in MSH3 gene.

The analysis of the damaged point mutations at the structural level is considered to be very important to understand the functional activity of the protein concerned. For this purpose we used the server PolyPhen (bibl), which is available at http://coot.embl.de/PolyPhen/, for missense mutations identified in this study. Moreover, we also used the bioinformatic analysis for the silent and intronic variants.

These variants were analyzed by the software "Human Splicing Finder", a tool to predict the effects of mutations on splicing signals or to identify splicing motifs in any human sequence. Most of these variants result in a polymorphism, which, however, can cause phenotypic variability, affecting the accuracy and efficiency of the protein function [24]. Interestingly, several patients were carriers of at least two genomic variants within the "minor" genes or a VUS in a major gene associated with a genetic variant in minor genes (Table 4).

Recently, the effect of polymorphisms and missense mutations in human MMR genes was studied in a *Saccharomyces cerevisiae*-based system. A number of weak alleles of MMR genes and MMR gene polymorphisms that are capable of interacting with other weak alleles of MMR genes to produce strong polygenic MMR defects, have been identified [46]. A similar situation found in our studies might support the hypothesis that weak MMR gene alleles are capable of polygenic interactions with other MMR gene alleles that might lead to tumour progression in Lynch syndrome.

PATIENTS	*MSH6*	*PMS2*	*MLH3*	*MSH3*	*PHENOTYPE*
9525	ex4 c.2633 T>C (Val>Ala)	ex14 c.2324 A>G (Asn>Ser)	ex1 c.2530 C>T (Pro>Ser) c.2533 T>C (Ser>Pro)	IVS7 -9 T>C	AM+
013		ex6 c.665G>C (Ser>Thr) IVS6 +16A>G	ex1 c.2533 T>C (Ser>Pro)		NO AM MSI-H
103	ex5 c.3261_62insC (Phe>stop)		ex1 c.2533 T>C (Ser>Pro)	ex12 c.1860G>A (Asp>Asn)	NO AM later onset MSI-H
423		IVS12-4G>A	ex1 c.2530 C>T (Pro>Ser) c.2533 T>C (Ser>Pro)		AM+ later onset MSI-L
015	ex5 c.3295_97delTT (Ile>stop)		ex1 c.666 G>A (Lys) c.2191 G>T (Val>Phe) c.2533A>G (Ser>Gly)		AM+ MSI-H
210	ex4 c.2941 A>G (Ile>Val)	IVS6+16A>G ex13 c.2324 T>C (Phe)	ex1 c.2530 C>T (Pro>Ser)	IVS6-64 C>T	AM+
211	ex4 c.2941 A>G (Ile>Val)	IVS12-4 G>A		IVS6-64 C>T	AM+
416		ex11 c.1714C>A (Thr>Lys)	ex 1 c.2027G>A (Arg>Lys)	IVS6-64 C>T	AM+ MSI-H
504*				ex4 c.693G>A (Pro) ex20 c.2732 T>G (Leu>Trp)	AM+ MSI-H

Table 4. Patients carrying variants in several MMR genes: MSH6, PMS2, MSH3, MLH3; *the patient shows also the UV in MSH2 gene (c.984 C>T)

In detail, we report the case of a Lynch family with mutations in several MMR genes. The index case of family 504 (II-5 in Figure 4), who had developed an adenocarcinoma of the left colon at the age of 34 years, an adenocarcinoma of the right colon at the age of 53 years and a new malignancy of the colon at 59 years of age, show two mutations in MSH3 gene, the c.2732 T>G in exon 20 and c.693 G>A in exon 4, and an UV within the MSH2 gene, the c.984 C>T in exon 6. The PolyPhen in silico analysis showed that the missense variant in MSH3 might alter the function of the protein, because it falls into a highly conserved region in different species, while the silent variant, analyzed by HSF could affect the splicing process.

To elucidate whether the mutation was associated with the disease in this family, we analysed another eight members. These variants was found in a brother of the index case, with the same phenotype. Instead, another brother (II-8 in Fig. 4) showed only a variant in the MSH2 gene and no genetic variants in the MSH3 gene. This patient had developed a polyp of the colon at 47 years of age. Today he is 59 years old, undergoes regular colonoscopy and so far has not presented other polyps. In the third generation (Fig. 4), we analysed four affected family members. Subjects III-1 and III-2, in Figure 4, showed a silent variant in MSH3 and a variant in MSH2; both subjects showed an early-onset right colon tumour. Subjects III-3 and III-4, in Figure 4, the sons of our proband, developed colon cancer at 36 years of age and a tubular adenoma of the colon at 34 years of age, respectively. Both subjects showed a silent variant in MSH2 and a missense variant and a silent variant in MSH3. The MSI analysis performed on DNA extracted from tumour tissues of patients II-5 and III-3 showed an MSI-H status. Thus, both subjects presented a strong mutator phenotype, probably due to an additive effect by several variants that leads to inefficiency of the MMR complex. The other family members analysed showed only one mutation in the MSH3 gene and they do not present a typical phenotype of Lynch syndrome (Tab.4). Therefore, it is clear that all subjects in this family with the Lynch phenotype showed the c.984T allele of MSH2 and a germ-line variant in the MSH3 gene (a missense and/or silent variant).

Patients belonging to other families showed mutations in several MMR genes; however, for these families it wasn't possible to perform segregation analysis of mutations with disease because no other family members were available for the analysis. In conclusion, several germ-line variants have been identified in several MMR genes using a DHPLC procedure; a method robust, automated, highly sensitive, fast, feasible and particularly useful for high-throughput analyses.

On the basis of this study, it is conceivable to hypothesize a model in which these genetic variants behave as low-risk alleles that contribute to the risk of colon cancer in Lynch families, mostly together with other low-risk alleles of other MMR genes. Therefore, if our assumptions are correct, these studies may indicate a novel inheritance model in the Lynch syndrome, and might suggest that the risk alleles identified to date represent just the tip of an iceberg of risk variants likely to include hundreds of modest effects and possibly thousands of very small effects. This could pave the way toward new diagnostic perspectives. Moreover, The same situation could occur in other forms of hereditary cancer and it may explain the large number of cases remained unresolved as well as the phenotypic heterogeneity that characterizes all hereditary cancer syndromes.

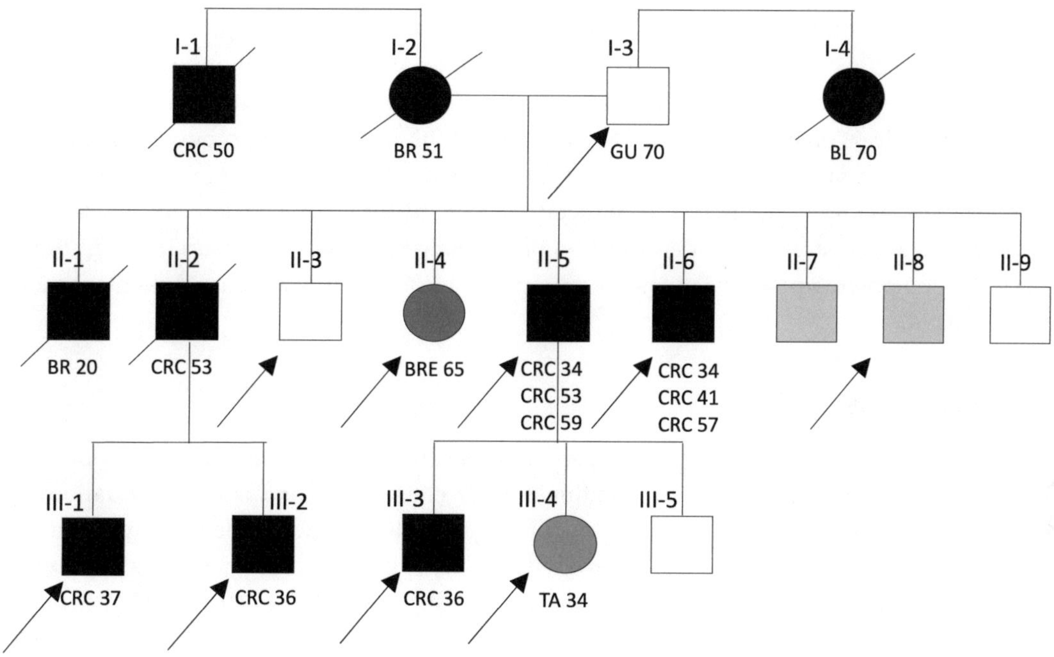

Figure 4. Pedegree of 504 family [53]. Symbols and abbreviations used are denoted as fellow: Arrows, analysed members of family; black symbol, colorectal cancer or cancer associate with HNPCC; gray symbols, adenomas or cancer not associated with HNPCC; CRC, colorectal cancer; Br, brain cancer; GU, gastric ulcer; BL, bladder cancer; Bre, breast cancer; TA, tubular adenoma. Number next to diagnosis denote age at oneset; l not detected.

PATIENT	c.984C>T EX6 MSH2	c.693G>A EX 4 MSH3	c.2732T>G EX20 MSH3
I-3	NO	YES	NO
II-3	NO	NO	YES
II-4	NO	YES	NO
II-5	YES	YES	YES
II-6	YES	YES	YES
II-8	YES	NO	NO
II-9	NO	YES	NO
III-1	YES	YES	NO
III-2	YES	YES	NO
III-3	YES	NO	YES
III-4	YES	YES	NO

Table 5. Genotypes of analysed patients; the patients are identified with number of pedigree (Fig.4).

4. Further research

The Lynch syndrome is associated mainly with germ-line mutations in MSH2 and MLH1 genes. However, mutational analysis of these two genes do not always provide informative results for genetic counseling of patients with a clinical diagnosis strongly predisposing to cancer development. Therefore, these subjects are considered candidates with simultaneous molecular analysis of all MMR genes. For this reason, high-throughput sequencing could be considered as an analytical approach that adapts better to clarify the molecular basis for each subject with a significant colorectal cancer history. In the future, these new technologies will enable faster identification of the molecular basis of cancer; it will improve the genotype-phenotype correlations the purpose of implementing a clinical treatment more personalized.

5. Conclusions

A field of biology where the "high-throughput technologies" is now widely applied is certainly the genetics of cancer for identification of constitutive and somatic mutations of putative genes associated with hereditary predisposition to cancer, particularly for those diseases characterized by genetic heterogeneity. Nowadays, we are witnessing a revolution in oncologic medicine, and the hope is that an increasing understanding of genetics will one day unlock the potential of personalized medicine. Clinical cancer genetics has traditionally been associated with risk estimation. Genome-wide germ-line mutation analysis will result in the identification of new cancer-associated alleles across the spectrum of risk. This may in time permit more precise estimation of development cancer risk. The new genetics will bridge the gap between germ-line and somatic genetics; prior analysis of the genetic makeup of the person and their tumour at time of diagnosis will be needed in order to tailor therapy. Central to this endeavour will be the increasing use of next-generation sequencers as whole cancer genomes become unravelled, revealing critical pathways that drive tumour progression and resistance. In the future these new technologies will enable faster identification of the molecular basis of cancer and thus improve the genotype-phenotype correlations, in order to implement more personalized monitoring and clinical treatment.

Nomenclature

den Dunnen JT, Antonarakis SE. *"Nomenclature for the description of human sequence variations"*. Hum Genet. *2001 Jul;109(1):121-4.*

Author details

Francesca Duraturo, Raffaella Liccardo, Angela Cavallo, Marina De Rosa and Paola Izzo
Department of Molecular Medicine and Medical Biotechnologie, University of Naples Federico II, Italy

Acknowledgement

Ministero Salute - Ricerca Oncologica - RECAM-2006-353005; PRIN 2007-prot. 2007EN8F7T-004

6. References

[1] van Wezel T, Middeldorp A, Wijnen JT, Morreau H. A review of the genetic background and tumour profiling in familial colorectal cancer. Wijnen JT, Morreau H. Mutagenesis. 2012; 27(2):239-45.

[2] Bodmer W., Tomlinson I. Rare genetic variants and the risk of cancer. Current Opinion in Genetics & Development 2010; 20:262–267

[3] Zhang J., Chiodinic R Badra A., Zhang G. The impact of next-generation sequencing on genomics. J Genet Genomics 2011; 38(3): 95-109.

[4] Mardis ER. Next-generation DNA sequencing methods. Annu Rev Genomics Hum Genet. 2008;9:387-402.

[5] Couch FJ., Rasmussen LJ., Hofstra R, Monteiro AN, Greenblatt MS, de Wind N; IARC Unclassified Genetic Variants Working Group. Assessment of functional effects of unclassified genetic variants. Hum Mutat. 2008;29(11):1314-26.

[6] Chung CC., Chanock SJ. Current status of genome-wide association studies in cancer. Hum Genet (2011) 130:59–78

[7] Galatola M, Paparo L, Duraturo F, Turano M, Rossi GB, Izzo P, De Rosa M. Beta catenin and cytokine pathway dysregulation in patients with manifestations of the "PTEN hamartoma tumor syndrome". BMC Med Genet. 2012; 13:28.

[8] Frank TS, Critchfield GC. Hereditary risk of women's cancers. Best Pract Res Clin Obstet Gynaecol. 2002;16(5):703-13.

[9] Bodmer W., Bonilla C. Common and rare variants in multifactorial susceptibility to common diseases Nat Genet 2008; 40:695 701

[10] Gorlov IP, Gorlova OY, Sunyaev SR, Spitz MR, Amos CI.. Shifting paradigm of association studies: value of rare single-nucleotide polymorphisms. Am J Hum Genet. 2008; 82(1):100-12.

[11] Chung CC., Magalhaes W., Gonzalez-Bosquet J., Chanock SJ. Genome-wide association studies in cancer—current and future directions. Carcinogenesis 2010; 31(1): 111–120.

[12] Barrett JC, Cardon LR. Evaluating coverage of genome-wide association studies. Nat Genet. 2006;38(6):659-62.

[13] Erichsen HC, Chanock SJ. SNPs in cancer research and treatment. Br J Cancer. 2004 Feb 23;90(4):747-51.

[14] Syngal S., Fox EA., Li C, Dovidio M, Eng C, Kolodner RD, Garber JE.Interpretation of genetic test results for hereditary nonpolyposis colorectal cancer: implications for clinical predisposition testing. JAMA. 1999; 282(3):247-53.

[15] Goldgar DE., Easton DF., Byrnes GB, Spurdle AB, Iversen ES, Greenblatt MS; IARC Unclassified Genetic Variants Working Group. Genetic evidence and integration of various data sources for classifying uncertain variants into a single model. Hum Mutat. 2008; 29(11):1265-72.

[16] Plon SE., Eccles DM., Easton D, Foulkes WD, Genuardi M, Greenblatt MS, Hogervorst FB, Hoogerbrugge N, Spurdle AB, Tavtigian SV; IARC Unclassified Genetic Variants Working Group. Sequence variant classification and reporting: recommendations for improving the interpretation of cancer susceptibility genetic test results. Hum Mutat. 2008; 29(11):1282-91.

[17] Hofstra RM., Osinga J, Buys CH.Mutations in Hirschsprung disease: when does a mutation contribute to the phenotype. Eur J Hum Genet. 1997; 5(4):180-5.

[18] Ou J., Niessen RC.,Lutzen A., Sijmons RH., Kleibeuker JH., deWind N., Rasmussen LJ., Hofstra RMW. Functional analysis helps to clarify the clinical importance of unclassified variants in DNA mismatch repair genes. Hum Mutat. 2007; 28(11):1047-54.

[19] Chan PA., Duraisamy S., Miller PJ, Newell JA, McBride C, Bond JP, Raevaara T, Ollila S, Nyström M, Grimm AJ, Christodoulou J, Oetting WS, Greenblatt MS. Interpreting missense variants: comparing computational methods in human disease genes CDKN2A, MLH1, MSH2, MECP2, and tyrosinase (TYR). Hum Mutat. 2007;28(7):683-93

[20] http://blocks.fhcrc.org/sift/SIFT.html

[21] http://genetics.bwh.harvard.edu/pph/

[22] Desmet FO, Hamroun D, Lalande M, Collod-Béroud G, Claustres M, Béroud C. Human Splicing Finder: an online bioinformatics tool to predict splicing signals. Nucleic Acids Res. 2009; 37(9):e67.

[23] www.umd.be/HSF/

[24] Duraturo F. Eterogeneità genetica e fenotipica nella Sindrome di Lynch: nuove implicazioni diagnostiche. Thesis of medical Genetics specialization. La Sapienza University of Rome; 2009.

[25] Pagenstecher C., Wehner M., Friedl W, Rahner N, Aretz S, Friedrichs N, Sengteller M, Henn W, Buettner R, Propping P, Mangold E.Aberrant splicing in MLH1 and MSH2 due to exonic and intronic variants. Hum Genet. 2006; 119(1-2):9-22.

[26] Naruse H., Ikawa N., Yamaguchi K, Nakamura Y, Arai M, Ishioka C, Sugano K, Tamura K, Tomita N, Matsubara N, Yoshida T, Moriya Y, Furukawa Y.Determination of splice-site mutations in Lynch syndrome (hereditary non-polyposis colorectal cancer) patients using functional splicing assay. Fam Cancer. 2009;8(4):509-17.

[27] Chanock S. Candidate genes and single nucleotide polymorphisms (SNPs) in the study of human disease. Dis Markers. 2011;17(2):89-98.

[28] Yeager M, Orr N, Hayes RB, Jacobs KB, Kraft P, Wacholder S, Minichiello MJ, Fearnhead P, Yu K, Chatterjee N, Wang Z, Welch R, Staats BJ, Calle EE, Feigelson HS, Thun MJ, Rodriguez C, Albanes D, Virtamo J, Weinstein S, Schumacher FR, Giovannucci E, Willett WC, Cancel-Tassin G, Cussenot O, Valeri A, Andriole GL, Gelmann EP, Tucker M, Gerhard DS, Fraumeni JF Jr, Hoover R, Hunter DJ, Chanock SJ, Thomas G. Genome-wide association study of prostate cancer identifies a second risk locus at 8q24. Nat Genet. 2007; 39(5):645-9.

[29] García-Closas M, Hein DW, Silverman D, Malats N, Yeager M, Jacobs K, Doll MA, Figueroa JD, Baris D, Schwenn M, Kogevinas M, Johnson A, Chatterjee N, Moore LE, Moeller T, Real FX, Chanock S, Rothman N. A single nucleotide polymorphism tags variation in the arylamine N-acetyltransferase 2 phenotype in populations of European background. Pharmacogenet Genomics. 2011;21(4):231-6.

[30] Cox A, Dunning AM, Garcia-Closas M, Balasubramanian S, Reed MW, Pooley KA, Scollen S, Baynes C, Ponder BA, Chanock S, Lissowska J, Brinton L, Peplonska B, Southey MC, Hopper JL, McCredie MR, Giles GG, Fletcher O, Johnson N, dos Santos Silva I, Gibson L, Bojesen SE, Nordestgaard BG, Axelsson CK, Torres D, Hamann U, Justenhoven C, Brauch H, Chang-Claude J, Kropp S, Risch A, Wang-Gohrke S, Schürmann P, Bogdanova N, Dörk T, Fagerholm R, Aaltonen K, Blomqvist C, Nevanlinna H, Seal S, Renwick A, Stratton MR, Rahman N, Sangrajrang S, Hughes D, Odefrey F, Brennan P, Spurdle AB, Chenevix-Trench G; Kathleen Cunningham Foundation Consortium for Research into Familial Breast Cancer, Beesley J, Mannermaa A, Hartikainen J, Kataja V, Kosma VM, Couch FJ, Olson JE, Goode EL, Broeks A, Schmidt MK, Hogervorst FB, Van't Veer LJ, Kang D, Yoo KY, Noh DY, Ahn SH, Wedrén S, Hall P, Low YL, Liu J, Milne RL, Ribas G, Gonzalez-Neira A, Benitez J, Sigurdson AJ, Stredrick DL, Alexander BH, Struewing JP, Pharoah PD, Easton DF. A common coding variant in CASP8 is associated with breast cancer risk. Nat Genet. 2007; 39(3):352-8.

[31] Grenet J, Teitz T, Wei T, Valentine V, Kidd VJ. Structure and chromosome localization of the human CASP8 gene. Gene. 1999;226(2):225-32.

[32] Sigurdson AJ, Bhatti P, Doody MM, Hauptmann M, Bowen L, Simon SL, Weinstock RM, Linet MS, Rosenstein M, Stovall M, Alexander BH, Preston DL, Struewing JP, Rajaraman P. Polymorphisms in apoptosis- and proliferation-related genes, ionizing radiation exposure, and risk of breast cancer among U.S. Radiologic Technologists. Cancer Epidemiol Biomarkers Prev. 2007;16(10):2000-7.

[33] McInerney NM, Miller N, Rowan A, Colleran G, Barclay E, Curran C, Kerin MJ, Tomlinson IP, Sawyer E. Evaluation of variants in the CHEK2, BRIP1 and PALB2 genes in an Irish breast cancer cohort. Breast Cancer Res Treat. 2010;121(1):203-10.

[34] Long J, Cai Q, Sung H, J, Zhang B, Choi JY, Wen W, Delahanty RJ, Lu W, Gao YT, Shen H, Park SK, Chen K, Shen CY, Ren Z, Haiman CA, Matsuo K, Kim MK, Khoo US, Iwasaki M, Zheng Y, Xiang YB, Gu K, Rothman N, Wang W, Hu Z, Liu Y, Yoo KY, Noh

DY, Han BG, Lee MH, Zheng H, Zhang L, Wu PE, Shieh YL, Chan SY, Wang S, Xie X, Kim SW, Henderson BE, Le Marchand L, Ito H, Kasuga Y, Ahn SH, Kang HS, Chan KY, Iwata H, Tsugane S, Li C, Shu XO, Kang DH, Zheng W.Genome-Wide Association Study in East Asians Identifies Novel Susceptibility Loci for Breast Cancer. PLoS Genet. 2012;8(2):e1002532.

[35] Smith TR., Liu-Mares W., Van Emburgh BO., Levine EA., Allen GO., Hill JW., Reis IM., Kresty LA., Pegram MD., Miller MS., Hu JJ. Genetic polymorphisms of multiple DNA repair pathways impact age at diagnosis and TP53 mutations in breast cancer. Carcinogenesis. 2011;32(9):1354-60.

[36] Wiklund FE, Adami HO Zheng SL, Stattin P, Isaacs WB, Gronberg H, Xu J.. Established prostate cancer susceptibility variants are not associated with disease outcome. Cancer Epidemiol Biomarkers Prev 2009; 18(5):1659–1662.

[37] Kim HC, Lee JY, Sung H, Choi JY, Park SK, Lee KM, Kim YJ, Go MJ, Li L, Cho YS, Park M, Kim DJ, Oh JH, Kim JW, Jeon JP, Jeon SY, Min H, Kim HM, Park J, Yoo KY, Noh DY, Ahn SH, Lee MH, Kim SW, Lee JW, Park BW, Park WY, Kim EH, Kim MK, Han W, Lee SA, Matsuo K, Shen CY, Wu PE, Hsiung CN, Lee JY, Kim HL, Han BG, Kang D .A genome-wide association study identifies a breast cancer risk variant in ERBB4 at 2q34: results from the Seoul Breast Cancer Study. Breast Cancer Res. 2012;14(2): R56

[38] Thomas G, Jacobs KB, Yeager M, Kraft P, Wacholder S, Orr N, Yu K, Chatterjee N, Welch R, Hutchinson A, Crenshaw A, Cancel-Tassin G, Staats BJ, Wang Z, Gonzalez-Bosquet J, Fang J, Deng X, Berndt SI, Calle EE, Feigelson HS, Thun MJ, Rodriguez C, Albanes D, Virtamo J, Weinstein S, Schumacher FR, Giovannucci E, Willett WC, Cussenot O, Valeri A, Andriole GL, Crawford ED, Tucker M, Gerhard DS, Fraumeni JF Jr, Hoover R, Hayes RB, Hunter DJ, Chanock SJ. Multiple loci identified in a genome-wide association study of prostate cancer. Nat Genet. 2008;40(3):310-5.

[39] Parikh H, Wang Z, Pettigrew KA, Jia J, Daugherty S, Yeager M, Jacobs KB, Hutchinson A, Burdett L, Cullen M, Qi L, Boland J, Collins I, Albert TJ, Vatten LJ, Hveem K, Njølstad I, Cancel-Tassin G, Cussenot O, Valeri A, Virtamo J, Thun MJ, Feigelson HS, Diver WR, Chatterjee N, Thomas G, Albanes D, Chanock SJ, Hunter DJ, Hoover R, Hayes RB, Berndt SI, Sampson J, Amundadottir L. Fine mapping the KLK3 locus on chromosome 19q13.33 associated with prostate cancer susceptibility and PSA levels. Hum Genet. 2011;129(6):675-85.

[40] Barnholtz-Sloan JS, Raska P, Rebbeck TR, Millikan RC. Replication of GWAS Hits by Race for Breast and Prostate Cancers in European Americans and African Americans. Front Genet. 2011;2:37.

[41] Tao S, Feng J, Jin G, Hsu FC, Chen SH, Kim ST, Wang Z, Zhang Z, Zheng SL, Isaacs WB, Xu J, Sun J. Genome-wide two-locus epistasis scans in prostate cancer using two European populations. Hum Genet. 2012, DOI: 10.1007/s00439-012-1148-4.

[42] Dai J, Gu J, Huang M, Eng C, Kopetz ES, Ellis LM, Hawk E, Wu X. GWAS-identified colorectal cancer susceptibility loci associated with clinical outcomes. Carcinogenesis. 2012 0 (0): 1–5.

[43] Fernandez-Rozadilla C, Cazier JB, Cazier JB, Moreno V, Crous-Bou M, Guinó E, Durán G, Lamas MJ, López R, Candamio S, Gallardo E, Paré L, Baiget M, Páez D, López-Fernández LA, Cortejoso L, García MI, Bujanda L, González D, Gonzalo V, Rodrigo L, Reñé JM, Jover R, Brea-Fernández A, Andreu M, Bessa X, Llor X, Xicola R, Palles C, Tomlinson I, Castellví-Bel S, Castells A, Ruiz-Ponte C, Carracedo A.. A. Pharmacogenomics in colorectal cancer: a genome-wide association study to predict toxicity after 5-fluorouracil or FOLFOX administration. Pharmacogenomics J. doi:10.1038/tpj.2012.2

[44] Zheng X, Wang L, Zhu Y, Guan Q, Li H, Xiong Z, Deng L, Lu J, Miao X, Cheng L. The SNP rs961253 in 20p12.3 Is Associated with Colorectal Cancer Risk: A Case-Control Study and a Meta-Analysis of the Published Literature. PLoS One. 2012;7(4):e34625.

[45] Tomlinson IP, Houlston RS, Montgomery GW, Sieber OM, Dunlop MG. Investigation of the effects of DNA repair gene polymorphisms on the risk of colorectal cancer. Mutagenesis. 2012;27(2):219-23.

[46] Martinez SL, Kolodner RD., Functional analysis of human mismatch repair gene mutations identifies weak alleles and polymorphisms capable of polygenic interactions. Proc Natl Acad Sci U S A. 2010;107(11):5070-5.

[47] Demogines A., Wong A., Aquadro C, Alani E. Incompatibilities involving yeast mismatch repair genes: a role for genetic modifiers and implications for disease penetrance and variation in genomic mutation rates. PLoS Genet. 2008;4(6):e1000103.

[48] Duraturo F. Analisi mutazionale dei geni del mismatch repair (MMR) mediante tecniche innovative in pazienti affetti da cancro ereditario non poliposico del colon-retto (HNPCC). PhD thesis. Federico II University, Naples; 2006.

[49] Carlomagno N, Duraturo F, Rizzo G, Cremone C, Izzo P, Renda A. Carcinogenesis. In: Renda A, ed. The Hereditary Syndromes. Springer-Verlag Italia, Inc., 2009. 107-128

[50] Boland CR, Goel A. Microsatellite instability in colorectal cancer. Gastroenterology 2010; 138(6):2073-84.

[51] Olschwang S., Bonaiti C. HNPCC syndrome (Hereditary Non Polyposis Colon Cancer) : identification and management. RevMed 2006; 54(4):215-29.

[52] Humar A, Boland CR. Revised Bethesda Guidelines for hereditary non polyposis colorectal cancer (Lynce Syndrome) and microsatellite instability. Journal Natl Cancer Inst. 2004; 18;96(4):261-8.

[53] Duraturo F, Liccardo R, Cavallo A, De Rosa M, Grosso M, Izzo P.. Association of low-risk MSH3 and MSH2 variant alleles with Lynch syndrome: probability of synergistic effects". Int J Cancer. 2011;129(7):1643-50.

[54] Jun S.-H., Kim TG., Ban C. DNA mismatch repair system. Classical and fresh roles. FEBS Journal 2006; 273: 1609-19.

Chapter 2

Binary System of Grading Epithelial Dysplasia in Oral Leukoplakias

Maria Auxiliadora Vieira do Carmo and Patrícia Carlos Caldeira

Additional information is available at the end of the chapter

http://dx.doi.org/10.5772/54466

1. Introduction

Cancers of the oral cavity and oropharynx account for approximatelly 3% of all malignancies among men and 2% among women in the United States, and oral squamous cell carcinoma represents 90% of these tumors. Despite great achievements concerning surgery, radiation and chemotherapy, survival rates in 5 years remain near 50 to 55%. As this survival time is directly related to the time of diagnosis of the lesion, prevention and early diagnosis remain important aspects to reduce incidence of the disease, as well as to enhance the survival rate of patients [1,2].

Oral squamous cell carcinoma can be preceded by potentially malignant alterations [1,3]. Such alterations are classified as potentially malignant due to the following evidence: 1) it was observed that these lesions evolved to malignant ones during follow-up; 2) typical alterations of potentially malignant lesions are seen co-existing in the margins of squamous cell carcinoma; 3) a proportion of these lesions show cytological and morphological alterations that are observed in malignant lesions; 4) some chromosomal, genomic, and molecular alterations are found in both, potentially malignant and malignant lesions [4].

1.1. Definition, epidemiology, and etiology of oral leukoplakias

In a recently published paper, leukoplakia has been defined as "a white plaque of questionable risk having excluded (other) known diseases or disorders that carry no increased risk for cancer" [5]. Nevertheless, the most used definition of leukoplakia is still the one proposed by the World Health Organization (WHO) in 1978, which states that "leukoplakia is a predominantly white patch that cannot be characterized clinically or histopathologically as any other definable lesion" [6,7].

Oral leukoplakia (OL) is the most common potentially malignant lesion of the oral mucosa [1,3]. In a published systematic review [8], the author estimated a global prevalence of OL of

2.6%, which is in accordance with the consensus that OL prevalence is between 1% and 5% [9,10]. However, isolated reports show variable rates from 0.5% to 26.92% [8].

OL is more frequent in middle-aged and elderly men, with higher indexes correlated with increased age. The most common sites are cheek, alveolar mucosa, and lower lip [1]. Nonetheless, lesions affecting the floor of the mouth, lateral border of tongue, and lower lip seem to present displastic or malignant alterations more frequently [1,9].

The main risk factor associated with OL is the use of tobacco. OL is six times more frquent among smokers than non-smokers [10]. The effects of alcohol, betel, human papiloma virus, and diet are associated as well, but their exact role is yet to be established [1,9-11]. In addition, there are some OL for which no obvious aetiological factor can be identified, and these lesions are named idiopathic leukoplakias. It is believed that such lesions are significantly more prone to develop into cancer than those OL with known causative factors [9].

1.2. Clinical and histological features

Clinically, OL can be classified as homogeneous and non-homogeneous lesions. Homogeneous OL arises as a white patch slightly elevated, thin, white to gray, uniform, and can present well defined borders or may gradually mix with normal adjacent mucosa (Figure 1 to 3). Non-homogeneous OL can be nodular, verrucous, or speckled (erythroplastic) (Figure 4) [4,10].

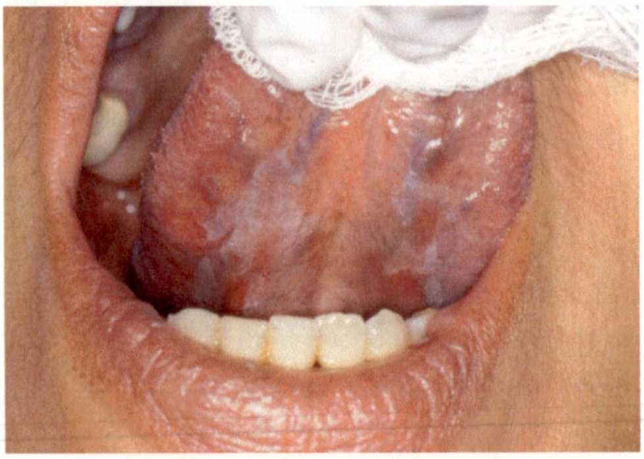

Figure 1. Homogeneous thin leukoplakia in the tongue.

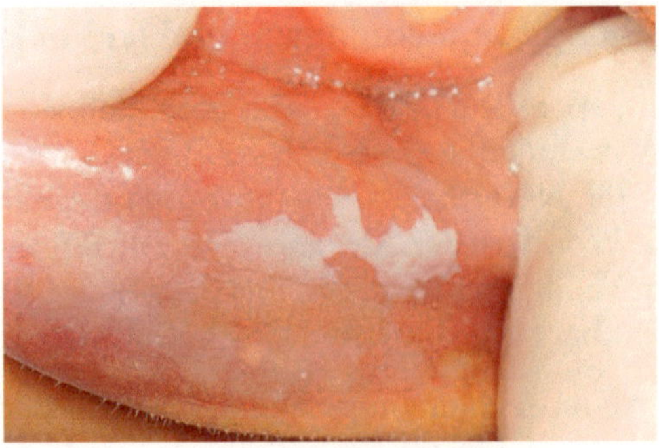

Figure 2. Homogeneous leukoplakia in the lower lip.

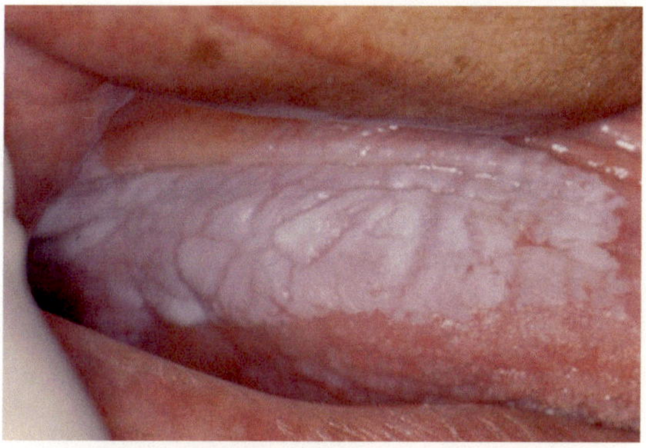

Figure 3. Homogeneous thick leukoplakia in the tongue.

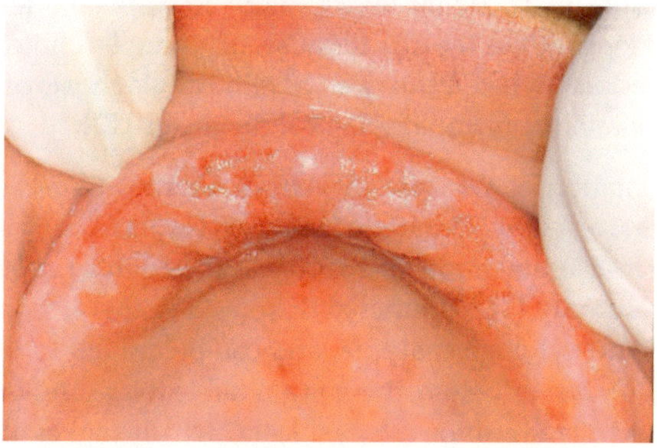

Figure 4. Non-homogeneous (speckled) leukoplakia in the upper alveolar ridge.

There is also the proliferative verrucous leukoplakia, characterized by multifocal evolvement, mainly in elderly female patients that do not present known risk factors (Figure 5 and 6). These lesions are usually resistant to treatment and show a high risk for malignant transformation [4,10].

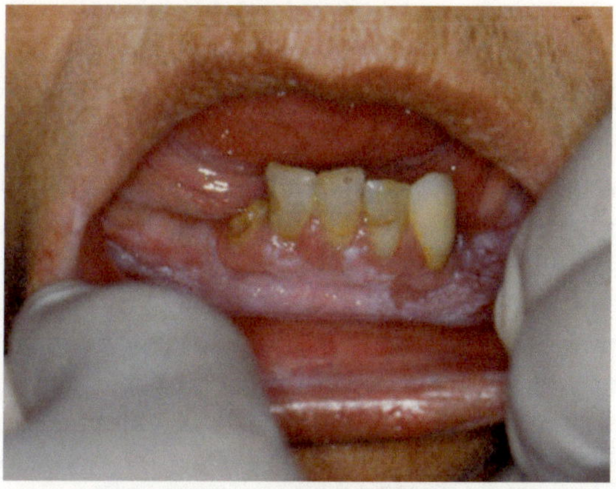

Figure 5. Proliferative verrucous leukoplakia. Notice the multifocal involvement in the lower gingiva.

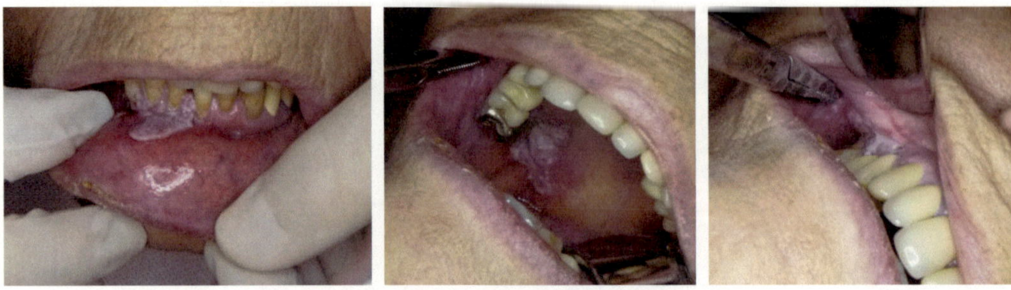

Figure 6. Proliferative verrucous leukoplakia. This elderly woman presented multiple lesions affecting different sites of the oral mucosa.

Many lesions must be excluded before formulating a diagnostic hypothesis of OL, such as chemical injuries, candidiasis, frictional lesion, hairy leukoplakia, leukoedema, linea alba, nicotinic stomatitis, among others [4,10]. Because of variable clinical presentation of the potentially malignant lesions, when a provisional clinical diagnosis of OL is made, a biopsy must be performed to obtain the histopathological diagnosis [12].

The microscopic presentation of OL can vary from slightly hyperkeratotic epithelium to lesions with severe dysplasia [13]. The frequencies of dysplastic or malignant alterations in OL vary from 15.6% to 39.2%, and a rate of 19.9% was found in a retrospective study of 3,300 white lesions of the oral cavity [14]. Epithelial dysplasia is characterized by the presence of architectural alteration and cytological atypia, and can be graded as mild, moderate, severe, and carcinoma *in situ* [10]. Nevertheless, there is a notable inter- and intra-observer variation in the interpretation and classification of dysplasia, which makes this method subjective with low reproducibility [12,15]. Thus, many different grading systems have been suggested to enhance the reproducibility and the predictive value for malignant transformation of OL.

It has been suggested a possible correlation between clinical and histopathological features of OL [16]. Following this proposal, thin and flat OL would show hyperkeratosis, acanthosis, and occasional lymphocytes. Thick fissured OL lesions would present, besides these microscopic alterations, mild to moderate dysplasia. The verrucous or granular OL would show irregular hyperkeratosis, drop-shaped rete ridges, a moderate amount of lymphocytes, and moderate to severe dysplasia. Finally, speckled OL and erythroplakia could show irregular hyperkeratosis, epithelial atrophy, numerous lymphocytes, and severe dysplasia or carcinoma *in situ*.

A research group published a proposal of a staging system for OL, in which a clinical feature of the lesion would be taken into account [17,18]. The lesion would be classified into one of the four stages (I, II, III, or IV), according to the association between two parameters. The first characteristic to be evaluated would be the size of the lesion, with four possible categories (L_1, L_2, L_3, and L_x). The second item concerned the histopathological presentation, focused on the presence of dysplasia, with three possible categories (P_0, P_1, and P_x). Therefore, a somehow similar strategy to that of TNM (extent of the tumor (T), spread to regional lymph nodes (N), and distant metastasis (M)) for oral cancer would be used to stage OL, and the authors intended to promote a uniform reporting of treatment or management of OL lesions.

1.3. Evolution and prognosis

OL may persist unchanged, progress, regress, or even disappear [9]. The malignant transformation risk varies from 3.6% to 36.0%, and some features such as the presence and degree of dysplasia, female gender, time of duration, non-smoker patient, location at floor of the mouth or tongue, size higher than 200mm^2, and non-homogeneous type, seem to be associated with a worse prognosis [10,19-22]. Surgical excision, cryosurgery, laser surgery, topical or systemic retinoids, therapy with mouth rinses with attenuated adenovirus, and photodynamic therapy are possible therapeutics [10,13,23]. Recurrence rates are highly variable among studies, from 0 to 30.0% [10].

Many efforts have attemped to identify molecular markers to predict cancer development in OL. However, the presence and degree of epithelial dysplasia in OL is yet regarded as the most relevant indicator of progression and prognosis, influencing the management of the patients [9,10,12].

2. Grading oral epithelial dysplasia

The term "dysplasia" is generally employed in the sense of a disordered development [24]. In a stratified squamous epithelium, architectural disturbances affecting normal maturation and stratification may occur. When such alterations are accompanied by cytological atypia, which can be detected as variations in the size and shape of the keratinocytes, the term "dysplasia" is applied [7,12].

Despite many efforts towards new evaluative methods, the histological analysis is still the most useful method for grading epithelial dysplasia in OL [12].

2.1. Relevance

The concept of a sequential developmental process from a normal epithelium through a dysplasia, ending in a carcinoma, was introduced from studying pathological changes in the uterine cervix [24]. It is believed that through this process there is an accumulation of genetic and epigenetic alterations and more and more layers of the epithelium are progressively involved, until it is replaced by atypical cells in full length. It is considered that the more severe the degree of dysplasia, the greater the likelihood of malignant transformation. Despite the imperfection of currently available systems, they remain essential, and the diagnosis is a prerequisite for the establishment of the treatment that provides the best prognosis [12,24].

2.2. Proposed systems

The elaboration of a classifying system is not a simple issue as the system may be, above all, an indicator of prognosis, guiding or at least helping in the establishment of the best treatment. Moreover, it should be reproducible, reliable, and as simple and objective as possible. Many classification schemes have been proposed over time, with variable acceptance and employment. Herein, three of the most mentioned systems will first be discussed, followed by the recently suggested binary system.

2.2.1. Squamous intraepithelial neoplasia (SIN)

This classification is a modification of a previously suggested system for cervical pre-malignant lesions, named cervical intraepithelial neoplasia [25]. After that, this concept has been adopted and extended to other sites, including oral mucosa, named "oral intraepithelial neoplasia" [12,26]. The term squamous intraepithelial neoplasia is also used to encompass all sites of the upper aerodigestive tract [26]. However, there is no evidence that many of the potentially malignant lesions of the oral mucosa are committed on a path to malignancy. Moreover, the SIN terminology would not clarify the knowledge concerning this issue, which would not justify replacing the widely accepted concept of dysplasia. Additionally, the WHO consensus group did not favour this system [12].

According to this system, lesions are classified as:

- SIN 1, would be similar to mild dysplasia
- SIN 2, would be similar to moderate dysplasia
- SIN 3, would combine severe dysplasia and carcinoma *in situ*

2.2.2. Ljubljana classification of squamous intraepithelial lesions

This classification system was proposed by laryngeal pathologists in 1971 and additionally formulated in 1997 by a Working Group of the European Society of Pathology [27,28]. Very detailed criteria have been published and this system is more complex than the concept of dysplasia, so that even experienced pathologists would require time to adapt to it. Moreover, despite some publications, the usefulness of this grading system for oral lesions is doubtful [12,24].

Briefly, lesions are classified into four groups according to this system:

- Simple hyperplasia, which is an increase in the stratum spinosum
- Basal/parabasal cell hyperplasia or abnormal hyperplasia, considered essentially a basal cell hyperplasia
- Atypical hyperplasia, also named risky hyperplasia, shows epithelial stratification, but with atypia
- Carcinoma *in situ*, characterized by loss of stratification throughout epithelium, but three to five layers of compressed cells may be present on the surface. Also, there is marked atypia and mitotic abnormalities

The first two degrees are considered mainly benign lesions, showing minimum risk for malignant transformation. The third degree would be a potentially malignant lesion, and the last one is actually considered a malignant lesion already. Additionally, the "atypical hyperplasia" and "carcinoma *in situ*" degrees are divided into basal cell type and spinous cell type [12,24].

2.2.3. World health organization

In 1997, the WHO published the "Histopathological Typing of Cancer and Precancer of the Oral Mucosa" and in the latest WHO's classification of Head and Neck Tumours, a grading system based on "thirds" was described [7,29]. This resembled the system described since the 1970's for lesions of the uterine cervix [24].

The WHO's classification system is truly widely accepted among pathologists. However, it is not able to reflect the clinical behaviour of every single lesion and does not provide a clear therapeutic guideline to clinicians [24]. Moreover, in spite of its wide acceptance, this system presents great variability and low reproducibility [10,12]. According to it, lesions are allocated into categories considering firstly the architectural features, followed by cytological alterations [7].

The architectural features that should be addressed are:

- Irregular epithelial stratification (Figure 7)
- Loss of polarity of basal cells (Figure 8)
- Drop-shaped rete ridges
- Increased number of mitotic figures
- Abnormally superficial mitoses
- Premature keratinisation in single cells (dyskeratosis) (Figure 9)
- Keratin pearls within rete pegs

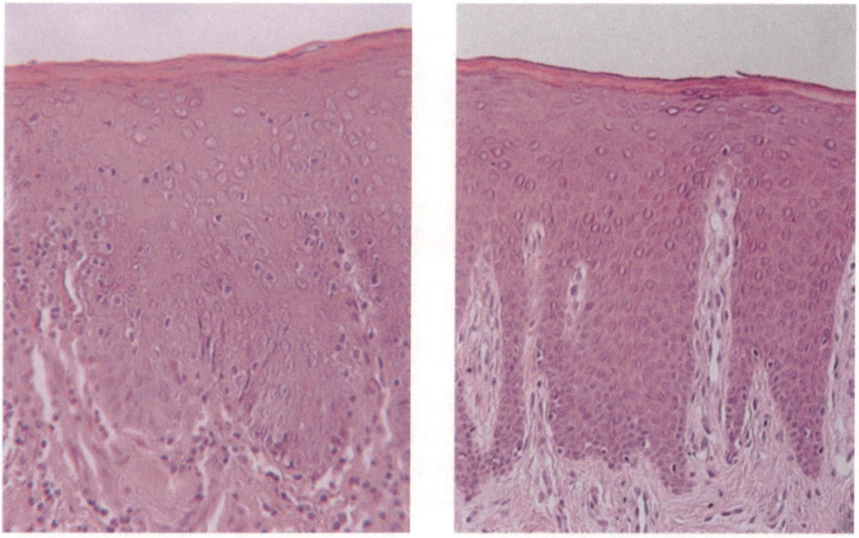

Figure 7. Left: specimen of an oral leukoplakia showing irregular epithelial stratification. Right: Normal oral mucosa. Hematoxylin and eosin, 200X magnification.

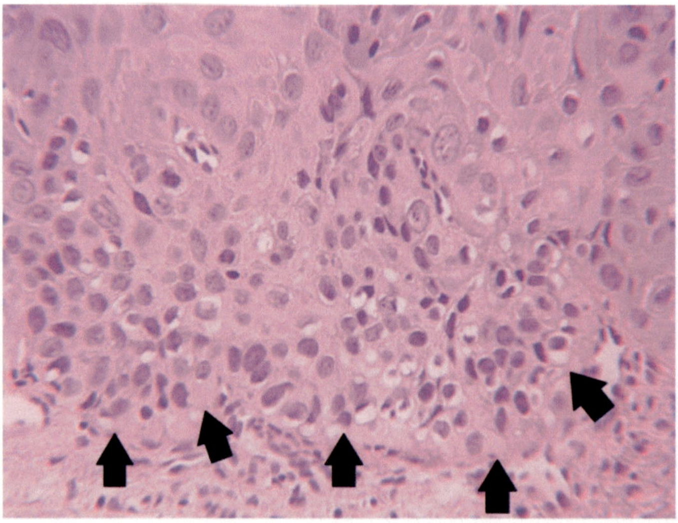

Figure 8. Loss of polarity of basal cells in a photomicrograph of an oral leukoplakia specimen (arrows). Hematoxylin and eosin, 400X magnification.

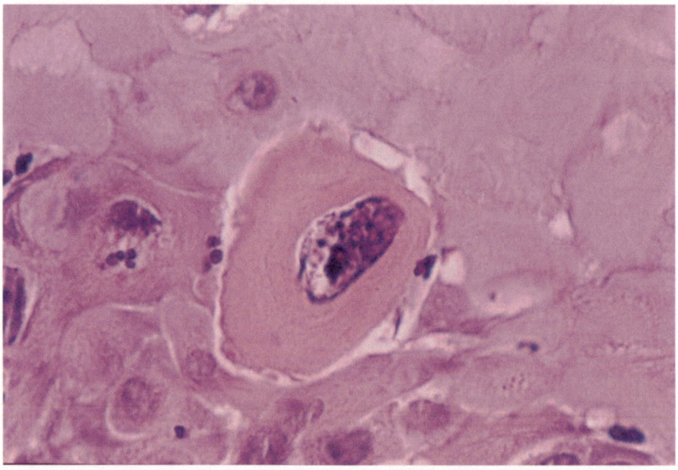

Figure 9. A keratinocyte showing dyskeratosis. Hematoxylin and eosin, 1000X magnification.

The cytological alterations to be observed are as follows:

- Nuclear pleomorphism: abnormal variation in nuclear shape (Figure 10)
- Cellular pleomorphism: abnormal variation in cell shape (Figure 10)
- Anisonucleosis: abnormal variation in nuclear size (Figure 10)
- Anisocytosis: abnormal variation in cell size (Figure 10)
- Increased nuclear size (Figure 10)
- Increased nuclear-cytoplasm ratio (Figure 10)
- Atypical mitotic figures (Figure 11)
- Increased number and size of nucleoli (Figure 10 and 12)

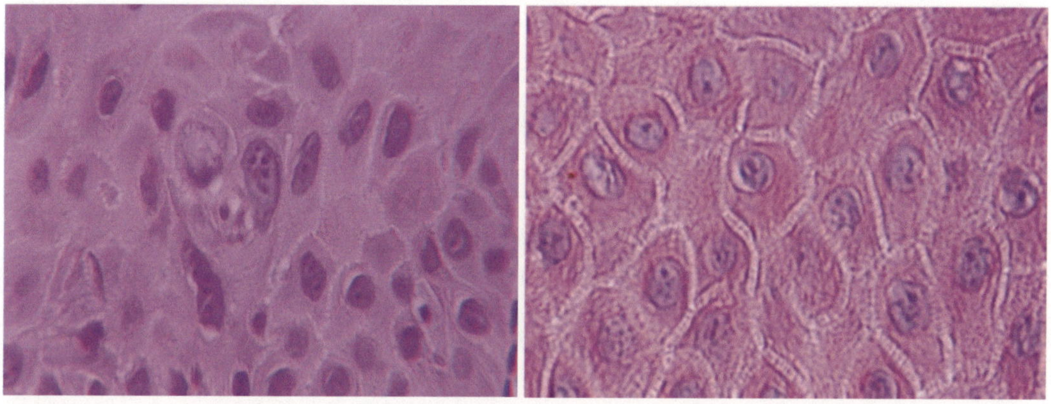

Figure 10. Left: in this specimen, it can be noticed anisonucleosis, anisocytosis, nuclear and cellular pleomorphism, increased nuclear size, increased nuclear-cytoplasm ratio, and increased number and size of nucleoli of keratinocytes in an oral leukoplakia. Right: normal keratinocytes. Hematoxylin and eosin, 1000X magnification.

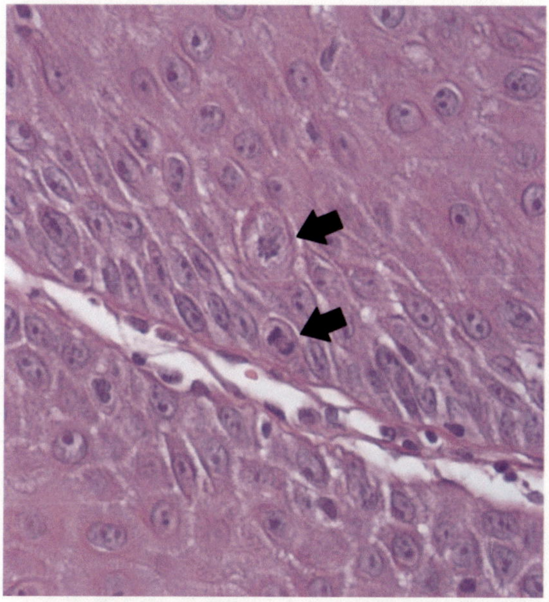

Figure 11. Keratinocytes exhibiting atypical mitotic figures (arrows). Hematoxylin and eosin, 400X magnification.

The observation of these alterations should be done considering the epithelium divided into "thirds". Accordingly, lesions should be classified into five categories, as described below:

1. Hyperplasia (Figure 13): describes a lesion showing an increase in cell number in the spinous layer and/or in the basal/parabasal cell layers. There is regular stratification and no cellular atypia.
2. Mild dysplasia (Figure 14): architectural disturbance only in the lower third of the epithelium with cytological atypia.

3. Moderate dysplasia (Figure 15): architectural disturbance extending into the middle third of the epithelium is the initial criteria, but the degree of cytological atypia may require upgrading it to "severe".
4. Severe dysplasia (Figure 16): architectural disturbance affecting greater than two thirds of the epithelium, with cytological atypia.
5. Carcinoma *in situ* (Figure 17): theorically, indicates that malignant transformation has occurred but invasion has not. Full or almost full thickness architectural disturbance in viable cellular layers with pronounced cellular atypia. Atypical mitotic figures and abnormal superficial mitoses are common.

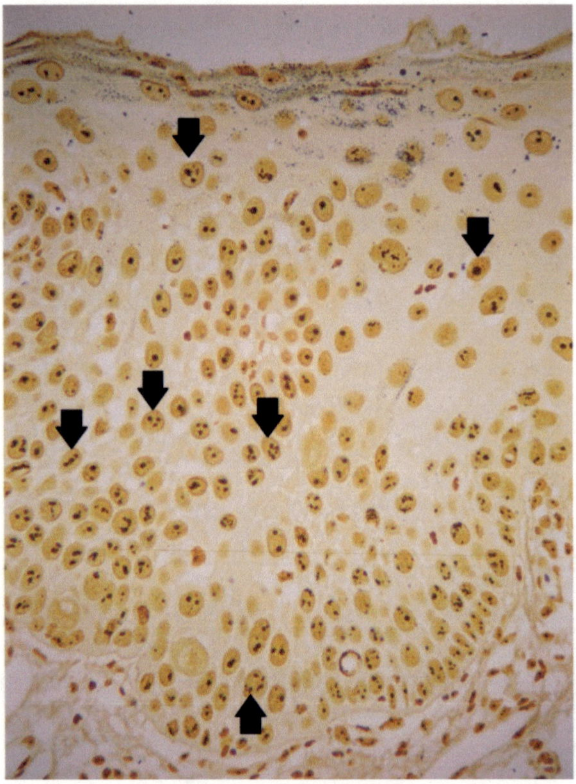

Figure 12. Oral leukoplakia specimen exhibiting increased number and size of nucleoli (arrows). AgNOR staining, 200X magnification.

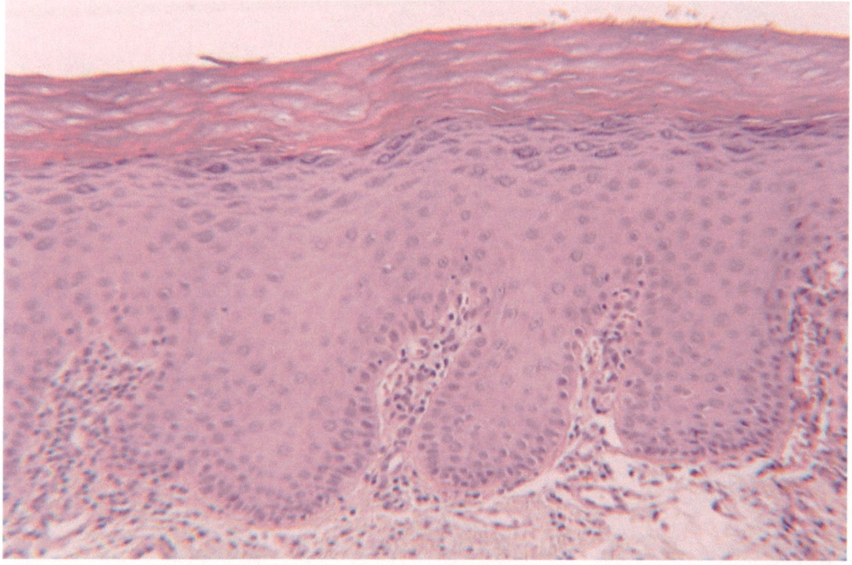

Figure 13. Sample of an oral leukoplakia showing hyperplasia. Note an increased number of basal / parabasal cells and a hyperkeratotic surface. Regular stratification is observed, as well as no cytological atypia. Hematoxylin and eosin, 200X magnification.

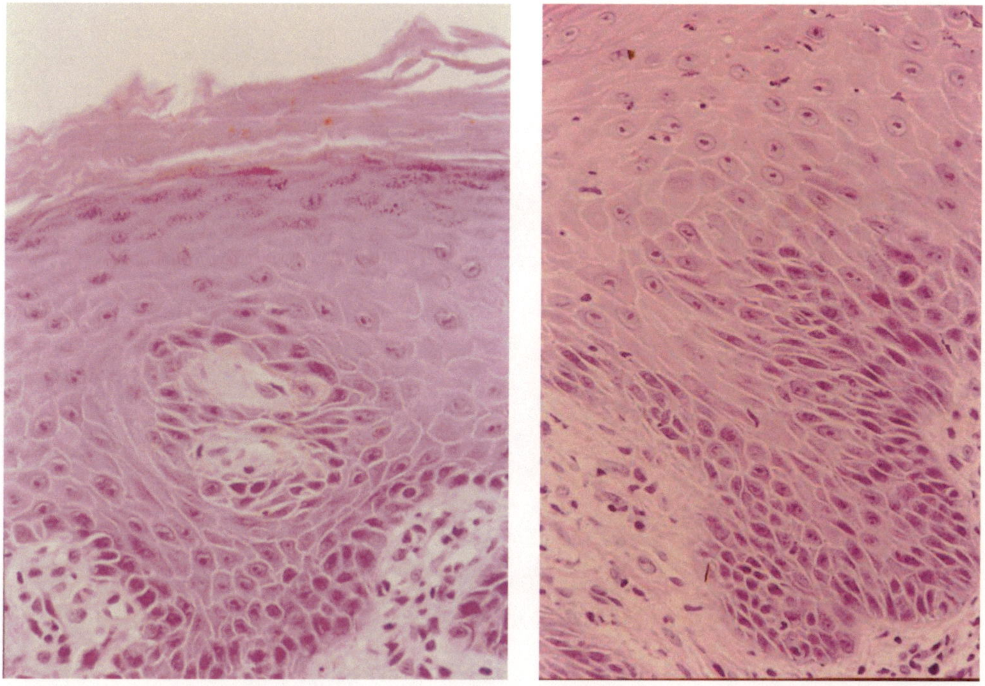

Figure 14. These specimens of oral leukoplakia exhibited mild dysplasia. Observe architectural disturbances affecting the lower third of the epithelium and cytological atypia. Hematoxylin and eosin, 200X magnification (left), 400X magnification (right).

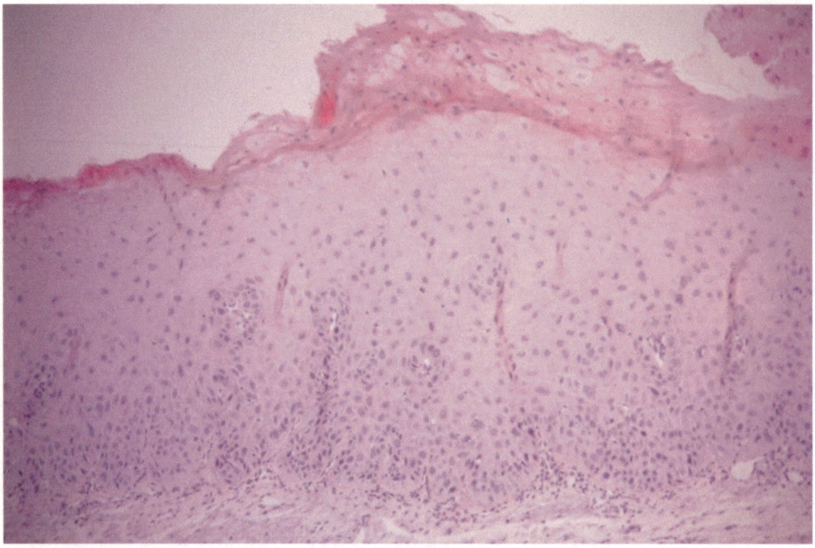

Figure 15. Microscopic presentation of an oral leukoplakia showing moderate dysplasia. Architectural disturbances extending into the middle third of epithelium, along with cytological atypia. Hematoxylin and eosin, 100X magnification.

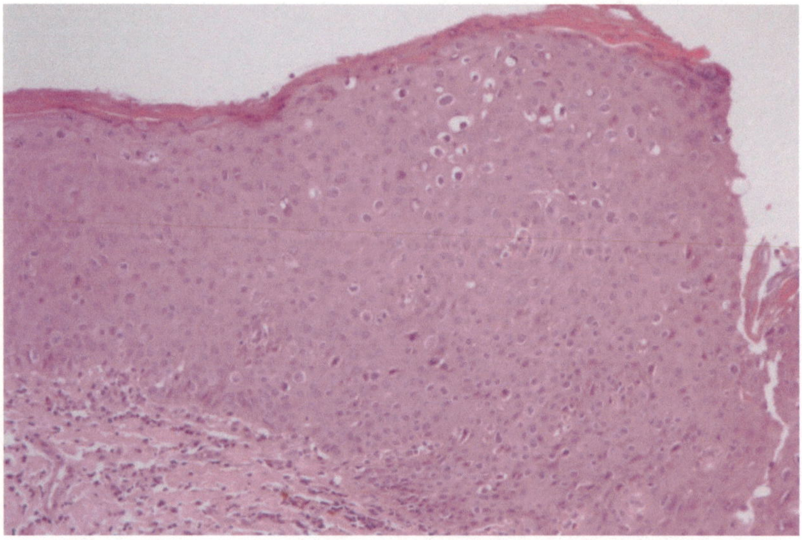

Figure 16. Histological section of oral leukoplakia exhibiting severe dysplasia. Architectural disturbances affecting greater than two thirds of the epithelium. Pronounced cytological atypia is evident. Hematoxylin and eosin, 100X magnification.

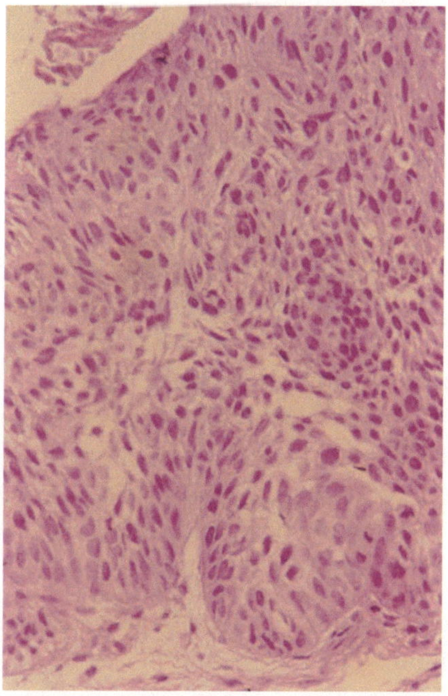

Figure 17. An oral leukoplakia that showed microscopic features of carcinoma *in situ*: architectural disturbances are observed in the full thickness of epithelium with pronounced cellular atypia. No superficial keratinisation can be observed. Hematoxylin and eosin, 200X magnification.

2.2.4. *Binary system*

As mentioned above, the proposed systems to grade epithelial dysplasia published so far, including the WHO's proposal, showed some shortcomings, such as great variability and low reproducibility. Thus, studies concerning classification criteria are being performed, looking for an enhancement for grading epithelial dysplasia in OL. In 2006, a new binary system was proposed, which could be a more feasible and reliable tool for grading epithelial dysplasia in OL [15]. According to this system, pathologists would observe the same morphological criteria used in the WHO classification, but lesions would be classified as low-risk OL (former "no/ mild / questionable" dysplasia) or as high-risk OL (former "moderate/ severe" dysplasia) [15,10,12]. This would provide more reliable criteria upon which to rely for the selection of patient treatment.

Interestingly, in 1988 the "Bethesda classification" for cervical cytopathology, already included only two grades [30]. According to this, lesions would be classified as low-grade squamous epithelial lesions, corresponding to former cervical intraepithelial neoplasia grade 1, and high-grade squamous epithelial lesions, corresponding to grades 2 and 3. This system has also been mentioned in some reports for oral lesions [26].

After the publication of those papers on the binary system for grading epithelial dysplasia in OL, a study was performed with 218 patients with OL, from which 39 (17.9%) developed into cancer [31]. The authors reported that high-risk OL was associated with a 4.57-fold increased risk for malignant transformation, compared with low-risk OL. Those authors suggested that high-risk dysplasia would be a significant indicator for evaluating malignant transformation risk in OL.

Subsequently, the same research group published a study in which they identified significant risk factors for malignant transformation in a long-term follow-up cohort of patients with oral epithelial dysplasia [32]. Of the 138 patients with histologically confirmed oral dysplasia, 115 had OL and 23 had lichen planus. From these 138 lesions, 37 (26.8%) developed into cancer and the "high-risk" degree of dysplasia was an independent risk factor for transformation. Moreover, high-risk degree of dysplasia was associated with a 2.78-fold increased risk of transformation compared with low-risk degree. The authors then suggest the utilization of high-risk dysplasia as a significant indicator for evaluating malignant transformation risk in patients with potentially malignant lesions. According to them, this would also help guiding treatment in clinical practice. In spite of these great achievements, it must be mentioned that malignancy also developed in some patients previously presenting low-risk potentially malignant lesions [32].

In our first paper [33], we investigated the immunoexpression of hMLH1 (a protein of the mismatch repair system) (Figure 18) in OL with different degrees of dysplasia, according to the WHO grading system. We evaluated lesions showing no, mild, moderate, and severe dysplasia, and we found that the greater difference in the hMLH1 immunoexpression was detected comparing OL with mild and moderate dysplasia, with decreasing indexes. Therefore, we suggested that this result would be in accordance with the proposed binary system of grading dysplasia in OL, as the morphological dysplastic alterations observed in routinely stained slides may be related to molecular changes.

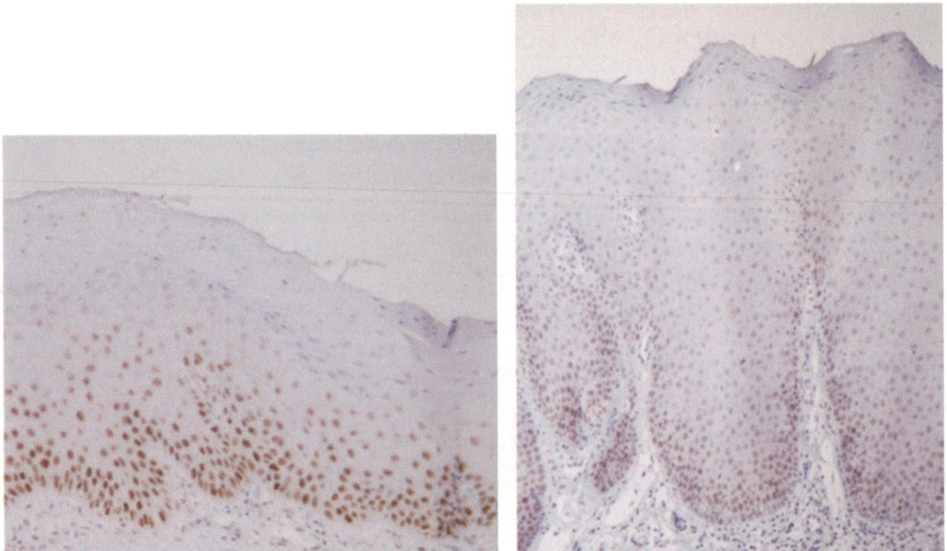

Figure 18. Immunoexpression of hMLH1 in oral leukoplakia showing no dysplasia (left) and severe dysplasia (right). Advance HRP, 200X magnification.

After that, we conducted a comparative immunohistochemical and histochemical study encompassing those same samples of OL [34]. At that time, the hMLH1 immunoexpression was compared to p53 immunoexpression (Figure 19) and AgNOR counting. Thus, we could assess the possible association between a protein of DNA repair, a tumor suppressor protein, and the cellular proliferation in OL with different degrees of dysplasia, *i.e.* no, mild, moderate, and severe. We concluded that it seemed reasonable that other molecular alterations may take place in early phases of carcinogenesis, related to tumor suppressor genes, like p53, as well as modifications in proliferation rates.

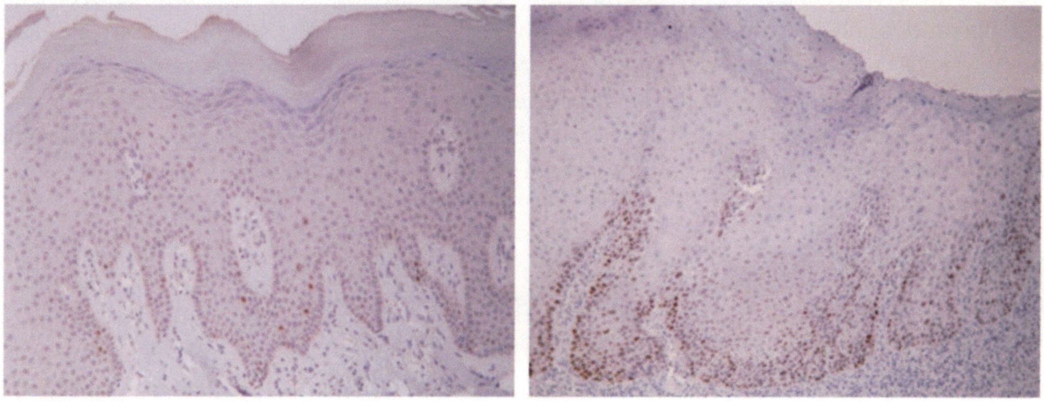

Figure 19. Immunoexpression of p53 in oral leukoplakia with mild dysplasia (left) and severe dysplasia (right). Streptoavidin-biotin, 100X magnification.

Recently, we decided to reevaluate those previous results in the light of the binary system to grade epithelial dysplasia in OL [35]. Therefore, we grouped OL formerly classified as showing no and mild dysplasia into low-risk lesions. Accordingly, OL previously classified as having moderate and severe dysplasia were defined as high-risk lesions. After that, we performed the statistical analyses again. Our findings showed statistically significant differences for hMLH1, p53, and AgNOR indexes between low- and high-risk OL. This suggests that the biological processes linked to the impairment of those proteins remain enhancing from low-risk OL to high-risk OL. Thus, the use of the binary system would give support to a more reliable clinical approach involving the removal of high-risk OL. Moreover, we could speculate that OL classified as low-risk may be reasonably named this way, since comparisons between hMLH1 and AgNOR indexes of this group and normal oral mucosa did not reach statistical significance, despite their different median values.

2.2.5. *Other proposals*

Apart from those investigations pointing towards an adaptation of the WHO classification to a binary system, there are also other recently published papers on different proposals to evaluate epithelial dysplasia.

As reviewed before, the Japanese Society for Oral Pathology reported a definition of carcinoma *in situ* and proposes the term "oral intraepithelial neoplasia", which in turn could be classified as differentiated and basaloid type [24]. The main difference between them would be the presence of keratinisation in the epithelium surface in the differentiated type. Additionally, some authors analyzed individual features of dysplasia in oral lesions and determined the reproducibility of scoring each one [36]. They suggested that those data might be used to improve or to develop simpler routine diagnostic methods.

3. Conclusion

To date, no system is free of presenting failures in identifying those OL prone to evolve to oral squamous cell carcinoma. Furthermore, the reproducibility and subjectivity are still key points to be addressed. Therefore, robust research on the predictive value, relevance, applicability, and feasibility of the binary system for grading epithelial dysplasia are clearly warranted. Such research should aim to establish of a reliable and reproducible method that, above all, could provide a better and less empiric clinical management of the patient.

Author details

Maria Auxiliadora Vieira do Carmo and Patrícia Carlos Caldeira
School of Dentistry, Universidade Federal de Minas Gerais, Brazil

Acknowledgement

The authors acknowledge National Council of Technological and Scientific Development (CNPq), Coordenação de Aperfeiçoamento de Pessoal de Nível Superior (CAPES), and Fundação de Amparo à Pesquisa do Estado de Minas Gerais (FAPEMIG) for the received grants and research funding.

4. References

[1] Neville BW, Day TA. Oral cancer and precancerous lesions. CA: A Cancer Journal for Clinicians 2002;52(4):195-215.

[2] Scully C, Bagan J. Oral squamous cell carcinoma: overview of current understanding of aetiopathogenesis and clinical implications. Oral Diseases 2009;15(6):388-99.

[3] Haya-Fernández MC, Bagán JV, Murillo-Cortés J, Poveda-Roda R, Calabuig C. The prevalence of oral leukoplakia in 138 patients with oral squamous cell carcinoma. Oral Diseases 2004;10(6):346-8.

[4] Warnakulasuriya S, Johnson NW, van der Waal I. Nomenclature and classification of potentially malignant disorders of the oral mucosa. Journal of Oral Pathology & Medicine 2007;36(10):575-80.

[5] van der Waal I. Potentially malignant disorders of the oral and oropharyngeal mucosa; present concepts of management. Oral Oncolology 2010;46(6):423-5.

[6] Kramer IR, Lucas RB, Pindborg JJ, Sobin LH. Definition of leukoplakia and related lesions: an aid to studies on oral precancer. Oral Surgery, Oral Medicine, Oral Pathology 1978;46(4):518-39.
[7] World Health Organization. Tumours of the Oral Cavity and Oropharynx. In: Barnes L, Eveson JW, Reichart P, Sidransky D, editors. Pathology & genetics. Head neck tumors. Lyon: IARC Press; 2005. p. 177-9.
[8] Petti S. Pooled estimate of world leukoplakia prevalence: a systematic review. Oral Oncology 2003;39(8):770-80.
[9] Napier SS, Speight PM. Natural history of potentially malignant oral lesions and conditions: an overview of the literature. Journal of Oral Pathology & Medicine 2008;37(1):1-10.
[10] van der Waal I. Potentially malignant disorders of the oral and oropharyngeal mucosa; terminology, classification and present concepts of management. Oral Oncology 2009;45(4-5):317-23.
[11] Campisi G, Panzarella V, Giuliani M, Lajolo C, Di Fede O, Falaschini S, et al. Human papillomavirus: its identity and controversial role in oral oncogenesis, premalignant and malignant lesions (review). International Journal of Oncology 2007;30(4):813-23.
[12] Warnakulasuriya S, Reibel J, Bouquot J, Dabelsteen E. Oral epithelial dysplasia classification systems: predictive value, utility, weaknesses and scope for improvement. Journal of Oral Pathology & Medicine 2008;37(3):127-33.
[13] Brennan M, Migliorati CA, Lockhart PB, Wray D, Al-Hashimi I, Axéll T, et al. Management of oral epithelial dysplasia: a review. Oral Surgery, Oral Medicine, Oral Pathology, Oral Radiology, and Edodontics 2007;103(Supp l):S19e1-12.
[14] Waldron CA, Shafer WG. Leukoplakia revisited. A clinicopathologic study 3256 oral leukoplakias. Cancer 1975;36(4):1386-92.
[15] Kujan O, Oliver RJ, Khattab A, Roberts SA, Thakker N, Sloan P. Evaluation of a new binary system of grading oral epithelial dysplasia for prediction of malignant transformation. Oral Oncology 2006;42(10):987-93.
[16] Bouquot JE, Gnepp DR. Laryngeal precancer: a review of the literature, commentary, and comparison with oral leukoplakia. Head & Neck 1991;13(6):488-97.
[17] van der Waal I, Schepman KP, van der Meij EH. A modified classification and staging system for oral leukoplakia. Oral Oncolology 2000;36(3):264-6.
[18] van der Waal I, Axéll T. Oral leukoplakia: a proposal for uniform reporting. Oral Oncolology 2002;38(6):521-6.
[19] Cruz I, Napier SS, van der Waal I, Snijders PJ, Walboomers JM, Lamey PJ, et al. Suprabasal p53 immunoexpression is strongly associated with high grade dysplasia and risk for malignant transformation in potentially malignant oral lesions from Northern Ireland. Journal of Clinical Pathology 2002;55(2):98-104.
[20] Holmstrup P, Vedtofte P, Reibel J, Stoltze K. Long-term treatment outcome of oral premalignant lesions. Oral Oncology 2006;42(5):461-74.
[21] Hsue SS, Wang WC, Chen CH, Lin CC, Chen YK, Lin LM. Malignant transformation in 1458 patients with potentially malignant oral mucosal disorders: a follow-up study based in a Taiwanese hospital. Journal of Oral Pathology & Medicine 2007;36(1):25-9.

[22] Smith J, Rattay T, McConkey C, Helliwell T, Mehanna H. Biomarkers in dysplasia of the oral cavity: a systematic review. Oral Oncology 2009;45(8):647-53.

[23] Lodi G, Porter S. Management of potentially malignant disorders: evidence and critique. Journal of Oral Pathology & Medicine 2008;37(2):63-9.

[24] Izumo, T. Oral premalignant lesions: from the pathological viewpoint. International Journal of Clinical Oncology 2011;16(1):15-26.

[25] Richart RM. Natural history of cervical intraepithelial neoplasia. Clinical Obstetrics & Gynecology 1967;10(4):748-784.

[26] Küffer R, Lombardi T. Premalignant lesions of the oral mucosa. A discussion about the place of oral intraepithelial neoplasia (OIN). Oral Oncology 2002;38(2):125-30.

[27] Kambic V, Lenart I. Notre classification des hyperplasies de l'epithelium du larynx au point de vue prognostic. Journal Français d'Oto-Rhino-Laryngologie, Audio-Phonologie et Chirurgie Maxillo-Faciale 1971;20(10):1145-50.

[28] Hellquist H, Cardesa A, Gale N, Kambic V, Michaels L. Criteria for grading in Ljubljana classification of epithelial hyperplastic laryngeal lesions. A study by members of the working group on epithelial hyperplastic laryngeal lesions of the European Society of Pathology. Histopathology 1999;34(3):226-233.

[29] World Health Organization. Pindborg JJ, Reichart PA, Smith CJ, van der Waal I, editors. Histological typing of cancer and precancer of the oral mucosa. Berlin: Springer; 1997.

[30] National Cancer Institute Workshop. The 1988 Bethesda System for reporting cervical/vaginal cytological diagnoses. JAMA 1989;262(7):931-4.

[31] Liu W, Wang YF, Zhou HW, Shi P, Zhou ZT, Tang GY. Malignant transformation of oral leukoplakia: a retrospective cohort study of 218 Chinese patients. BMC Cancer, 2010;16(10):685.

[32] Liu W, Bao ZX, Shi LJ, Tang GY, Zhou ZT. Malignant transformation of oral epithelial dysplasia: clinicopathological risk factors and outcome analysis in a retrospective cohort of 138 cases. Histopathology 2011;59(4):733-40.

[33] Caldeira PC, Abreu MH, Batista AC, Do Carmo MA. hMLH1 immunoexpression is related to the degree of epithelial dysplasia in oral leukoplakia. Journal of Oral Pathology & Medicine 2011;40(2):153-9.

[34] Caldeira PC, Aguiar MC, Mesquita RA, Do Carmo MA. Oral leukoplakias with different degrees of dysplasia: comparative study of hMLH1, p53, and AgNOR. Journal of Oral Pathology & Medicine 2011;40(4):305-11.

[35] Caldeira PC, Abreu MH, Carmo MA. Binary system of grading oral epithelial dysplasia: evidence of a bearing to the scores of an immunohistochemical study. Journal of Oral Pathology & Medicine 2012;41(6):452-3.

[36] Tilakaratne WM, Sherriff M, Morgan PR, Odell EW. Grading oral epithelial dysplasia: analysis of individual features. Journal of Oral Pathology & Medicine 2011;40(7):533-40.

Section 2

Cancer Development and Progression

Chapter 3

Human Papillomavirus and Carcinogenesis in the Upper Aero-Digestive Tract

Andrés Castillo

Additional information is available at the end of the chapter

http://dx.doi.org/10.5772/54800

1. Introduction

Infectious agents are suspected to play causal roles in a variety of human malignancies. The public health impact of the oncogenic effects of these infections is considerable. Infection is estimated to be responsible for about 17.8% of all incident cases of cancer worldwide, accounting for 26.3% of all malignancies in economically developing countries and 7.7% in developed countries [1].

The evaluation of causality for these infectious agents as human carcinogens is difficult given their ubiquitous nature, the substantial length of time between infection and the cancer event, the nature of cofactors, and the rarity of malignancy among those infected. Thus, a central problem for the epidemiologist is to define the natural history of infection and to identify those factors that are related to the development of cancer. Hence, informative biomarkers of the agent (such as viral load), of the host (such as abnormal antibody pattern), and of other oncogenic exposures (such as tobacco use) are required for understanding the viral-human interactions and for developing interventions [2].

Case-control studies have now recognized that human papilloma virus (HPV) infection in the oral cavity is a strong risk factor for head and neck squamous cell carcinoma (HNSCC), and mostly for oropharyngeal cancer. The risk is increased for high-risk HPV-16 infection [3]. Therefore, HPV infection in the oral cavity has important health consequences, requiring more studies about these aspects to clarify the implications of a diagnosis of HPV in the oral cavity and HNSCC.

2. Human papillomavirus (HPV)

HPVs are nonenveloped icosahedral viruses with a diameter of 55 nm, belonging to the *papillomaviridae* family. This epitheliotropic virus has 72 capsomers enclosing an 8 kbp-long circular DNA genome. Although its DNA is double-stranded, only one strand contains open reading frames (ORF) that are transcribed. The viral DNA has eight ORFs and an upstream regulatory region, also called the long control region (LCR), which contains an origin of replication and cis-acting transcriptional regulatory elements [4]. Figure 1 shows the genome organization of HPV-16, the HPV type most strongly related to cervical cancer. The early region of the HPV genome contains six ORFs corresponding to E1, E2, E4, E5, E6, and E7 genes, which encode proteins necessary for viral replication and cell transformation. The late region codes for the two proteins of the viral capside: L1, the major structural protein; and L2, the protein linking to encapsulated DNA [4].

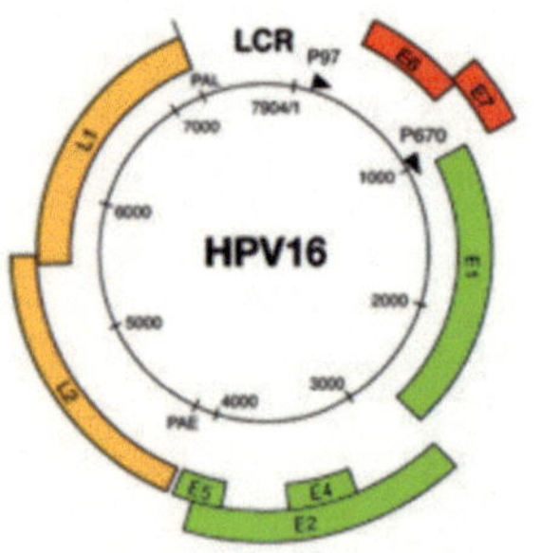

PROTEIN	FUNCTIONS
E6	Destruction of p53 tumor supressor protein (Accumulation of mutation and Apoptosis inhibition)
E7	Inactivation of pRb tumor supressor protein (Cell cycle progression and accumulation of p16INK4a)
E1	Viral DNA replication
E2	Viral DNA replication: repression of E6-E7 genes
E4	Assembly and release of the viral particle
E5	Interaction with the Epidermal Growth factor (EGF)
L1	Major capsid protein in the viral particle
L2	Minor capsid protein in the viral particle

Figure 1. HPV genomic organization. The early region of the HPV genome contains six ORFs corresponding to E1, E2, E4, E5, E6, and E7 genes, which encode proteins necessary for viral replication and cell transformation. The late region codes for the two proteins of the viral capside: L1, the major structural protein; and L2, the protein linking to encapsulated DNA.

3. Classification of papillomaviruses

The L1 ORF is the most conserved gene in the papillomavirus (PV) genome and has therefore been used for identifying new PV types over the past 15 years. A new PV isolate is recognized as a new PV type if the complete genome has been cloned and the DNA sequence of L1 ORF differs by more than 10% from any known PV types. A difference between 2% and 10% homology defines a subtype, and less than 2%, a variant [5].

HPV has more than 100 types, of which approximately 90 have already been characterized and assigned with numbers, and has five genuses: alpha-papillomavirus, beta-papillomavirus, gamma-papillomavirus, mu-papillomavirus, and nu-papillomavirus [5]. HPV is also subdivided into two major groups, cutaneous and mucosal, based on data from clinical manifestations [6]. Most mucosal HPV types exist in the genital area, which can be divided into high-risk and low-risk HPV types [7]. HPV of high-risk types increases the risk of cervical cancer, which is almost always associated with HPV infection. To this date, approximately 20 HPV types have been identified as high-risk. Among them, HPV-16 and HPV-18 are considered to be associated with 70% of all cervical cancer. In contrast, low-risk type HPV, such as HPV-6 and HPV-11, causes genital warts but not cancer.

Furthermore, HPVs have intratype variants. However, information on variants is limited to certain HPV types. Yamada *et al.* [8] showed five phylogenetic clusters with distinct geographic distributions, analyzing the sequences of E6, L1, and LCR of HPV-16 isolated from cervical samples collected worldwide. The AA (Asian American) variant was isolated mainly from Central and South America and Spain. The African variants 1 and 2 (Af1 and Af2) and Asian (As) variant were present mainly from Africa and Southeast Asia, respectively. In all regions other than Africa, the European-350T (E-350T) prototype as well as the European-350G (E-350G) variant were detected.

4. HPV life cycle and its carcinogenesis

The life cycle of HPV is linked to the differentiation program of the infected host cell, epidermal or mucosal epithelial cell. Cells in the basal layer consist of stem cells, which persist indefinitely, and a much larger number of "transit amplifying cells", which arise from the stem cells and divide a finite number of times until they become differentiated, providing a reservoir of cells for subrabasal regions [9].

HPV initially infects the basal layer of epithelia via minor abrasions. Viral entry into a cell is not clearly understood. It is suspected that the heparin sulfate mediates the initial attachment of virions to cells [10] and that HPV enters a cell via interaction with certain receptors such as alfa-6 integrin for HPV-16 [11].

The first HPV genes to be expressed are E7 and E6 (Figure 2). The virus protein E7 promotes cell division by binding to pRb, a tumor suppressor protein that usually binds to and inactivates E2F, a transcription factor. E2F released from pRb causes transcription of genes involved in DNA replication and cell division. E6 virus protein binds to and inhibits p53 protein, which is active in repressing the cell cycle in the event of DNA damage, and in triggering apoptosis in the case of damage too severe to be repaired. E6 virus protein also activates cellular telomerase that synthesizes the telomere repeat sequences in eukaryotic cells and allows their immortal replication [12]. The transforming activities of high-risk HPV type represent a consequence of a viral replication strategy that is driven by the necessity to replicate the HPV genomes in suprabasal cells [12]. During the early phases of infection, the copy number of viral genome is between 50 and 100, and the viral genome exists as extrachromosomal plasmid or an episomal form that replicates as the host cell chromosomes replicate. As the infected cells differentiate, the rest of the early viral genes, such as E1, E2, E4, and E5 genes, become switched on [13]. E1 and E2 proteins, a helicase and a transcription factor binding to LCR viral region, respectively, support viral DNA replication so that the infected stem cells can be maintained in the lesion for a long period. E4 viral protein is thought to be involved in activating the productive phase of the HPV life cycle. E5, another viral protein, is involved in transformation, enhancing the activity of EGF. As infected daughter cells migrate to the upper layers of the epithelium, viral L1 and L2 late gene products and the major and minor viral capsid proteins are produced to initiate the vegetative phase of the HPV life cycle, resulting in high-level amplification of the viral genome. In the upper layers of stratified squamous epithelia, viral DNA is packaged into capsids and produced virions are freed through normal desquamation processes, triggering little inflammation [14]. In addition, E6 and E7 proteins inactivate interferon regulatory factor [15] so that HPV infection can remain persistent and asymptomatic.

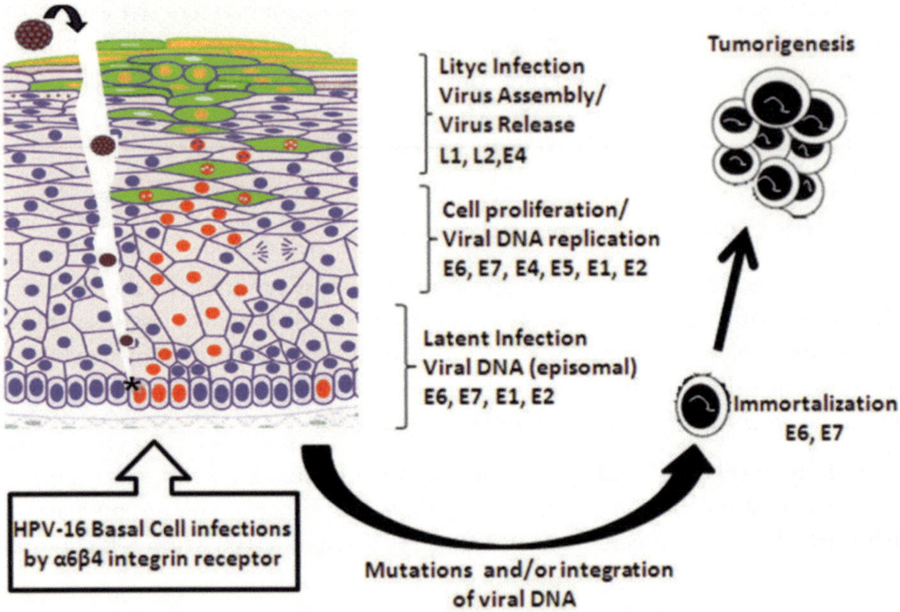

Figure 2. HPV life cycle. HPV establishes latent infection in the basal cells of the differentiating epithelium as episomal multicopy circular nuclear plasmids in order to support the viral life cycle via action of the viral replication proteins E1 and E2. Development of invasive cervical cancer is a stepwise process, which is associated with integration of the high risk HPV DNA into the host cell chromosome, upregulating the expression of viral oncoproteins E6 and E7.

The infection with high-risk HPV is associated with cervical dysplasia or cervical intraepithelial neoplasia (CIN). Long-term persistent HPV infection in these lesions is thought to give rise to cervical cancers. CIN I (mild dysplasia) and CIN II (moderate dysplasia) lesions, in which the viral genomes replicate episomally, show relatively low levels of E6 and E7 gene expression, and are, in most cases, resolved spontaneously by an effective immune response (Figure 3). In contrast, CIN III (severe dysplasia, carcinoma in situ) and invasive cancer lesions, where viral DNA is integrated into the host genome in most cases, often display high-level expression of E6 and E7 genes [16].

The integration of the viral genome into the host cell is a very rare event with a predilection for host chromosomal fragile sites [17], but after it has happened carcinogenic transformation progresses rapidly. HPV integration into the host genome induces the increased E6 and E7 protein expressions since integration results in disruption of HPV E2 gene, which is a negative regulator of HPV E6 and E7 transcription. In addition, once integrated, the E6 and E7 mRNA gains a longer half-life by using host genome poly (A) signals. However, the ultimate development of cervical cancer is rarely accompanied by high expression of E6 and E7 proteins [17]. High-risk HPV E6 and E7 oncoproteins can each independently induce genomic instability in normal human cells [18]. They cooperate to generate mitotic defects and aneuploidy through the induction of centrosome abnormalities in normal human epithelial cells, and the characteristic multipolar mitoses in cervical lesions are caused by centrosome abnormalities [19]. HPV oncoproteins expressing cells also exhibit centrosome-independent manifestations of genomic instability. These manifestations include anaphase bridges that may be caused by double-strand DNA breaks as well as lagging chromosomal material [20]. To date, information on co-factors of HPV-related carcinogenesis in extra-genital organs is quite limited. Muñoz et al. [21] proposed the following three groups of potential cofactors in the cervical carcinogenesis: i) environmental or exogenous cofactors, including hormonal contraceptives, tobacco smoking, parity, and co-infection with other sexually transmitted agents; ii) Viral cofactors: such as HPV types, multiple HPV type infections, HPV integration, HPV viral load, and HPV variants; and iii) Host cofactors: including endogenous hormones, genetic factors, and other factors related to the immune response.

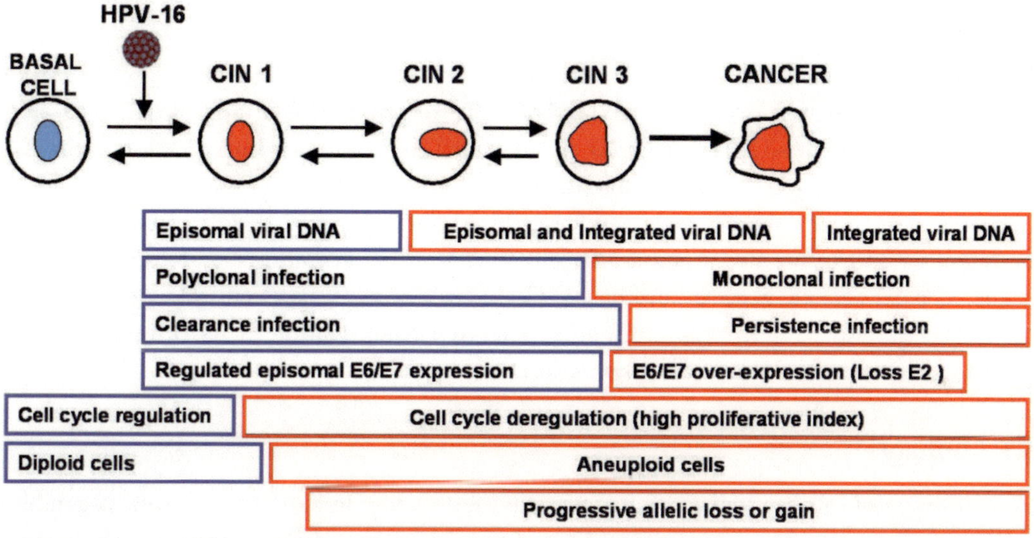

Figure 3. Cervical carcinogenesis. A long-term persistent HPV infection in cervical dysplasia or cervical intraepithelial neoplasia (CIN) could possibly lead to cervical cancer by integration of viral DNA into the host genome and overexpression of viral genes E6 and E7.

5. Squamous cell carcinomas (SCC) in the upper aero-digestive tract (UADT)

5.1. Epidemiology

Oral cancer is the 11th most common cancer in the world in terms of number of cases, while cancer of the pharynx ranks as 20th. Worldwide, about 389,000 new cases occurred in 2000, two-thirds of which were in economically developing countries, and these cancers are responsible for some 200,000 deaths each year [22]. The male-female ratio of its incidence varies from 2 to 15 depending on the anatomical sub-site. An extremely high ratio is a characteristic of cancers of the tongue, floor of mouth, and pharyngeal. Cancers of the mouth and anterior two-thirds of the tongue are predominant in economically developing countries, whereas pharyngeal cancers are common in developed countries and in Central and Eastern Europe. In most countries, oral/pharyngeal cancer incidence and mortality rates have either been stable or increasing in the last four decades [23]. Cancers of the esophagus are the sixth most frequent cancers worldwide. In 2000, the number of deaths due to esophageal cancer amounted to some 337,500 out of a total of 6.2 million cancer deaths worldwide [24]. About 412,000 cases of cancer of the esophagus occur each year, of which over 80% are in economically developing countries. The incidence of esophageal cancer shows a distinct geographical difference, which is more evident than in any other cancers. In certain regions in Asia, the incidence rates of esophageal squamous cell carcinomas (ESCC) are as high as 200 per 100,000. Even within these high risk areas, there are striking local variations in ESCC risk

5.2. Genetic alterations

The genetic alterations observed in the cancers of the UADT include activation of protooncogenes such as cyclin D1, MYC, RAS, EGF receptor, HST-1, and HST-2, as well as inactivation of tumor suppressor genes (TSGs), such as those encoding p53 and p16INK4a [25]. Likewise, in cancer of the esophagus, the mutation of the p53 gene is detected in 35-70% of tumors, depending on geographic origin. Mutations in p53 have also been observed in dysplasia and in normal mucosa adjacent to cancer lesions, and considered as an early event. The p16INK4a gene is another TSG that plays an important role in the UADT development, and p16INK4a is often subject to hypermethylation of its promoter region, resulting in down-regulation of its expression [26].

5.3. Etiology

Consumption of tobacco and alcohol, associated with a low intake of fresh fruit, vegetables, and meat, is causally associated with SCCs of the UADT worldwide. However, the relative contribution of these risk factors varies from one geographic area to another [27]. Smoking is estimated to be responsible for about 41% of oral/pharyngeal cancers in men, and 15% in women worldwide. In more economically developed countries, it is estimated that 90% of ESCCs are attributable to tobacco and alcohol, with a multiplicative increase in risk when individuals are exposed to both factors. In addition, it has been reported that a genetic polymorphism of aldehyde dehydrogenase 2 (ALDH2), which plays a role in ethanol metabolism, is significantly associated with ESCC in the Japanese population [28].

Other environmental risk factors include nitrosamines, deficiency of vitamins A and C, copper, and zinc, poor nutrition, and ingestion of pickled and preserved foods contaminated with fungi such as *Aspergillus flavum, Geotrichum candidum* and *Fusarium sp*. Infectious agents, such as HPV and EBV, have also been suggested to be involved in the development of cancer of the UADT [22].

5.4. HPV infection

The International Agency for Research on Cancer considers that there is convincing evidence that infection with HPV-16, -18, -31, -33, -35, -39, -45, -51, -52, -56, -58, -59 and -66 can lead to cervical cancer [29]. Regarding HPV-16, evidence supports its causal role in cancers of the vulva, vagina, penis, and anus. The association of HPV with cancers of the UADT is also suspected. The UADT consists of a complex mucosa-covered conduit for food and air that extends from the vermilion surface of the lips to the esophagus. Major malignancies observed in the UADT are cancers of the oral cavity, oropharynx, larynx, and esophagus. Among them, HPV-16 is strongly suspected to cause cancers of the oral cavity and oropharynx. Limited evidence is available for the association of HPV with cancers of the larynx and periungual skin, but there is insufficient evidence for roles of HPVs in cancer of the esophagus [30].

In our current research, we found HPV infections in 21 ESCC specimens (29%) [31]. Sequencing analysis of an amplified L1 fragment identified HPV-16 genotype in six Colombian cases (13%) and in five Chilean cases (19%). We also found that a large proportion of ESCC specimens harbour HPV-16 genotype in the integrated form in a certain geographical area with a high ESCC incidence in China [32]. In addition, studies on the association of HPV with cancers of the oral cavity, oropharynx, and esophagus, using cancer specimens from Japan, Pakistan, and Colombia found HPV DNA in around half of the cases in SCCs of the oral cavity and oropharynx, and in a smaller proportion of ESCCs. The high-risk type HPV-16 was the most prevalent type with a viral load in SCC of the tonsil similar to that of cervical cancer (Table 1). The HPV-16 genomes detected in SCCs of the oral cavity, oropharynx and esophagus were frequently integrated in the host genome [33].

The most recent systematic review that included 5,046 SCC of head and neck cancers cases from 60 studies employing PCR-based methods showed that the presence of HPV DNA was 25.9%, being significantly higher in oropharyngeal SCC (35.6%; range 11–100%) than in oral (23.5%; range 4–80%) or laryngeal SCC (24.0%; range 0–100%). HPV-16 accounted for a larger majority of HPV-positive oropharyngeal SCC (86.7%) than HPV-positive oral (68.2%) and laryngeal SCC (69.2%) [34]. Another meta-analysis of 4,680 samples from 94 reports published during the period between 1982 and 1997 showed that HPV was between 2 and 3 times more likely to be detected in precancerous oral mucosa and 4.7 times more likely to be detected in oral carcinoma than in normal mucosa [35]. Among the studies used in their meta-analysis, the largest-scale and most well designed study was the one by Maden *et al.* [36]. They examined 112 normal mucosa specimens and 118 oral carcinomas, and detected HPV-16 in six cases of oral carcinomas but only one sample of normal mucosa. On the other hand, HPV-6 was detected in 12 and 10 oral carcinomas and normal mucosa, respectively. A recent hospital-based case-control study of oropharyngeal cancer in the US detected HPV-16 DNA in 72% of 100 paraffin-embedded tumor specimens, and showed an association of oral HPV-16 infection with oropharyngeal cancer. The study also showed that 64% of patients with cancer were seropositive for the HPV-16 oncoproteins E6 or E7, or both [37]. HPV DNA in situ hybridization clearly showed its presence in the nuclei of cancer cells and not in

COUNTRY	Cancer site		HPV-16	HPV-16 viral load	HPV-16 physical status		
		N	Positive(%)	GM (95% C.I.)	Integrated	Mixed	Episomal
JAPAN							
	Tonsil	24	10(42)	17.76 (1.44 - 216.9)	6(60)	4(40)	-
	Tongue	4	1(25)	0.09	1(100)	-	-
	Others OC	13	6 (46)	0.04(0.02 - 0.07)	6(100)	-	-
	Esophagus	75	9(12)	0.07(0.02 - 0.22)	9(100)	-	-
			P* = 0.002	**P** < 0.001**			P*** = 0.083
PAKISTAN							
	Tongue	28	15(54)	0.01(0.002 - 0.08)	13(87)	-	2(13)
	Others OC	20	12 (60)	0.16(0.03 - 0.95)	11(92)	1(8)	-
	Esophagus	42	9(21)	0.12(0.02 - 0.80)	5(56)	4(44)	-
			P* = 0.003	**P** = 0.031**			**P*** = 0.010**
COLOMBIA							
	Tongue	5	4(80)	2.1(0.01 - 348.4)	2(50)	2(50)	-
	Others OC	1	1 (100)	1.29	1(100)	-	-
	Esophagus	49	6(12)	0.25(0.04 - 1.73)	3(50)	1(17)	2(22)
			P* = 0.001	P** = 0.438			P*** = 0.844
Total							
	Tonsil	24	10(42)	17.76(1.44 - 216.9)	6(60)	4(40)	-
	Tongue	37	20(54)	0.03(0.01-0.23)	16(80)	2(10)	2(10)
	Others OC	34	19(56)	0.12(0.04-0.37)	18(95)	1(5)	-
	Esophagus	166	24(14)	0.12(0.05-0.27)	17(71)	5(21)	2(8)
			P* < 0.001	**P** < 0.001**			P*** = 0.141

* Fisher's exact test value for difference of HPV-16 detection rate among cancer sites
** Kruskal-Wallins test value for difference of HPV-16 geometric mean copies per cell
*** Fisher's exact test value for difference of HPV-16 genomic status

Table 1. HPV-16 genomes detected in SCCs of the oral cavity, oropharynx and esophagus.

surrounding normal cells. Another case-control study in the US found high-risk HPV, mainly HPV-16, more frequently in exfoliated oral cells from cancer patients than in those specimens from controls, suggesting an association of oral HPV infection with an increased risk of SCC in the head and neck [38]. In addition, elevated antibodies against L1 and/or E6/E7 were shown in an international study [39].

A review also showed that 15.2% of the 2,020 Esophageal SCC cases tested by PCR until the year 2002 were HPV positive [40]. However, the role of HPV in esophageal carcinomas remains unclear and controversial. European prospective serologic studies that used stored serum specimens [41] as well as a Chinese case-control study [42] found a strong association between the risk of ESCCs and seropositivity to HPV-16. In contrast, other retrospective studies conducted in Europe [43] and a large prospective serologic study in China [44] found no significant association of HPV-16 or HPV-18 with SCCs or adenocarcinomas of the esophagus.

Recently, in United State, Gillison [45] showed that HPV is a causal factor for a distinct group of UADT cancers particularly in oropharyngeal cancers that occur more frequently in men than women, where oral sex appear to be the principal risk factor for HPV-associated oral cancers in adolescents [46]. Also, the tumor HPV status may be a strong and independent prognostic factor for survival among patients with oropharyngeal cancer [47].

One important question is the route of HPV infection in the oral cavity, oropharynx, and esophagus tract. HPV is known to be sexually transmitted in the case of the anogenital organs. However, limited available data suggest that HPV infection in oral cavity is possibly sexually acquired: a history of sexually transmitted disease and number of oral sexual partners are associated with both oral HPV infection [48] and HPV-positive oropharyngeal cancer. Some data suggest that the presence and persistence of an oral high-risk HPV infection is associated with a persistent oral infection in a spouse [49] as well as with an increased risk for oral cancer among women with a history of cervical cancer and their husbands [50]. In addition, other several conceivable ways have been proposed for acquiring HPV infection in oral and pharyngeal cavities. These include intrapartum infection during passage through the infected birth canal, transplacental infection in uterus prior to birth, and postnatal infection by contact. For instance, HPV can be transmitted from a mother to her newborn baby during vaginal delivery resulting in recurrent respiratory papillomatosis. In addition, HPV DNA has been detected in the foreskin of normal newborn and in a high percentage of neonates vaginally delivered by HPV-infected mothers as well as in the amniotic fluid [51].

5.5. Etiological role of HPV

Studies on prevalence of HPV infections in premalignant and malignant lesions of the oral cavity suggested the implication of HPV during the early stages of oral neoplasia and a role in malignant progression [52].Studies in oral keratinocytes immortalized by HPV-16 have demonstrated an accumulated progression of chromosomal aberrations as well as high levels of cellular differentiation [53], however, in nude mice model, the tumorigenic activity is possible if there is a chronic exposure to the carcinogen benzopyrene of tabacco [54]. Both benzopyrene stimulation and the HPV-16 infection in cultured oral epithelial cells have been shown to confer anti-apoptotic characteristics, such as downregulation in the expression of the Fas and Bax proteins, as well as overexpression of Bcl2 via p53 deregulation. Consequently, HPV alone is not sufficiently to induce malignant transformation in several oral anatomic locations. Therefore further studies are needed.

6. Methods for HPV detection

As HPVs cannot be cultured easily, HPV detection and genotype assays are based on the detection of viral nucleic acids, usually viral DNA. HPV-DNA is detected by target amplification methods and/or signal amplification methods. The most used target amplification-based method is the polymerase chain reaction (PCR) using conserved sequences of the HPV genome, almost exclusively within the L1 open reading frame (ORF). In our studies in UADT using formalin-fixed and paraffin-embedded specimens [31], we detected HPV-DNA by GP5+/GP6+ primer pair for PCR [55] that amplified 150 base pair regions within L1, and the results were confirmed by southern blot analysis. Also, sequencing of an amplified L1 gene fragment was used to identify HPV genotype. In other studies in the UADT using formalin-fixed and paraffin-embedded specimens [32,33], we used an ultrasensitive short-fragment PCR assay, the SPF10, which amplifies a 65 base pair region within L1 [56]. The HPV types were determined using the INNO-LiPA HPV genotyping v2 kit (Innogenetics NV, Belgium), which is based on the reverse hybridization principle. In brief, part of the L1 gene region of the HPV genome is amplified using SPF10 primers tagged with a biotin at the 5′ and denatured. Biotinylated amplicons are hybridized with specific oligonucleotides probes immobilized on the strip. In total 25 genotypes (HPV-6, -11, -16, -18, -31 -33, -35, -39, -40, -42, -43, -44, -45, -51, -52, -53, -54, -56, -58, -59, -66, -68, -70, -73 and -74) were examined. Recently, real-time PCR assays have been used to determine the number of viral copies of HPV as well as to determine its integration status [57]. HPV-16 physical status is determined on the assumption that the E2 gene is disrupted in the integrated viral genome. On the other hand, episomal viral genome has equivalent copy numbers of the E2 and the E6 genes. In addition, mixed viral genome for HPV-16 shows both integrated form and episomal forms (figure 4).

Other target amplification-based methods such as reverse-transcriptase (RT-) PCR assays can be applied to detect HPV mRNAs in fresh-frozen specimens or samples in which RNA is well preserved (i.e. liquid-based cytology samples of cervical scrapings). Signal amplification methods are based on an initial hybridization step of nucleic acids in the specimen with target-specific probes in liquid phase or in situ on cells or tissue slides, after which the signal (i.e. the hybridization event) is amplified and ultimately visualized with one of the various available methodologies. The liquid-phase signal amplification method the Digene Hybrid Capture 2 (HC2) assay [58] (Qiagen, Gaithersburg, MD, USA), is the first

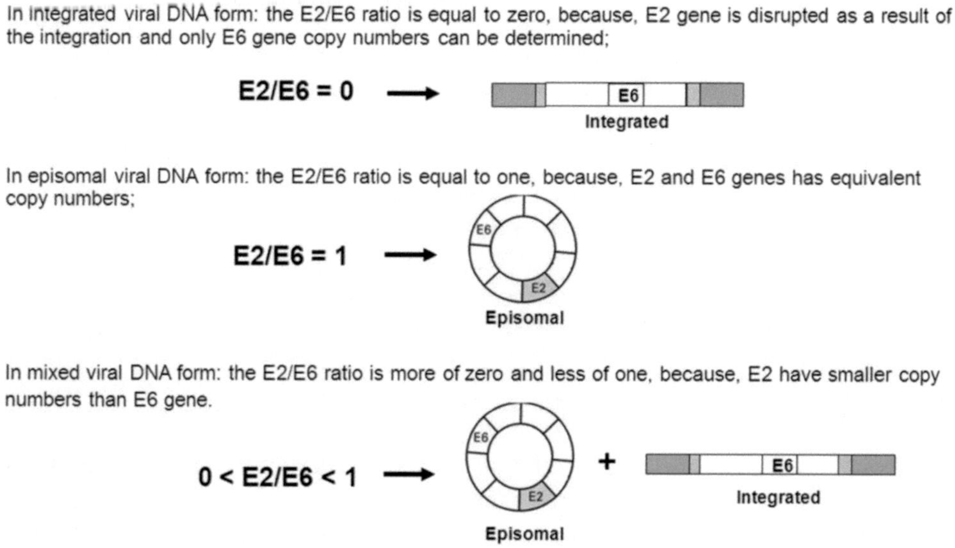

Figure 4. HPV Physical status by real-time PCR assay.

Food and Drug Administration (FDA) approved test that screens for the presence or absence of oncogenic HPV types. The HC2 assay uses a mixture of RNA probes representing 13 HPV genotypes (HPV-16, -18, -31, -33, -35, -39, -45, -51, -52, -56, -58, -59 and -68) to hybridize to HPV-DNA positive samples. DNA–RNA hybrids are subsequently captured in microplate wells coated with antibodies that specifically recognize DNA–RNA hybrids. For clinical validation of a new HPV tests a clinical equivalence analysis is necessary that compare the new test with a clinically validated reference for HPV using samples that originate from a population-based screening cohort.

Our studies showed that the HPV genome was detected in 56% and 19% of SCCs of the oral cavity and esophagus, respectively, in cases collected from Japan, Pakistan and Colombia and the HPV prevalence in both oral cancers (OCs) and esophageal cancers (ECs) did not significantly differ by country [33]. HPV16 was frequently integrated into the host genome in patients with OCs and ECs, however, the viral loads in these malignancies were much lower than those found in cancer of the cervix [33]. It should be noted, however, that human cancer is often regarded as a stem cell-like disease originating from a small fraction of cancer cells that show self-renewal and pluripotency and are capable of initiating and sustaining tumor growth [59]. This means that HPV may be present in only a small fraction of cancer cells with a stem cell-like nature present even in advanced tumors.

On the other hand, there was a significant geographical difference in the distribution of HPV16 E6 variants, which was also related to the viral load. HPV-16-positive OC cases with the E-350G variant showed a higher viral load than those with non-E-350G variants. Similar trends were observed in ECs although the difference was not statistically significant. Among HPV-16 intratypes, there is one polymorphism in the sequence of the E6 probe at nucleotide 145, and the Asian-American variant harbors this nucleotide substitution (C to T) [33]. However, this polymorphism is unlikely to cause a difference in viral load because the copy number of HPV-16 in the Asian-American variant was similar to other intratypes except E-350G. The HPV-16 E-350G variant contains a polymorphism at residue 83, leucine to valine (L83V), which is associated with the risk of invasive cancers of the cervix in European studies [60,61]. Only the E-350T prototype and the E-350G variant were detected in Japan. On the other hand, in Pakistan, E-350G was the predominant HPV16 variant. In Colombia, the Asian-American variant was the most commonly found type, but this variant was not found at all in Japan and Pakistan. Our findings are similar to those of Yamada et al [25], who detected the E-350G, E-350T, and Asian-American variants in 52%, 25%, and 20%, respectively, of 228 HPV16-positive cervical cancer specimens from Central and South America. No particular HPV16 E6 variant predisposed those infected to OCs or ECs.

7. HPV vaccine

Preventive HPV vaccines are based on empty virus-like particles (VLPs) assembled from recombinant HPV coat proteins. Two prophylactic HPV vaccines are currently on the market: Gardasil and Cervarix. The vaccine works by making recipient immune to two key strains of the HPV (HPV-16 and -18). Together, the two strains are known to cause approximately 70% of all cervical cancer cases worldwide and some other genital cancers. Gardasil also protects against the two HPV types (HPV-6 and HPV-11) that cause 90% of genital warts [62]. In UK, the Joint Committee on Vaccination and Immunization recommended routine vaccination for 11 to 12-year olds, including the possibility of a catch-up campaign but only up to the age of 16. Similar recommendations on vaccination of young women against HPV to prevent cervical cancer were made by Public health officials in Australia, Canada, Europe, and the United States [63]. It is suggested that vaccinating most teenage girls could save hundreds of lives a year, although, the benefits would not be seen until those receiving the vaccine enter middle age.

In 2009, the Food and Drug Administration (FDA) licensed to Gardasil for use in males aged 9 through 26 years for prevention of genital warts caused by HPV-6 and -11. HPV-6 and -11 cause approximately 90% of genital warts and most cases of recurrent respiratory papillomatosis [63]. HPV-associated cancers in males include certain anal, penile, and oropharyngeal and oral cavity cancers caused primarily by HPV 16 [45, 64, 65]. Mathematical modeling suggests that adding male HPV vaccination to a female-only HPV vaccination program is not the most cost-effective vaccination strategy for reducing the overall burden of HPV-associated conditions in males and females when vaccination coverage of females is high (>80%) [66]. Since the health burden is greater in females than males, and numerous models have shown vaccination of adolescent girls to be a cost-effective use of public health resources, improving coverage in females aged 11 and 12 years could potentially be a more effective and cost-effective strategy than adding male vaccination.

Men who have sex with men (MSM) are particularly at risk for conditions associated with HPV-6, -11, -16, and -18; diseases and cancers that have a higher incidence among MSM include anal intraepithelial neoplasias, anal cancers, and genital warts [67]. Gardasil has high efficacy for prevention of anal intraepithelial neoplasias in MSM [68]. The 3-dose series of gardasil may be given to fenales and males aged 9 through 26 years to reduce their likelihood of acquiring genital warts and gardasil would be most effective when given before exposure to HPV through sexual contact.

On the other hand, laboratory research and clinical trials are focused on the development of therapeutic vaccines against HPV oncogenes, such as E6 and E7. It is hoped that immune responses against the two oncogenes might eradicate established tumors [69, 70].

8. Conclusions

Currently, the HPV vaccines potentially hold promise for the prevention of a greater majority of HPV-positive cervical cancers in woman. Thus, studies that attempt to clarify the association between HPV with cancers of the oral cavity and esophagus are important. They give us reason to be optimistic that HPV vaccines may be protective against UADT HPV infection, and consequently, effective in preventing HPV-associated UADT cancers in both men and women.

Author details

Andrés Castillo
School of Basic Sciences, Faculty of Health, Universidad del Valle, Cali, Colombia

Acknowledgement

To Dr. Suminori Akiba and Dr. Chihaya Koriyama from Department of Epidemiology and Preventive Medicine at Kagoshima University-Japan, and Dr. Yoshito Eizuru from Division of Oncogenic and Persistent Viruses at Kagoshima University-Japan.

To Japanese Government (Monbukagakusho) Scholarship and the Grants-in-Aid for Scientific Research on Priority Areas (17015037) of the Ministry of Education, Culture, Sports, Science and Technology, Japan.

9. References

[1] Parkin DM. The global health burden of infection-associated cancers in the year 2002 (2006) Int. J. Cancer. 118:3030-3044.

[2] Mueller NE, Birmann B, Parsonnet J, Schiffman M, Stuver S (2005) Infectious agents. In: Schottenfeld D, Fraumeni JF Jr, editors. Cancer epidemiology and prevention 3rd ed. Oxford University Press. Chapter 26.

[3] D'Souza G, Kreimer AR, Viscidi R, Pawlita M, Fakhry C, Koch WM, et al. (2007) Case-control study of human papilloma virus and oropharyngeal cancer. N. Engl. J. Med. 356: 1944-1956.

[4] zur Hausen H (2002) Papillomaviruses and cancer: from basic studies to clinical application. Nat. Rev. Cancer. 2:342-350.

[5] de Villiers EM, Fauquet C, Broker TR, Bernard HU, zur Hausen H (2004) Classification of papillomaviruses. Virology. 324:17-27.

[6] Van Ranst M, Kaplan JB, Burk RD (1992) Phylogenetic classification of human papillomaviruses: correlation with clinical manifestations. J. Gen. Virol. 73:2653-2660.

[7] Muñoz N, Bosch FX, de Sanjosé S, Herrero R, Castellsagué X, Shah KV, et al. (2003) Epidemiologic classification of human papillomavirus types associated with cervical cancer. N. Engl. J. Med. 348:518-527.

[8] Yamada T, Manos MM, Peto J, Greer CE, Munoz N, Bosch FX, et al. (1997) Human papillomavirus type 16 sequence variation in cervical cancers: a worldwide perspective. J. Virol. 71:2463-2472.

[9] Longworth MS, Laimins LA (2004) Pathogenesis of human papillomaviruses in differentiating epithelia. Microbiol. Mol. Biol. Rev. 68:362-372.

[10] Joyce JG, Tung JS, Przysiecki CT, Cook JC, Lehman ED, Sands JA, et al. (1999) The L1 major capsid protein of human papillomavirus type 11 recombinant virus-like particles interacts with heparin and cell-surface glycosaminoglycans on human keratinocytes. J. Biol. Chem. 274:5810-5822.

[11] Yoon CS, Kim KD, Park SN, Cheong SW (2001) alpha (6) Integrin is the main receptor of human papillomavirus type 16 VLP. Biochem Biophys Res Commun. 283:668-673.

[12] Doorbar J (2005) The papillomavirus life cycle. J. Clin. Virol. 32:S7-S15.

[13] Münger K, Baldwin A, Edwards KM, Hayakawa H, Nguyen CL, Owens M, et al. (2004) Mechanisms of human papillomavirus-induced oncogenesis. J. Virol. 78:11451-11460.

[14] Moscicki AB, Schiffman M, Kjaer S, Villa LL (2006) Chapter 5: Updating the natural history of HPV and anogenital cancer. Vaccine. 24:S42-S51.

[15] Um SJ, Rhyu JW, Kim EJ, Jeon KC, Hwang ES, Park JS (2002) Abrogation of IRF-1 response by high-risk HPV E7 protein in vivo. Cancer Lett. 179:205-212.

[16] Wentzensen N, Vinokurova S, von Knebel Doeberitz M (2004) Systematic review of genomic integration sites of human papillomavirus genomes in epithelial dysplasia and invasive cancer of the female lower genital tract. Cancer Res. 64:3878-3884.

[17] Pett M, Coleman NJ (2007) Integration of high-risk human papillomavirus: a key event in cervical carcinogenesis?. J. Pathol. 212:356-367.

[18] Duensing S, Münger K (2004) Mechanisms of genomic instability in human cancer: insights from studies with human papillomavirus oncoproteins. Int. J. Cancer.109:157-162.

[19] Duensing S, Münger K (2003) Human papillomavirus type 16 E7 oncoprotein can induce abnormal centrosome duplication through a mechanism independent of inactivation of retinoblastoma protein family members. J. Virol.77:12331-12335.

[20] Duensing S, Münger K (2002) The human papillomavirus type 16 E6 and E7 oncoproteins independently induce numerical and structural chromosome instability. Cancer Res. 62:7075-7082.

[21] Muñoz N, Castellsagué X, de González AB, Gissmann L (2006) Chapter 1: HPV in the etiology of human cancer. Vaccine. 24:S1-S10.

[22] Stewart BW, Kleihues P, editors. (2003) World Cancer Report. Lyon: IARC Press.

[23] Schwartz JL (2000) Biomarkers and molecular epidemiology and chemoprevention of oral carcinogenesis. Crit Rev Oral Biol Med. 11:92-122.
[24] Montesano R, Hollstein M, Hainaut P (1996) Genetic alterations in esophageal cancer and their relevance to etiology and pathogenesis: a review. Int. J. Cancer. 69:225-35.
[25] Mandard AM, Hainaut P, Hollstein M (2000) Genetic steps in the development of squamous cell carcinoma of the esophagus. Mutat Res. 462:335-342.
[26] Ruesga MT, Acha-Sagredo A, Rodríguez MJ, Aguirregaviria JI, Videgain J, Rodríguez C, et al. (2007) p16(INK4a) promoter hypermethylation in oral scrapings of oral squamous cell carcinoma risk patients. Cancer Lett. 250:140-145.
[27] Guha N, Boffetta P, Wünsch Filho V, Eluf Neto J, Shangina O, Zaridze D, et al. (2007) Oral health and risk of squamous cell carcinoma of the head and neck and esophagus: results of two multicentric case-control studies. Am. J. Epidemiol. 166:1159-1173.
[28] Yokoyama A, Muramatsu T, Ohmori T, Yokoyama T, Okuyama K, Takahashi H, et al.(1998) Alcohol-related cancers and aldehyde dehydrogenase-2 in Japanese alcoholics. Carcinogenesis. 19:1383-1387.
[29] Cogliano V, Baan R, Straif K, Grosse Y, Secretan B, El Ghissassi F (2005) WHO International Agency for Research on Cancer. Carcinogenicity of human papillomaviruses. Lancet Oncol. 6:204.
[30] Gillison ML, Shah KV (2003) Chapter 9: Role of mucosal human papillomavirus in nongenital cancers. J. Natl. Cancer Inst. Monogr. 31:57-65.
[31] Castillo A, Aguayo F, Koriyama C, Torres M, Carrascal E, Corvalan A, et al. (2006) Human papillomavirus in esophageal squamous cell carcinoma in Colombia and Chile. World J. Gastroenterol. 12:6188-6192.
[32] Shuyama K, Castillo A, Aguayo F, Sun Q, Khan N, Koriyama C, et al. (2007) Human papillomavirus in high- and low-risk areas of oesophageal squamous cell carcinoma in China. Br. J. Cancer. 96:1554-1559.
[33] Castillo A, Koriyama C, Higashi M, Anwar M, Bukhari MH, Carrascal E, et al (2011) Human papillomavirus in upper digestive tract tumors from three countries. World J. Gastroenterol. 17:5295-5304.
[34] Kreimer AR, Clifford GM, Boyle P, Franceschi S. (2005) Human papillomavirus types in head and neck squamous cell carcinomas worldwide: a systematic review. Cancer Epidemiol Biomarkers Prev. 14:467-475.
[35] Miller CS, Johnstone BM (2001) Human papillomavirus as a risk factor for oral squamous cell carcinoma: a meta-analysis, 1982-1997. Oral Surg. Oral Med. Oral Pathol. Oral Radiol. Endod. 91:622-635.
[36] Maden C, Beckmann AM, Thomas DB, McKnight B, Sherman KJ, Ashley RL, et al. (1992) Human papillomaviruses, herpes simplex viruses, and the risk of oral cancer in men. Am J Epidemiol. 135:1093-1102.
[37] D'Souza G, Kreimer AR, Viscidi R, Pawlita M, Fakhry C, Koch WM, et al. (2007) Case-control study of human papillomavirus and oropharyngeal cancer. N. Engl. J. Med. 356:1944-1956.

[38] Smith EM, Ritchie JM, Summersgill KF, Hoffman HT, Wang DH, Haugen TH, Turek LP. (2004) Human papillomavirus in oral exfoliated cells and risk of head and neck cancer. J. Natl. Cancer Inst. 96:449-455.

[39] Herrero R, Castellsagué X, Pawlita M, Lissowska J, Kee F, Balaram P, et al. (2003) Human papillomavirus and oral cancer: the International Agency for Research on Cancer multicenter study. J. Natl. Cancer Inst. 95:1772-1783.

[40] Syrjanen KJ (2002) HPV infections and oesophageal cancer. J. Clin. Pathol. 55:721-728.

[41] Bjorge T, Hakulinen T, Engeland A, Jellum E, Koskela P, Lehtinen M, et al. (1997) A prospective, seroepidemiological study of the role of human papillomavirus in esophageal cancer in Norway. Cancer Res. 57:3989-3992.

[42] Han C, Qiao G, Hubbert NL, Li L, Sun C, Wang Y, et al. (1996) Serologic association between human papillomavirus type 16 infection and esophageal cancer in Shaanxi Province, China. J. Natl. Cancer Inst. 88:1467-1471.

[43] Van Doornum GJ, Korse CM, Buning-Kager JC, Bonfrer JM, Horenblas S, Taal BG, et al. (2003) Reactivity to human papillomavirus type 16 L1 virus-like particles in sera from patients with genital cancer and patients with carcinomas at five different extragenital sites. Br. J. Cancer 88:1095-1100.

[44] Kamangar F, Qiao YL, Schiller JT, Dawsey SM, Fears T, Sun XD, et al. (2006) Human papillomavirus serology and the risk of esophageal and gastric cancers: Results from a cohort in a high-risk region in China. Int. J. Cancer. 119: 579-84.

[45] Gillison ML (2009) HPV and prognosis for patients with oropharynx cancer. Eur. J. Cancer 45:383-385.

[46] Gillison ML (2008) Human papillomavirus-related diseases: oropharynx cancers and potential implications for adolescent HPV vaccination. J Adolesc Health. 43:S52-S60.

[47] Ang KK, Harris J, Wheeler R, Weber R, Rosenthal DI, Nguyen-Tân PF, et al. (2010) Human papillomavirus and survival of patients with oropharyngeal cancer. N. Engl. J. Med. 363:24-35.

[48] Scardina GA, Pisano T, Messina P (2009) Oral and cervical lesions associated with human papillomavirus. Recenti Prog Med. 100:261-266.

[49] Rintala M, Grenman S, Puranen M, Syrjanen S (2006) Natural history of oral papillomavirus infections in spouses: a prospective Finnish HPV Family Study. J. Clin. Virol. 35:89-94.

[50] Hemminki K, Dong C, Frisch M (2000). Tonsillar and other upper aerodigestive tract cancers among cervical cancer patients and their husbands. Eur. J. Cancer Prev. 9:433-437.

[51] Puranen M, Yliskoski M, Saarikoski S, Syrjänen K, Syrjänen S (1996) Vertical transmission of human papillomavirus from infected mothers to their newborn babies and persistence of the virus in childhood. Am. J. Obstet. Gynecol. 174:694-699.

[52] Tsantoulis PK, Kastrinakis NG, Tourvas AD, Laskaris G, Gorgoulis VG (2007) Advances in the biology of oral cancer. Oral Oncol. 43:523-534.

[53] Oda D, Bigler L, Mao EJ, Disteche CM (1996). Chromosomal abnormalities in HPV-16-immortalized oral epithelial cells. Carcinogenesis. 17:2003–2008.

[54] Park NH, Gujuluva CN, Baek JH, Cherrick HM, Shin KH, Min BM (1995) Combined oral carcinogenicity of HPV-16 and benzo(a)pyrene: an in vitro multistep carcinogenesis model. Oncogene 10:2145–2153.

[55] De Roda Husman AM, Walboomers JM, van den Brule AJ, Meijer CJ, Snijders PJ (1995) The use of general primers GP5 and GP6 elongated at their 3′ ends with adjacent highly conserved sequences improves human papillomavirus detection by PCR. J. Gen. Virol. 76:1057–1062.

[56] Kleter, B., L. J. Van Doorn, L. Schrauwen, A. Molijn, S. Sastrowijoto, J. ter Schegget, J. Lindeman, B. et al. (1999) Development and clinical evaluation of a highly sensitive PCR-reverse hybridization line probe assay for detection and identification of anogenital human papillomavirus. J Clin Microbiol. 37:2508-2517.

[57] Peitsaro P, Johansson B, Syrjanen S (2002) Integrated human papillomavirus type 16 is frequently found in cervical cancer precursors as demonstrated by a novel quantitative real-time PCR technique. J Clin Microbiol. 40:886-891.

[58] Clavel C, Masure M, Putaud I, Thomas K, Bory JP, Gabriel R, et al. (1998) Hybrid capture II, a new sensitivetest for human papillomavirus detection. Comparison with hybrid capture I and PCR results in cervical lesions. J Clin Pathol. 51:737–740.

[59] Boman BM, Wicha MS (2008) Cancer stem cells: a step toward the cure. J. Clin. Oncol. 26:2795-2799.

[60] Zehbe I, Wilander E, Delius H, Tommasino M (1998) Human papillomavirus 16 E6 variants are more prevalent in invasive cervical carcinoma than the prototype. Cancer Res. 58:829-833

[61] Grodzki M, Besson G, Clavel C, Arslan A, Franceschi S, Birembaut P, Tommasino M, et al. (2006) Increased risk for cervical disease progression of French women infected with the human papillomavirus type 16 E6-350G variant. Cancer Epidemiol Biomarkers Prev. 15:820-822.

[62] Allen JD, Coronado GD, Williams RS, Glenn B, Escoffery C, Fernandez M, Tuff RA, et al. (2010) A systematic review of measures used in studies of human papillomavirus (HPV) vaccine acceptability. Vaccine. 28:4027-4037.

[63] Hu D, Goldie S. (2008) The economic burden of noncervical human papillomavirus disease in the United States. Am J Obstet Gynecol 98:500-507.

[64] Hartwig S, Syrjänen S, Dominiak-Felden G, Brotons M, Castellsagué X. (2012) Estimation of the epidemiological burden of human papillomavirus-related cancers and non-malignant diseases in men in Europe: a review. BMC Cancer 20:12:30.

[65] Joseph DA, Miller JW, Wu X, Chen VW, Morris CR, Goodman MT, Villalon-Gomez JM, Williams MA, Cress RD. (2008) Understanding the burden of human papillomavirus-associated anal cancers in the U.S. Cancer 113:2892-2900.

[66] Brisson M, Van de Velde N, Boily MC. (2009) Economic evaluation of human papillomavirus vaccination in developed countries. Public Health Genomics12:343-351.

[67] Jin F, Prestage GP, Kippax SC, Pell CM, Donovan B, Templeton DJ, Kaldor JM, Grulich AE. (2007) Risk factors for genital and anal warts in a prospective cohort of HIV-negative homosexual men: the HIM study. Sex Transm Dis 34:488-493.

[68] Palefsky J, Male Quadrivalent HPV Vaccine Efficacy Trial Team. Quadrivalent HPV vaccine efficacy against anal intraepithelial neoplasia in men having sex with men (2010). 9th International Multidisciplinary Congress, Monte Carlo, Monaco. Abstract 17-20.

[69] Lin K, Doolan K, Hung CF, Wu TC (2010) Perspectives for preventive and therapeutic HPV vaccines. J Formos Med. Assoc. 109:4-24.

[70] Garland SM, Smith JS (2010) Human papillomavirus vaccines: current status and future prospects. Drugs. 70:1079-1098.

Chapter 4

Oestrogens, Xenoestrogens and Hormone-Dependent Cancers

Anna Ptak and Ewa Lucja Gregoraszczuk

Additional information is available at the end of the chapter

http://dx.doi.org/10.5772/54464

1. Introduction

The hormonal microenvironment surrounding endocrine-sensitive tissues may play an important role in the carcinogenesis of these tissues. Epidemiological evidence strongly suggests that steroid hormones, primarily oestrogens (E2), are implicated in ovarian and breast carcinogenesis.

The breast is an endocrine-sensitive organ. The development of the breast from puberty through the cycles of pregnancy, lactation and involution is regulated through hormonal controls. Epidemiological studies have demonstrated that 50% or more of breast cancers are environmental in origin. Epidemiological evidence linking breast cancer incidence to oestrogen exposure and the ability of oestrogen to drive the growth of breast tumours in vivo is well documented in clinical studies. In addition, the mechanism of oestrogen action on the growth of breast cancer cells in animal models and in vitro has been extensively described in experimental studies. The involvement of oestrogen in the progression of breast cancer is the basis for the successful use of endocrine therapy as a treatment for breast cancer. In addition to the physiological steroidal oestrogens, many compounds have been found to have oestrogenic activity such that the human breast can be exposed to environmental oestrogens from a variety of sources. The link between breast cancer and the use of the oral contraceptive pill has been extensively studied, and a study involving a million women has documented an increase in breast cancer following the use of hormone replacement therapy (HRT). Such findings demonstrate that the development of breast cancer can be influenced at all stages of life after puberty through the voluntary exposure to exogenous oestrogens.

Ovarian cancer is the fourth-ranking cause of cancer-related death in women from Western countries. The natural history of this cancer is characterised by the potential for particularly aggressive local invasion. Unfortunately, these tumours are often diagnosed at an advanced stage (i.e., 70% of tumours are discovered at stage III). Although all cell types of the human ovary may undergo neoplastic transformation, the vast majority (80-90%) of tumours are derived from ovarian surface epithelium (OSE). One of the hypotheses regarding the causes of ovarian cancer argues that the repeated cycles of ovulation-induced trauma and repair of the OSE during ovulation, without pregnancy-induced rest periods, contribute to ovarian cancer development. This "incessant ovulation" hypothesis suggests that regenerative repair of OSE cells that occurs during ovulation results in the accumulation of mutations, which predisposes this cell layer to tumourogenesis. There is also growing experimental evidence that oestrogens may play an important role in ovarian carcinogenesis. Use of HRT for menopause-related symptoms could be associated with an increased risk of ovarian cancer incidence or mortality.

2. Endogenous oestrogens

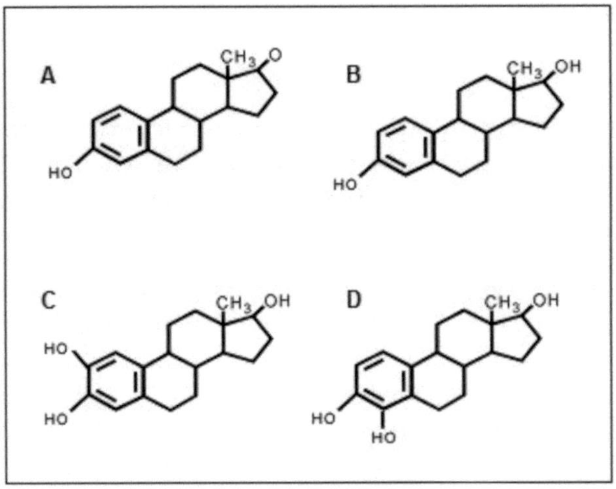

Figure 1. A) Oestrone (E1); B) Oestradiol (E2); C) 2-hydroxyoestradiol (2-OH-E2); D) 4-hydroxyoestradiol (4-OH-E2)

2.1. Carcinogenesis of oestrogens

Oestrogens are believed to play a critical role in the etiology of breast and ovarian cancer through two distinct pathways. First, the products of oestrogen metabolism damage DNA by forming adducts and oxidised bases, leading to mutations in oncogenes and tumour suppressor genes that normally control cell growth and proliferation [1]. Second, oestrogens may alter the expression of specific genes, which stimulate growth and proliferation of epithelial cells in the breast and ovary. Notably, oestradiol-17β has been classified as a carcinogen by the International Agency for Research on Cancer. Thus, natural oestrogens levels in men and women have the potential to act as carcinogens. For example, early menarche and late menopause are risk factors for breast cancer, due to longer oestrogen exposures. It is well established that chronic exposure to elevated oestrogen levels contributes to carcinogenesis of multiple reproductive organs. Ovaries are not only the principal source of oestrogens in premenopausal women but are the key target tissue of oestrogen activity. Oestradiol and oestrone are mainly produced by follicular cells. Ovarian tissue oestrogen levels are at least 100-fold higher than the circulating levels and those in the follicular fluid of ovulatory follicles are even higher [2]. Additionally, active oestrogens are formed from circulating oestrone sulphate or oestradiol sulphate, as the result of de-conjugation by sulphatase [3]. The local release of biologically active oestrogens from conjugates and their further metabolism prolong the effect of oestrogen on peripheral tissues [4]. Oestrogen is essential to the function of the female reproductive system and a major regulator of growth and differentiation in normal ovaries. Furthermore, oestrogens are required for the proliferation and differentiation of healthy breast epithelium.

2.2. Classic ER mediated activity

The classic oestrogen receptors (ERs) are nuclear hormone receptors that act as transcription factors, regulating genes involved in homeostasis, development and metabolism. Two forms of ER have been identified, ERα and ERβ. While ERβ is predominantly expressed by granulosa cells, theca cells, surface epithelium, and CL, oocytes have also been reported to express the receptor. Both receptors are ligand-inducible nuclear hormone receptors. The classic mechanism of ER action involves binding of the ER to its ligand, resulting in receptor dimerisation, interaction with consensus oestrogen-response elements (EREs), and recruitment of transcriptional co-regulators, resulting in the formation of a complex that modulates the transcription of oestrogen target genes. The best-described nuclear receptor cofactors are the p160 family of co-activators, namely, SRC-1, SRC-2, and SRC-3; however, the cofactor complexes that mediate the ultimate outcome of ER signalling are complicated with more than 300 cofactors described in the literature [5]. Numerous genes with diverse functions in energy production, cell growth, cell cycle regulation, and cytoskeleton organisation, whose expression is induced or repressed by oestrogen, have been identified by microarray analysis. Oestrogen receptors have been shown to interact with other transcription factors, co-activator proteins, and tyrosine kinase growth-factor receptors and to cross–talk with other signal transduction pathways [6]. Through regulating gene expression, oestrogen functions as a potent stimulus for proliferation and inhibition of apoptosis, which may lead to the development of cancer.

2.3. Non-genomic ER mediated activity

ER signalling may occur in a ligand-dependent, non-genomic (extra-nuclear) pathway. This pathway involves the activation of other signal transduction pathways that lead to rapid responses, generally within minutes, to oestrogen exposure. The mechanism of non-genomic ER signalling is not clear, but is potentially mediated by a membrane-associated receptor. A G-protein coupled receptor known as GPR30 mediates rapid oestrogen signalling independent of ERs, which can lead to activation of the MAPK or phosphoinositide-3-kinase (PI3) kinase signalling cascades, fluctuations in intracellular calcium, or stimulation of cAMP production [7]. E2 mediation activates the MAPK and PI3 pathways that are the major effectors of cell proliferation and cell survival. Deregulations of cell proliferation, differentiation, and apoptosis may allow cells that have harboured mutations in proto-oncogenes and tumour suppressor genes to survive and expand clonally.

2.4. Metabolism of oestrogens

There is growing evidence that E2 and its metabolites may be involved in breast cancer development. Endogenous E2 metabolites may play an important role by influencing the growth of oestrogen-sensitive target cells, both stimulating and inhibiting proliferation [8]. It is generally known that both the biosynthesis and metabolism of E2 occur in cancerous breast tissues. The cytochrome P450-dependent monooxygenases (CYP) are responsible for the biosynthesis and metabolism of endogenous compounds such as steroid hormones. 2-hydroxyestadiol (2-OH-E2) and 4-hydroxyestradiol (4-OH-E2) are two major hydroxylated metabolites of E2 formed by cytochrome P450 1A1 and 1B1, respectively. The catechols 2-OH-E2 and 4-OH-E2 can be oxidised to quinones, which are putative tumour initiators, and the 4-hydroxylated form of E2 appears to be one of the most genotoxic metabolites of E2 in the breast epithelium. The 4-OH-E2 to 2-OH-E2 concentration ratio has been reported to be 4:1 in a human breast cancer extract [9]. The catechol-*O*-methyltransferase (COMT), which methylates catechol estrogens, prevents their conversion to quinones. There are reports that 2-hydroxylated E2/E1 are better substrates for COMT than their 4-hydroxylated isomers [10,11]. Thus, the 2OH-E2/4OH-E2 ratio may be a critical parameter of the carcinogenicity of E2.

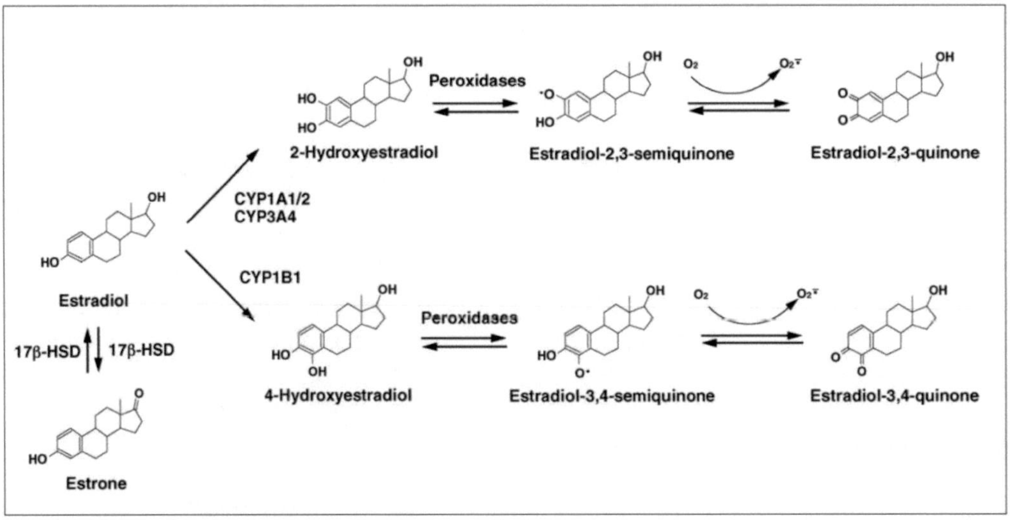

Figure 2. Major metabolic pathway in cancer initiation by oestrogens

We propose that local activation of the cytochrome P450 enzymes CYP1A1 and CYP1B1 by E2 may generate active metabolites that affect apoptosis and thereby promote mammary carcinogenesis. To test this hypothesis, we measured the ability of E2 to induce CYP1A1 and CYP1B1 and assessed the influence of the parent compounds and their hydroxylated metabolites on apoptosis.

The previously published results demonstrated that E2 increased CYP1B1 protein expression after 48 h of cell culture but had no effect on CYP1A1 protein levels [12], Figure 3. CYP1B1 has been suggested to play key roles in initiating breast cancers in humans, as this enzyme is active in catalysing oestradiol to a 4-hydroxylated metabolite. Cytochrome P450 enzymes, the products of the *CYP* genes, are components of the oestrone hydroxylase enzyme system. Elevated 4-hydroxyoestrogen production has been associated with breast tumours [13].

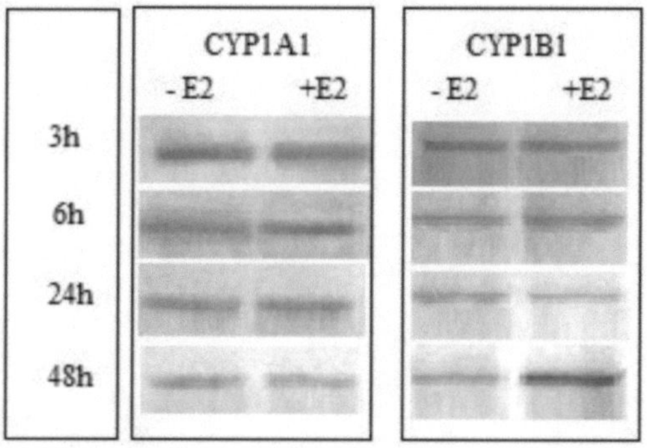

Figure 3. The effect of oestradiol (1nM) on expression of the CYP 1B1 protein in MCF-7 cells [12]

2.5. Action of E2 and its hydroxylated metabolites (2-OH-E2 and 4-OH-E2) on MCF-7 breast cancer cell proliferation

In our previously published data [12], we demonstrated that E2 can be locally metabolised to their hydroxylated derivatives via cytochrome P450 enzymes in breast cancer MCF-7 cells. Additionally, E2 hydroxylated metabolites had a time-dependent affect on MCF-7 cell proliferation [14]. While E2 and 4-OH-E2 elicited a significant increase in cell proliferation over the entire time of exposure, 2-OH-E2 resulted in an increase of cell proliferation only after a long incubation period, Figure 4.

Our observations were consistent with the results of [15], who demonstrated that 4-OH-E2 is more oestrogenic than 2-OH-E2. In [16] it was indicated that certain oestradiol metabolites, i.e., 4-OH-E2 and 16-OH-E2, are able to mimic the effects of 17β-oestradiol on proliferation and markers of tumour metastasis. The effect was more pronounced for 16-OH-E2. In contrast, the metabolite 2-OH-E2 did not show any significant effect on these parameters. The effect of the various oestrogen metabolites appears to be dependent on their ability to bind to the oestrogen-receptor. The most potent oestrogen regarding an influence on proliferation, apoptosis and metastasis is 17β-oestradiol. As this oestrogen appears to be metabolised intracellularly, the direction of oestradiol metabolism may influence breast cancer risk in certain predisposed women. Enhanced metabolism towards 2-OH-E2 may even be protective, as this metabolite is rapidly converted into 2-methoxyestradiol, which has been shown to be a potent anti-proliferative and anti-angiogenic agent in various tumour cells [17].

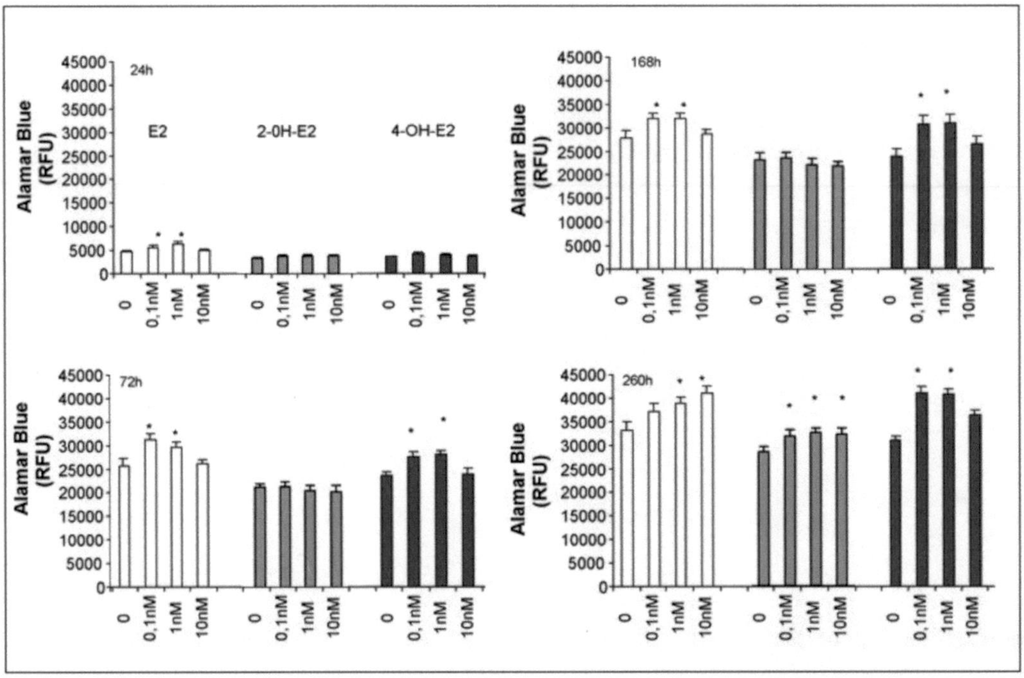

Figure 4. Action of E2 and its hydroxylated metabolites 2-OH-E2 and 4-OH-E2 on MCF-7 cell proliferation after 24, 72, 168, and 260 h of exposure to 0.1, 1.0 or 10nM concentrations of these compounds. (*) $p < 0.05$ [14]

2.6. Molecular mechanisms of E2 and its hydroxylated metabolites (2-OH and 4-OH)

The human sex hormone-binding globulin (SHBG), a glycoprotein that specifically binds plasma androgens and oestradiol, participates in the mechanism of action of oestradiol in breast cancer cells. The SHBG protein has been detected, using reverse transcriptase-polymerase chain reaction (RT-PCR), in ZR-75-1, MCF-7 and MDA MB 231 cells, as well as in 11 breast tissue samples [18]. Although the data concerning the cell lines were convincing, no evidence for mRNA translation has been presented. Due to its unique property to regulate bioavailable oestradiol, several epidemiological studies have implicated SHBG as having a role in breast cancer, and it has been suggested that plasma SHBG levels are inversely associated with breast cancer risk in post-menopausal women. According to [19], for SHBG to be biologically relevant, the interaction of SHBG with its membrane-binding site (SHBG-R) requires the occurrence of a precise sequence of events. First, SHBG must bind to a membrane (through SHBG-R), and a ligand must then interact with the SHBG bound to the membrane. It is only at this point that the biological effect is elicited. If the ligand binds to SHBG before the protein binds to the membrane, it is blocked from interacting with membranes, Figure 5. In breast cancer MCF-7 cells, SHBG binds to the membrane, and through cyclic adenosine monophosphate (cAMP) induction and protein kinase A (PKA) activation, it inhibits oestradiol-induced cell proliferation [20].

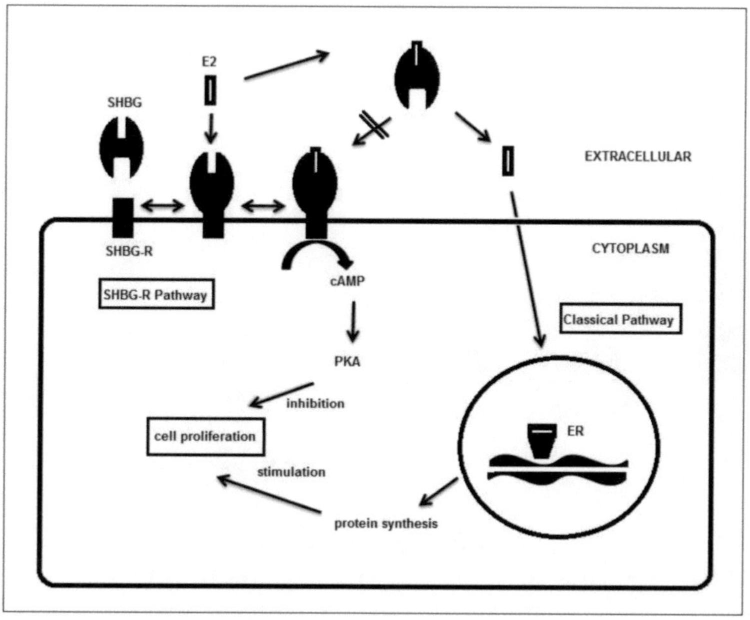

Figure 5. Model for SHBG-mediated signalling pathway

Despite extensive years of research, the action of hydroxylated metabolites of E2 (2-OH-E2 and 4-OH-E2) on SHBG intra/extracellular secretion as well as gene and protein expression in extrahepatic tissue has not yet been investigated. Our data demonstrated that hydroxylated metabolites of E2, with a potency of E2 > 4-OH-E2 > 2-OH-E2, increased intracellular and had no effect on extracellular SHBG levels [21], Figure 6.

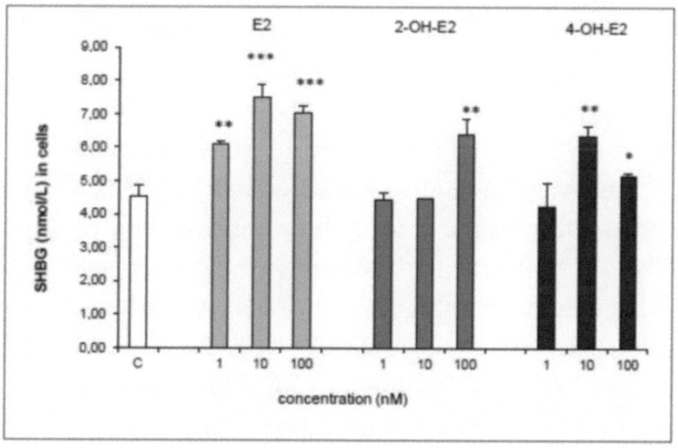

Figure 6. The effect of E2, 2-OH-E2 and 4-OH-E2 on intracellular SHBG levels in MCF-7 cells. (*) $p<0.05$, (**) $p<0.01$, (***) $p<0.001$ [21]

Additionally, we demonstrated that E2, 2-OH-E2 and 4-OH-E2 increased SHBG mRNA and protein expression [21], Figure 7.

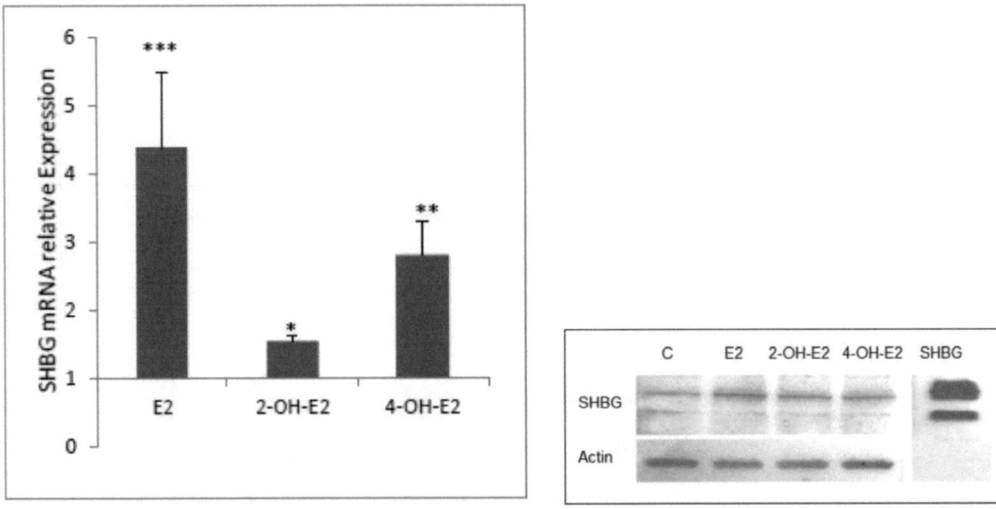

Figure 7. The effects of E2, 2-OH-E2 and 4-OH-E2 on SHBG mRNA and protein expression in MCF-7 cells. SHBG mRNA determined by real time PCR. (*) $p<0.05$, (**) $p<0.01$, (***) $p<0.001$ [21]

In addition to classical transcriptional actions, oestrogens also trigger rapid intracellular signalling events typically associated with membrane receptors. Oestradiol, a biologically potent oestrogen, can induce rapid activation of many signalling molecules, including cAMP/PKA and MAPK pathways [22]. An increasing number of studies indicate that the cellular action of E2 can be initiated at the plasma membrane, through membrane versions of oestrogen receptors (mERs) or via other membrane-resident E2-binding proteins [23]. The binding of E2 to the membrane receptor causes an increase of intracellular cAMP levels [23]. As a second messenger, cAMP is involved in a variety of intracellular signalling pathways that lead to diverse physiological effects, including the control of cell proliferation. The majority of cAMP signalling in eukaryotic cells is through PKA. It has been reported that activation of the cAMP/PKA pathway induces growth inhibition in a variety of human cancer cells, including the MCF-7 cell line [23]. Mitogen-activated protein kinases (MAPKs), such as extracellular signal-regulated kinases (ERK1 and ERK2), are also rapidly stimulated by oestrogens in various cell types, including breast cancer cells. Additionally, it has been reported that the cAMP/PKA and the MAPK pathways are connected in MCF-7 cells [23,24]. Notably, ERK can be activated or inhibited by cAMP and E2, although activation of the cAMP/PKA suppresses the activity of ERK1/2 [25]. However, controversies also exist regarding the extent to which E2 may influence ERK1/2 activation [26]. We have shown that E2 and its hydroxylated metabolites do not activate cAMP/PKA and ERK1/2 in breast cancer cells and confirmed previously published data, which demonstrated a lack of ERK1/2 activation in a breast cancer cell line [27], Figure 8, 9. The observed reversible action of PD98059 on cell proliferation can be explained via the actions of hydroxylated estrogens, which similarly to E2, stimulate secretion of a number of growth factors that affect MAPK activity [28].

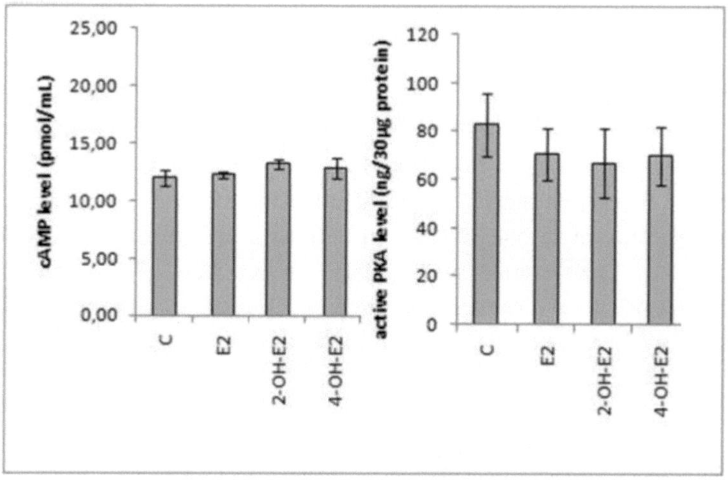

Figure 8. The effects of E2, 2-OH-E2 and 4-OH-E2 on cAMP and PKA levels in MCF-7 cells. [27]

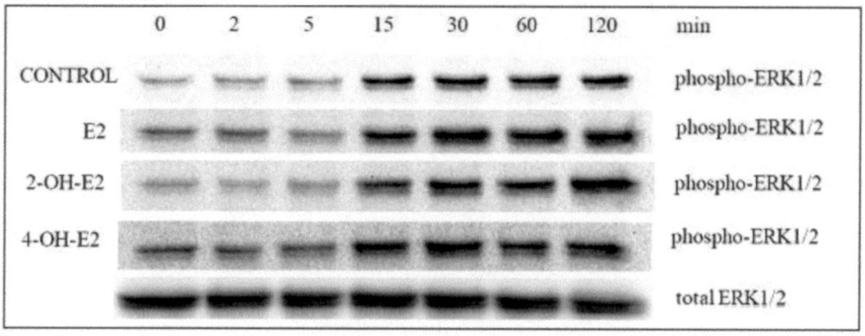

Figure 9. Time-dependent effects of E2, 2-OH-E2 and 4-OH-E2 on phospho- and total ERK1/2 protein expression in MCF-7 cells. [27]

3. Xenoestrogens

Xenoestrogens form a diverse group of man-made chemicals that have been released into the environment from agricultural spraying (herbicides, pesticides), by-products of industrial processes and waste disposal of polychlorinated biphenyls (PCBs) and dioxins or as discharges from treatment systems (alkyl phenols). They are also found in household products in daily use, such as plastics (bisphenol A, phthalates) and flame retardants (polybrominated organics) and cosmetic products (e.g., parabens, cyclosiloxanes). They may be present in diets, and because they are lipophilic, they can pass up the food chain dissolved in animal fat and accumulate in humans at the top of the food chain.

3.1.1. Polychlorinated biphenyls and breast cancer

Polychlorinated biphenyls (PCBs) are industrial chemicals that have been used as hydraulic fluids, dielectric fluids for transformers and cooling fluids for capacitors in the formulation of lubricating and cutting oils and as plasticisers in prints, copy paper, adhesives, sealants and plastics. PCBs are complex chemical mixtures that comprise theoretically 209 congeners. Although the production and use of these compounds were banned in the late 1970s, a significant portion of the PCBs purchased by industry are still in use, mostly within capacitors and transformers. These compounds remain in our environment and are routinely found in human serum, breast milk and adipose tissue, including breast tissue. PCB exposure has been classically thought to alter normal endocrine signalling by mimicking endogenous hormone action by binding to hormone receptors, blocking receptors, or through interference with steroid metabolism. The relationship between exposure to PCBs and breast cancer has been addressed in numerous epidemiological studies since the early 1990s [29].

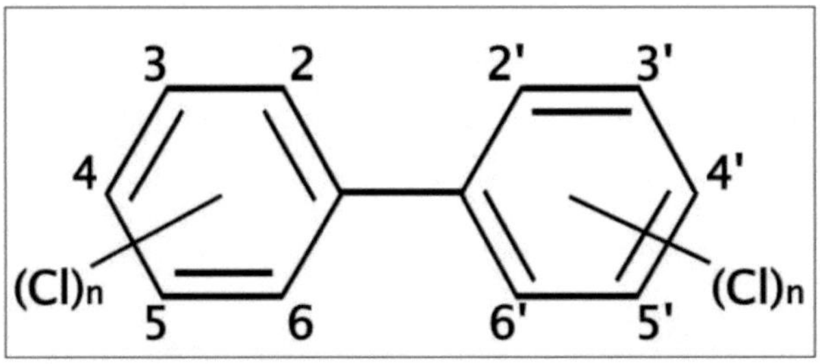

Figure 10. Polychlorinated biphenyls (PCBs)

3.1.2. Metabolism of polychlorinated biphenyls

PCBs are not only efficacious inducers but also substrates for cytochrome P450 enzymes. This enzyme metabolises PCBs, as well as other environmental compounds that enter the body, into by-products that are mutagenic and carcinogenic. Notably, lower chlorinated PCBs (such as PCB3) are rapidly metabolised and therefore called "episodic congeners" [30]. One member of the CYP1 family, CYP1A1, has been shown to play an important role in the metabolism of PCBs [31,32].

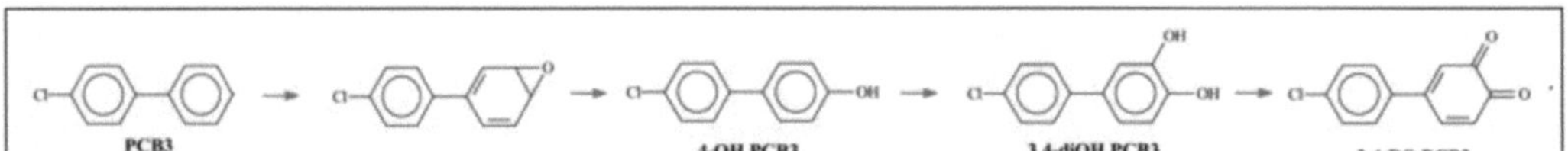

Figure 11. The metabolic activation of the 4-chlorobiphenyl (PCB3)

We demonstrated previously in MCF-7 breast cancer cells that PCB3 modestly increases CYP1A1 but not CYP1B1, protein levels and activity, Figure 12. This alteration may change metabolic activation pathways of PCB3 itself or local oestrogen metabolism and excretion [32]. The metabolic activation of PCBs and/or E2 by CYPs leads to the formation of arene oxide intermediates and reactive quinones, which can bind covalently to macromolecules such as DNA, RNA and proteins [33].

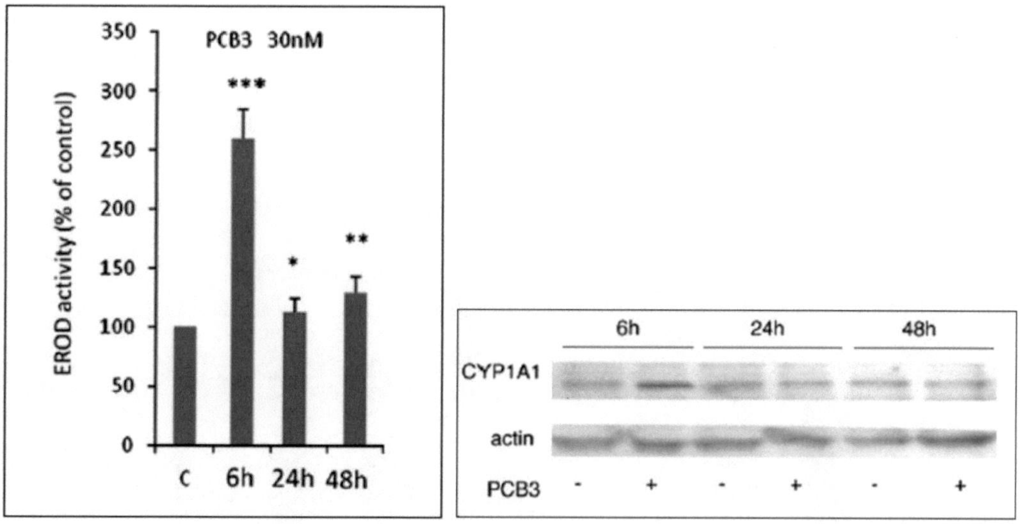

Figure 12. The effects of PCB3 on CYP1A1 activity (EROD assay) and protein levels in MCF-7 cells (*) p<0.05, (**) p<0.01, (***) p<0.001 [32]

3.1.3. Action of PCB3 (4-chlorobifenyl) and its metabolites (4-diOH-PCB3 and 3,4-diOH-PCB3) on MCF-7 human breast cancer cell proliferation and apoptosis

The balance between proliferation and apoptosis determines tissue homeostasis under physiological conditions. Apoptosis is recognised as a major barrier that must be circumvented by tumour cells to survive and proliferate under stressful conditions. Apoptosis can be initiated via two different types of signals: intracellular stress signals (intrinsic pathway) and extracellular ligands (extrinsic pathway). Previous studies have provided conflicting data regarding the proliferation and apoptosis effects of PCBs on breast cancer cells. As opposed to the action of oestrogen on MCF-7 proliferation, we showed that PCB3 and its metabolite 4-OH-PCB3 had no effect on cell proliferation at any time during exposure, while at the highest concentration, 3,4-diOH-PCB3 decreased cell proliferation [14]. Additionally, we showed that PCB3 and both of its hydroxylated metabolites had no effect on caspase-8 (extrinsic pathway) and caspase-9 (intrinsic pathway) activity when cells were grown in medium deprived of oestrogen, but they reduced caspase-9 activity when cells were grown in medium supplemented with serum containing oestradiol, Figure 13. Interestingly, a decrease in DNA fragmentation was observed upon treatment with 3,4-diOH-PCB3 in both culture conditions, suggesting that 3,4-diOH-PCB3 inhibits a caspase-independent pathway of cell death [34].

3.1.4. Molecular mechanisms of PCB3 and its hydroxylated metabolites (4-diOH-PCB3 and 3,4-diOH-PCB3)

Similarly to endogenous oestrogens, xenoestrogens can also contribute to the activity of the SHBG pathway and the MAP kinase pathways. Several studies have demonstrated that human SHBG binds phytoestrogens, fatty acids and 4-OH-2′,3′,4′,5′-PCB and 4-OH-2,2′,3′,4′,5′-PCB [35]. Our previously published data indicated that 3,4-diOH-PCB3 does not interact with SHBG through the membrane-binding site or directly. However, an increase in intracellular SHBG levels was noted under the influence of 3,4-diOH-PCB3 in MCF-7 cells [34], Figure 14.

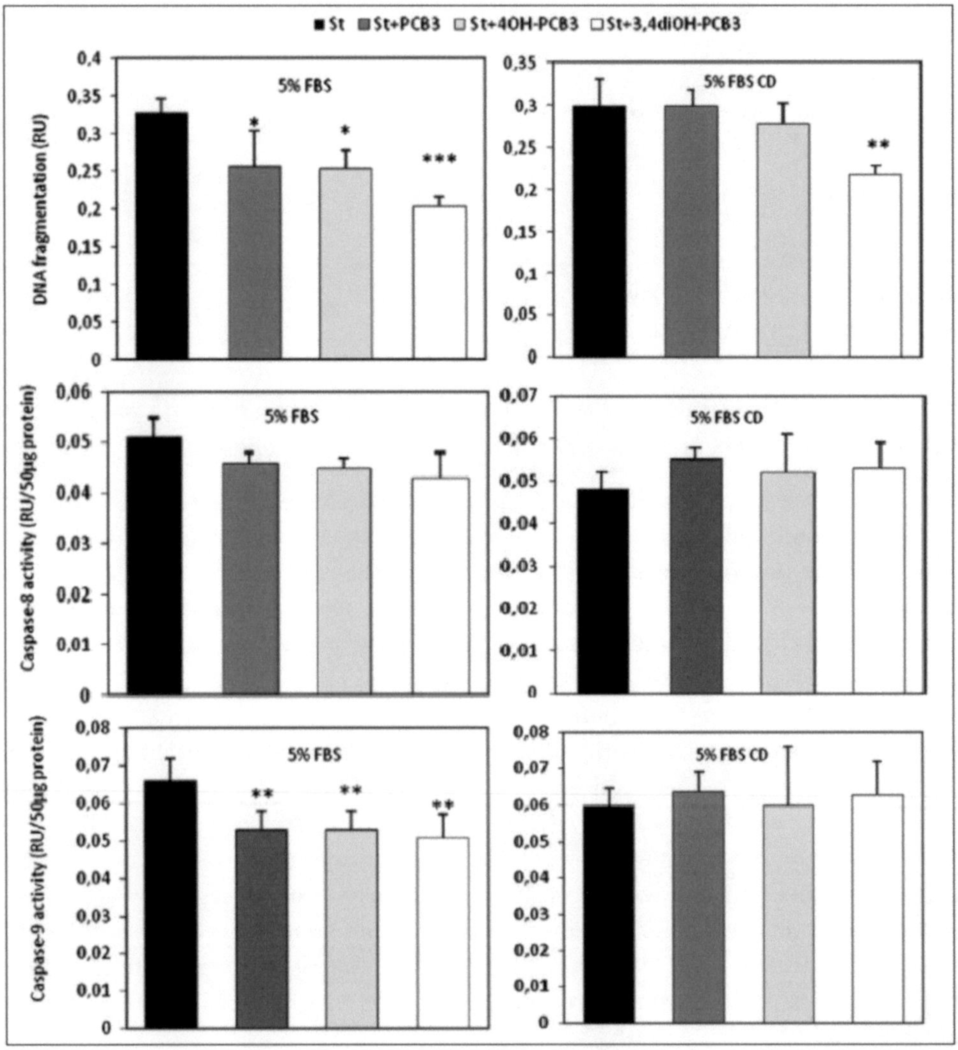

Figure 13. Effects of PCB3 (300 nM) and its metabolites on DNA fragmentation, as determined by ELISA; caspase-8 activity and, caspase-9 activity after 24 h of growth in medium supplemented with 5% FBS (left panel) or deprived of estrogen and by treatment with activated charcoal-dextran (5% FBS CD) (right panel). Staurosporine (St; 0.1 μM) was added during the last 3 h to induce apoptosis. (*) $p<0.05$, (**) $p<0.01$, (***) $p<0.001$ [32]

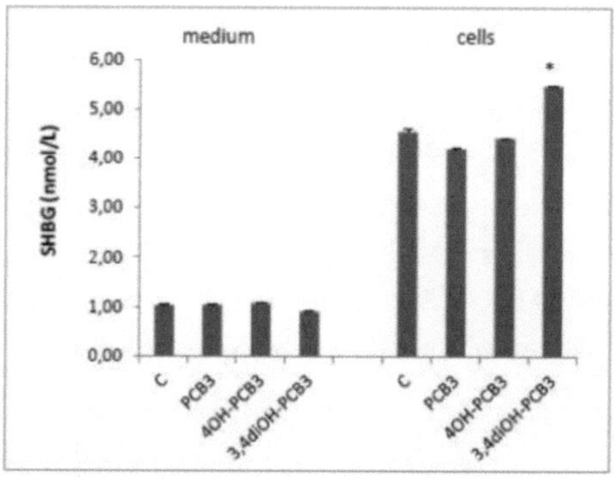

Figure 14. The effects of PCB3, 4-OH-PCB3 and 3,4-di-OH-PCB3 on extracellular (medium) and intracellular (cells) SHBG levels' in MCF-7 cells. (*) p<0.05 [34]

Furthermore, 3,4-diOH-PCB3 is ineffective in the activation of cAMP. Moreover, using a PKA inhibitor, we demonstrated that neither PCB3 nor its metabolites act through PKA [34], Figure 15.

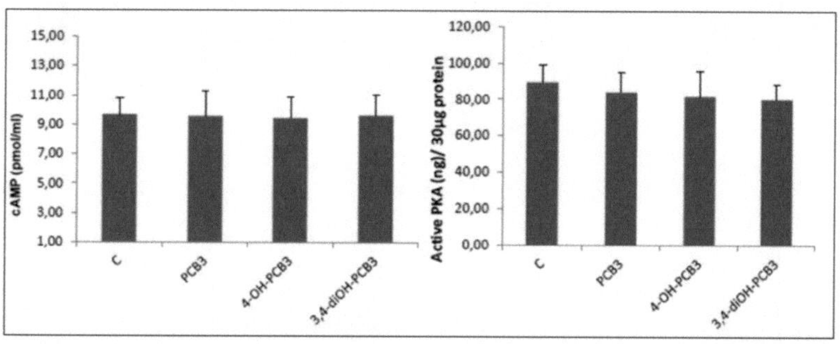

Figure 15. The effects of PCB3, 4-OH-PCB3 and 3,4-di-OH-PCB3 on cAMP and PKA levels in MCF-7 cells. ($p < 0.05$) [34]

Thus, the anti-proliferative action of 3,4-diOH-PCB3 is not due to inhibition of the ERK1/2 pathway via the SHBG/AMP/PKA pathway, but rather a direct inhibitory action on the ERK1/2 system [34], Figure 16.

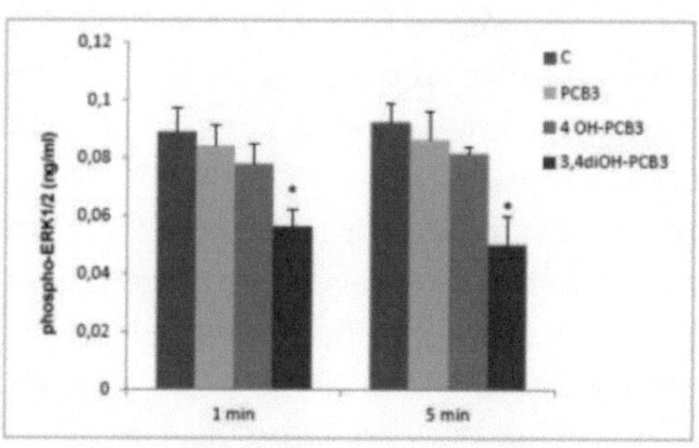

Figure 16. The effect of PCB3, 4-OH-PCB3 and 3,4-di-OH-PCB3 on phospho- ERK1/2 levels in MCF-7 cells. (*) p<0.05 [34]

Others have demonstrated that xenoestrogens can lead to the oscillating activation of ERK. Compounds from different classes of endocrine disruptors such as phytoestrogen (coumestrol), organochlorinated pesticides and their metabolites (endosulfan, dieldrin, DDE) and detergents (p-nonylphenol) can produce the same time-dependent activation pattern for ERKs [36]. These xenoestrogens produced rapid (3–30 min after application), concentration-dependent ERK1/2 phosphorylation. In addition, [37] demonstrated that the mitogenic effect of PCB153 was ERK1/2-mediated. Moreover, they showed that inhibition of ERK1/2 with PD98059 completely blocks the mitogenic effect of PCBs.

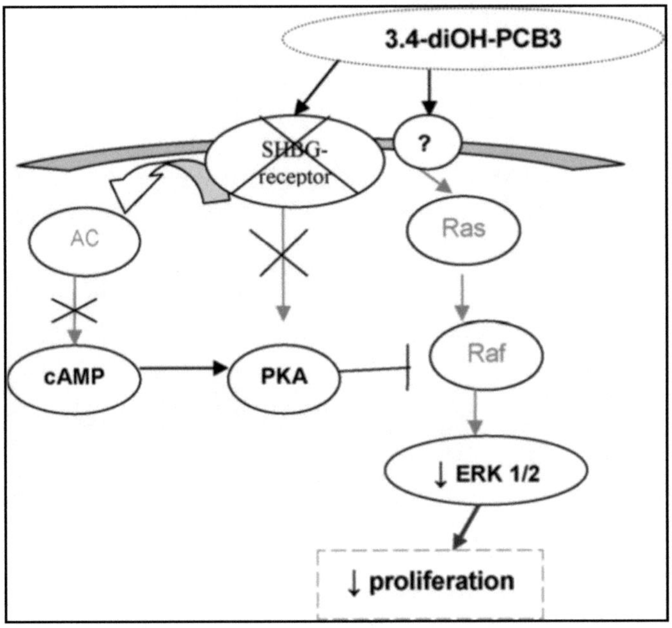

Figure 17. Proposed mechanism of antiproliferative action of 3,4-di-OH-PCB3 in MCF-7 cells [34]. The down arrow indicates a ERK1/2 decrease and proliferations decrease. AC, adenylyl cyclase; Ras-Raf, mitogen-activated protein kinase; ERK, extracellular signal-regulated kinase.

3.2. Bisphenol A and ovarian cancer

Bisphenol A (BPA) is a small monomer (228 Da) commonly used as plasticiser in the manufacture of polycarbonate plastics and epoxy resins. It is present in a multitude of products, including the interior coatings of food cans, milk containers, and baby formula bottles, as well as in dental composites and sealants. BPA was found in the serum, milk, saliva, and urine of humans at nanomolar concentrations. Many studies in the United States, Europe, and Japan have documented BPA levels ranging from 0.2 to 18.9 ng/mL (0.5–100 nM) in adult and foetal human serum [38]. Epidemiological studies have highlighted the correlation between the increase of BPA levels in the environment and the incidence of cancer in humans. BPA can act as an endocrine disruptor and a mitogenic substance inducing cell proliferation. As a mitogen, BPA induces susceptibility to neoplastic transformation [39].

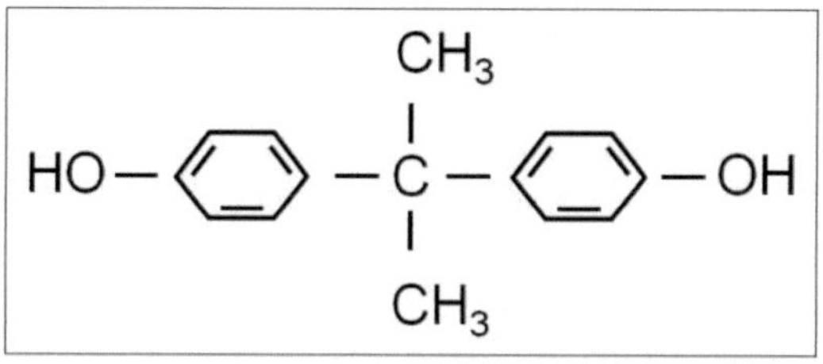

Figure 18. Bisphenol-A (BPA)

3.2.1. BPA action on cell proliferation

BPA can increase cell proliferation in a dose-dependent manner in OVCAR- 3 human ovarian cancer cells [40], MCF-7 breast cancer cells [41] and HeLa cells [42], Figure 19.

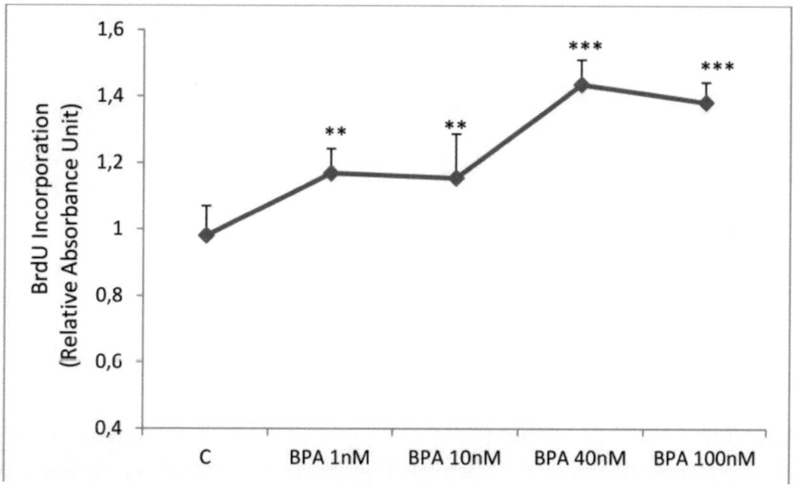

Figure 19. The effect of BPA on the proliferation of OVCAR-3 cells. (**) $p<0.01$, (***) $p<0.001$ [40]

Alterations in the mechanisms controlling cell cycle progression play a relevant role in the pathogenesis of different types of human neoplasia. As the cell cycle is regulated by the coordinate action of cyclin-dependent kinases (cdk), specific cyclin proteins and cdk inhibitors, we focused on cell cycle associated gene analysis. The cell cycle has four sequential phases: the S phase, when DNA replication occurs, and the M phase, when the cell divides into two daughter cells, as well as two gap phases referred to as G1 and G2. The G1-S transition in normal cells requires phosphorylation of the retinoblastoma protein (Rb) by cyclin D/Cdk4 or cyclin D/Cdk6 in mid G1 and by cyclin E/Cdk2 complexes later in G1. As cells progress into the S phase, cyclin A is expressed and becomes the primary cyclin associated with Cdk2. Progression from G2 into mitosis requires the activity of the Cdk and Cdc2 (also known as Cdk1) complexed with cyclin B, which has been shown to phosphorylate proteins regulated during mitosis. Basal and mitogen-induced cell growth is regulated by cell cycle inhibitors, which can bind to and inhibit the Cdks (such as p15, p16, p21, p27, p57). The results of our study [40] demonstrated that BPA promotes G1 to S-phase progression by stimulating the expression of cyclin D1, CDK4, E2F1, E2F3 and PCNA while inhibiting the expression of inhibitors (p21WAF1/CIP1, Weel-1 and GADD45 alpha) and progression from G2 into mitosis by stimulating the expression of cyclin A in ovarian cancer cells OVCAR-3, Figure 20. The results of our study [40] additionally demonstrated that the suppression of p21/WAF mRNA, a marker of poor overall survival in ovarian cancer patients, was under the influence of BPA.

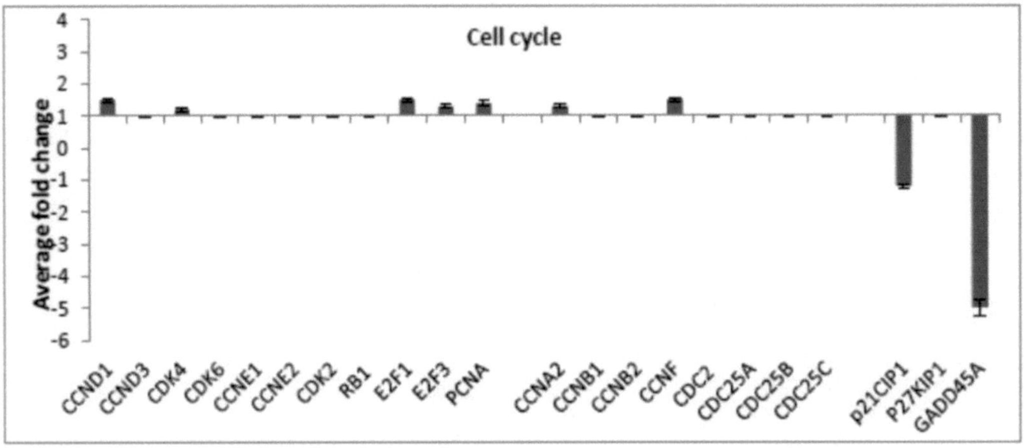

Figure 20. Selected cell cycle gene expression changes in OVCAR-3 cells exposed to BPA identified by real-time PCR [40]

3.2.2. BPA action on apoptosis

Studies on the effects of BPA on apoptosis have generated conflicting results, largely due to the micromolar concentrations of BPA utilised by most studies. BPA, in doses of 10, 1 and 0.1 mM, was a potent inhibitor of apoptosis in MCF-7 cells [43]. In contrast, BPA increased the expression of Bax (pro-apoptotic) and concomitantly decreased the expression of Bcl2 (pro-survival) at both protein and mRNA levels in granulosa cells [44]. In addition, BPA at a concentration of 100 μM decreased cell viability and increased necrosis in human endometrial endothelial cells (HEECs) [45].

A hallmark of apoptosis is the fragmentation of nuclear DNA. The intrinsic apoptosis pathway is activated when intracellular stress signals lead to the release of cytochrome c and other pro-apoptotic proteins within the mitochondria, which is regulated by members of the Bcl-2 family of proteins. The consequent release of cytochrome C leads to the formation of the apoptosome (cytochrome C, Apaf-1 and procaspase-9) in which procaspase-9 is auto-activated, thereby activating the executioner caspases. The extrinsic pathway is activated when extracellular ligands (such as Fas ligand, TNFα, TRAIL) bound to the death receptor domains of these receptors, recruit adaptor proteins (such as FADD and TRADD) and initiator caspase-8 and -10 (DISC). Both apoptotic pathways lead to the activation of the executioner caspases-3, -6 and -7, which are the main proteases that degrade the cell. A hallmark of apoptosis is the fragmentation of nuclear DNA. Endonuclease G is essential for DNA fragmentation during caspase-independent apoptosis. In response to apoptotic stimuli, it is also released from the mitochondria into the cytosol, where it translocates to the nucleus and generates oligonucleosomal DNA fragmentation.

In our previously published study, we demonstrated that inhibition of the caspase-3 activity had no effect on DNA fragmentation in cells exposed to BPA [40]. We demonstrated that BPA acts by suppressing the expression of pro-apoptotic genes, such as FAS, FADD, RAIDD, caspase-8, -10, -3, -6, -7, CAD, Bax, Bak, Bok and Apaf-1, and inducing the expression of pro-survival genes, such as Bcl-x and Mcl-1. Moreover, BPA activates the caspase-independent apoptotic pathway via the induction of endonuclease G gene expression, Figure 21. The absence of an effect of BPA on DNA fragmentation is hypothesised to result from the simultaneous activation of the caspase-independent pathway and an inhibition of caspase-dependent DNA fragmentation. The observed induction of p53 (a nuclear transcription factor that accumulates in response to cellular stress, including DNA damage and oncogene activation) and suppression of caspase-3 and -7 is thought to activate the DNA repair process. Therefore, despite the observed induction of endo G gene expression, an action of BPA on DNA fragmentation was not observed [40].

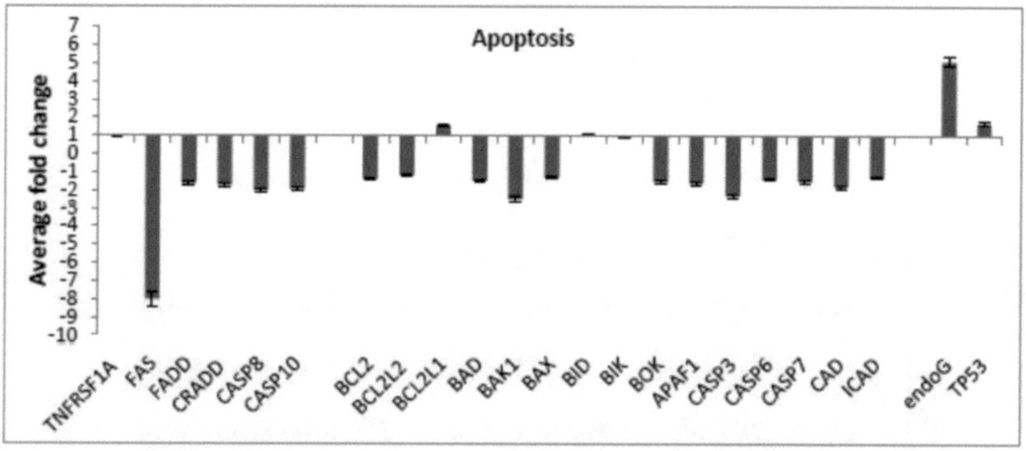

Figure 21. Selected apoptosis gene expression changes in OVCAR-3 cells exposed to BPA identified by real-time PCR [40]

3.2.3. Mechanism of action of BPA in OVCAR-3 cell cycle regulation

BPA can elicit rapid responses in cells via the involvement of a non-genomic signalling pathway though the activation of second messenger systems. Our data demonstrated that BPA stimulated proliferation of ovarian epithelial cancer cells via the induction of a rapid activation of ERK1/2, Stat3, and Akt signalling systems [46], Figure 22, 23. Previous studies demonstrate that BPA triggers a rapid biological response through the phosphorylation of Stat3, ERK1/2 and Akt in 3T3-L1 cells [47] and ERα/β-positive and -negative breast cancer cells [48].

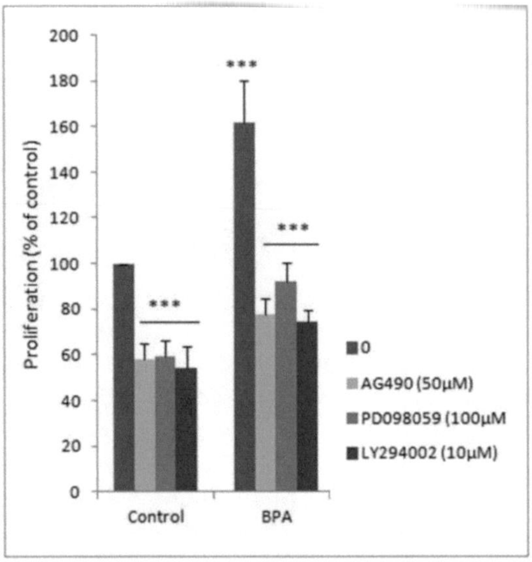

Figure 22. The effect of BPA on cell proliferation. OVCAR-3 cells were pretreated with AG490 (50 μM), PD098059 (100 μM) or LY294002 (10 μM) for 1 hr, then the cells were treated BPA (8 ng/ml) and an alamarBlue assay was performed. (***) p<0.001 [46]

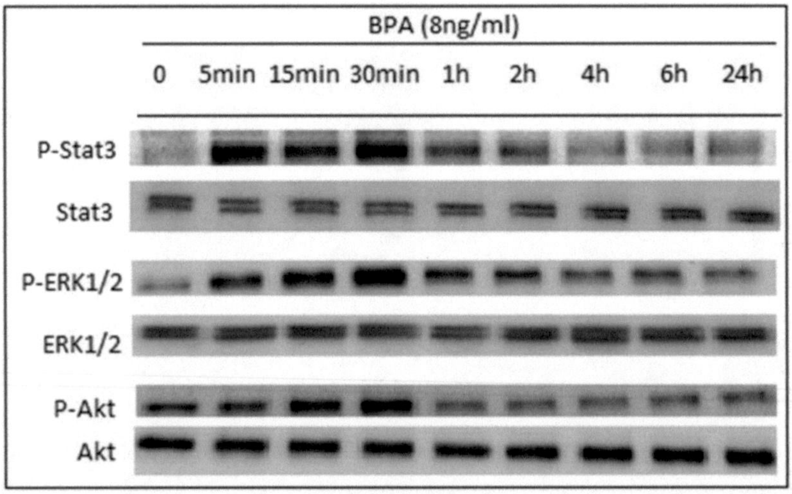

Figure 23. The effects of BPA on the activation of Stat-3, ERK1/2 and Akt in OVCAR-3 cells. Western blot analysis was performed following BPA treatment in a time-dependent manner (5, 15, and 30 min and 1, 2, 4, 6 and 24 hrs). Total Stat-3, ERK1/2 and Akt were used to normalise the level of phosphorylated Stat-3, ERK1/2 and Akt, respectively [46]

3.3. Combinatory effects of endo- and exogenous oestrogens.

Recently, an increasing amount of data has demonstrated that xenoestrogens can interfere with endogenous oestrogens. In our previously published data, we investigated the contribution of specific representative PCBs and PBDEs on the oestrogenic action of endogenous oestradiol on the proliferation and apoptosis of the breast cancer cell line MCF-7. The structure of polybrominated diphenyl ethers (PBDEs) is similar to that of PCBs. PBDEs are a series of 209 possible congeners that differ in the number and position of bromine atoms. These chemicals are widely used as flame retardants in plastic foams, textiles, electronic devices, and building materials. As a result, they are widely found in the environment and can be found in human blood and milk. Some of the PBDE congeners most commonly found in human samples are BDE-47, BDE-99, and BDE-153 [49].

Our data demonstrated that all PCB congeners (118, 138, 153 and 180) and all concentrations tested increased MCF-7 cell proliferation while decreased cell apoptosis to a greater extent than oestradiol. However, in co-treatment experiments with oestradiol, cell proliferation decreased in comparison to the cell proliferation observed for cells exposed to PCB congeners alone, and no additional effect on cell apoptosis was observed [50], Figure 24.

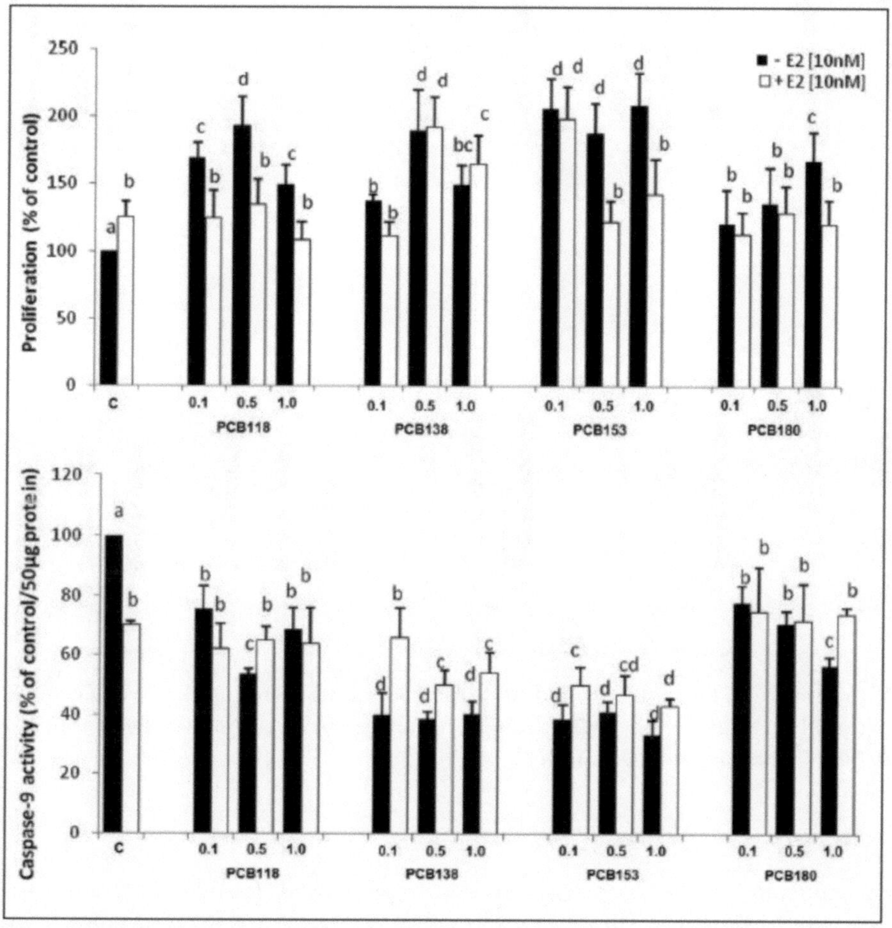

Figure 24. The effects of PCB (0.1, 0.5 and 1 mM) and oestradiol, alone (black bar) and combination treatment (open bar) on proliferation after 72 hours of culture and on caspase-9 activity after 24 hours of culture in MCF-7 cells. (a<b<c<d) $p < 0.05$ [50]

Despite the similarity in structure, PCBs and PBDEs had different effects on proliferation and apoptosis in MCF-7 breast cancer cells. None of the PBDE congeners tested (47, 99, 100, 209) had an effect on basal cell proliferation; however, all PBDE congeners tested significantly decreased basal cell apoptosis. In the presence of oestradiol, additive anti-apoptotic activity and an ability to induce cell proliferation were observed [51], Figure 25.

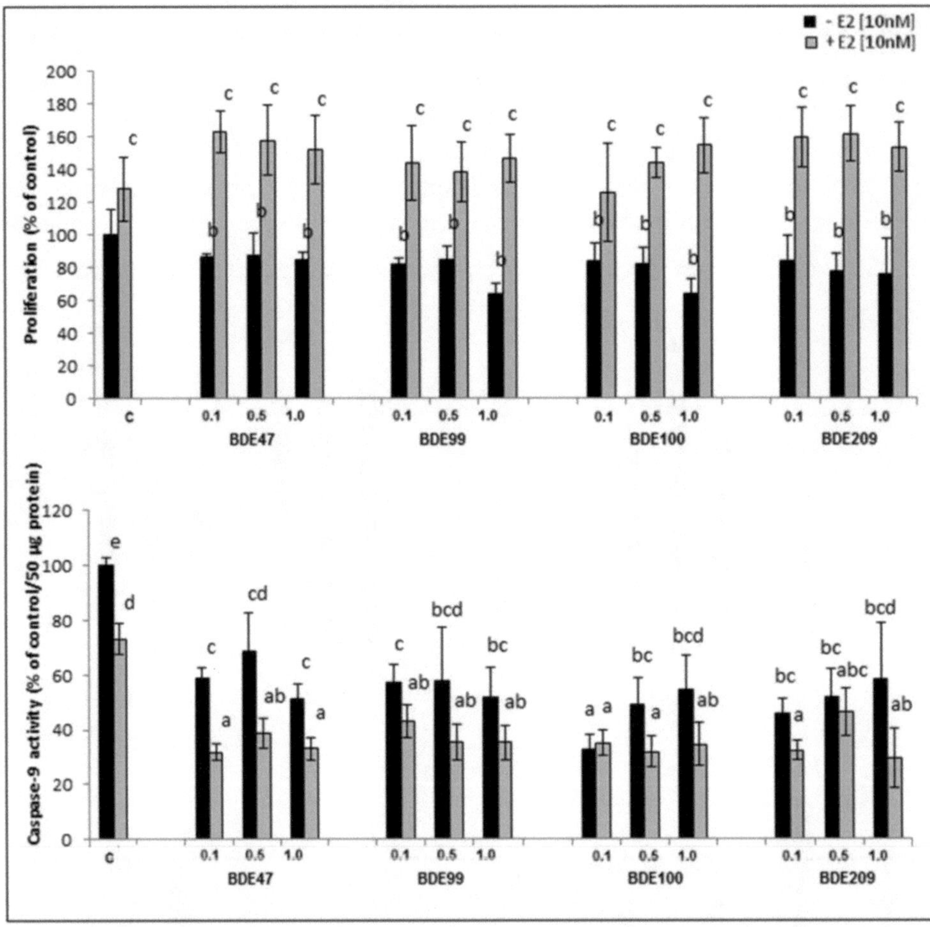

Figure 25. The effects of PBDE (0.1, 0.5 and 1 mM) and oestradiol, alone (black bar) and combination treatment (gray bar) on proliferation after 72 hours of culture and on caspase-9 activity after 24 hours of culture in MCF-7 cells. (a<b<c<d) $p < 0.05$ [51]

4. Conclusion

Despite a reduction in the doses of natural oestrogens used in HRT and contraceptives, as well as the production and use of environmental oestrogens, these compounds remain in our environment and are routinely found in human serum, breast milk and adipose samples, including breast tissue. Importantly, differences in activity as potential carcinogens are being studied. The potencies of these compounds in nuclear transcription reporter assays, compared with the endogenous oestrogens, range from very weak (e.g., PCBs) to somewhat weak (e.g., bisphenol A) to strong (DDE). Moreover, both endogenous and exogenous oestrogens form metabolites during metabolism that act more strongly than their corresponding parental compounds. The results of a published study suggest that the genomic and nongenomic actions of the parent endogenous and exogenous oestrogens lead to the activation of secondary messenger systems responsible for proliferation and apoptosis. The results of our study indicate that it is necessary to consider local metabolism in peripheral tissues, such as ovary and breast. Therefore, an accurate assessment of the carcinogenicity of oestrogens and xenoestrogens requires an understanding of not only the potential mode of action of the parent compounds but also their hydroxylated metabolites. These include the promotion of tumorigenic progression, genotoxicity, and the developmental reprogramming that increases susceptibility to other carcinogenic events.

Author details

Anna Ptak and Ewa Lucja Gregoraszczuk
Department of Physiology and Toxicology of Reproduction, Institute of Zoology, Jagiellonian University, Cracow, Poland

Acknowledgement

This research was supported by the Polish Committee for Scientific Research as a project 0050/B/PO1/2010/38 from 2010 to 2013 (Poland).

5. References

[1] Russo J, Russo IH (2006) The role of estrogen in the initiation of breast cancer. J Steroid Biochem Mol Biol. 102: 89-96.
[2] Lindgren PR, Bäckström T, Cajander S, Damber MG, Mählck CG, Zhu D, Olofsson JI (2002) The pattern of estradiol and progesterone differs in serum and tissue of benign and malignant ovarian tumors. Int J Oncol. 21 :583-589.
[3] Eliassen AH, Hankinson SE (2008) Endogenous hormone levels and risk of breast, endometrial and ovarian cancers: prospective studies. Adv Exp Med Biol 630:148–165
[4] Zhu BT (1998) Functional role of estrogen metabolism in target cells: review and perspectives. Carcinogenesis 19: 1–27.
[5] Lonard DM, O'Malley BW (2007) Nuclear receptor coregulators: Judges, juries, and executioners of cellular regulation. Mol Cell. 27: 691–700.
[6] Acconcia F, Kumar R (2006) Signaling regulation of genomic and nongenomic functions of estrogen receptors. Cancer Lett. 238: 1-14.
[7] Warner M, Gustafsson JA (2006) Nongenomic effects of estrogen: why all the uncertainty? Steroids. 71: 91-95.
[8] Lippert C, Seeger H, Mueck AO (2003) The effect of endogenous estradiol metabolites on the proliferation of human breast cancer cells. Life Sci 72: 877-883.

[9] Liehr JG (2000) Is estradiol a genotoxic mutagenic carcinogen? Endocr Rev. 21: 40-54.

[10] Gerstner S, Glasemann D, Pfeiffer E, Metzler M (2008) The influence of metabolism on the genotoxicity of catechol estrogens in three cultured cell lines. Mol Nutr Food Res. 52: 823-829.

[11] Bai HW, Shim JY, Yu J, Zhu BT (2007) Biochemical and molecular modeling studies of the O-methylation of various endogenous and exogenous catechol substrates catalyzed by recombinant human soluble and membrane-bound catechol-O-methyltransferases. Chem Res Toxicol. 20: 1409-1425.

[12] Gregoraszczuk E, Ptak A (2011) Involvement of caspase-9 but not caspase-8 in the anti-apoptotic effects of estradiol and 4-OH-Estradiol in MCF-7 human breast cancer cells. Endocrine Regul. 45: 3-8.

[13] Cavalieri EL, Rogan EG (2011) Unbalanced metabolism of endogenous estrogens in the etiology and prevention of human cancer. J Steroid Biochem Mol Biol. 125: 169-180.

[14] Gregoraszczuk EL, Rak A, Ludewig G, Gasinska A (2008) Effect of estradiol, PCB3 and their hydroxylated metabolitem on proliferation, cell cycle and apoptosis of human breast cancer cells. Environ Toxicology and Pharmacol 25: 227-233.

[15] Hoogenboom LAP, de Haan L, Hooijerink D, Bor G, Murk AJ, Brouwer A (2001) Estrogenic activity of estradiol and its metabolites in the ER-CALUXassay with human T47D breast cells. APMIS 109: 101-107.

[16] Seeger H, Wallwiener D, Kraemer E, Mueck AO (2006) Comparison of possible carcinogenic estradiol metabolites: Effects on proliferation, apoptosis and metastasis of human breast cancer cells Maturitas 54: 72–77.

[17] Zhu BT, Connery AH (1998) Is 2-methoxyestradiol an endogenous metabolite that inhibits mammary carcinogenesis? Cancer Res 58: 2269–2277.

[18] Moore KH, Bertram KA, Gomez RR, Styner MJ, Matej LA (1996) Sex hormone binding globulin mRNA in human breast cancer: detection in cell lines and tumor samples. J Steroid Biochem Mol Biol 59: 297-304.

[19] Hryb DJ, Khan MS, Romas NA, Rosner W (1990). The control of the interaction of sex hormone-binding globulin with its receptor by steroid hormones. J. Biol. Chem. 15: 6048–6054.

[20] Fortunati N, Fissore F, Fazzari A, Becchis M, Comba A, Catalano MG, Berta L, Frairia R (1996) Sex steroid binding protein exerts a negative control on estradiol action in MCF-7 cells (human breast cancer) through cyclic adenosine 3′,5′-monophosphate and protein kinase A. Endocrinology 137: 686–692.

[21] Gregoraszczuk EL, Ptak A, Wrobel A (2011) The ability of hydroxylated estrogens (2-OH-E2 and 4-OH-E2) to increase of SHBG gene, protein expression and intracellular levels in MCF-7 cells line. Endocr Regul. 45: 125-130.

[22] Sutter-Dub MT (2002) Rapid non-genomic and genomic responses to progestogens, estrogens, and glucocorticoids in the endocrine pancreatic B cell, the adipocyte and other cell types. Steroids 67: 77-93.

[23] Zivadinovic D, Gametchu B, Watson CS (2005) Membrane estrogen receptor-alpha levels In MCF-7 breast cancer cells predict cAMP and proliferation responses. Breast Cancer Res. 7: 101–112.

[24] Houslay MD, Kolch W (2000) Cell-type specific integration of cross-talk between extracellular signal-regulated kinase and cAMP signaling. Mol Pharmacol 58: 659-668.

[25] Filardo EJ, Quinn JA, Frackelton A, Bland KI (2002) Estrogen action via the G protein-coupled receptor, GPR30: stimulation of adenylyl cyclase and cAMP-mediated attenuation of the epidermal growth factor receptor-to-MAPK signaling axis. Mol Endocrinol 16: 70-84.

[26] Brower SL, Roberts JR, Antonini JM, Miller MR (2005) Difficulty demonstrating estradiol-mediated Erk1/2 phosphorylation in MCF-7 cells. J Steroid Biochem Mol Bio 96: 375-385.

[27] Kwiecinska P, Ptak A, Wrobel A, Gregoraszczuk EL (2012) Hydroxylated estrogens (2-OH-E2 AND 4-OH-E2) do not activate cAMP/PKA and ERK1/2 pathways activation in a breast cancer MCF-7 cell line. Endocr Regul. 46: 1-12.

[28] Lobenhofer E, Marks J (2000) Estrogen-induced mitogenesis of MCF-7 cells does not require the induction of mitogen-activated protein kinase activity. J Steroid Biochem Mol Biol 75: 11-20.

[29] Güttes S, Failing K, Neumann K, Kleinstein J, Georgii S, Brunn H (1998) Chlororganic pesticides and polychlorinated biphenyls in breast tissue of women with benign and malignant breast disease. Arch Environ Contam Toxicol 35: 140–147

[30] Hansen LG (1998) Stepping backward to improve assessment of PCB congener toxicities. Environ Health Perspect. 106: 171-189.

[31] Ptak A, Ludewig G, Kapiszewska M, Magnowska Z, Lehmler HJ, Robertson LW, Gregoraszczuk EL (2006) Induction of cytochromes P450, caspase-3 and DNA damage by PCB3 and its hydroxylated metabolites in porcine ovary. Toxicol Lett. 166: 200-211.

[32] Ptak A, Ludewig G, Rak A, Nadolna W, Bochenek M, Gregoraszczuk EL (2010) Induction of cytochrome P450 1A1 in MCF-7 human breast cancer cells by 4-chlorobiphenyl (PCB3) and the effects of its hydroxylated metabolites on cellular apoptosis. Environ Int. 36: 935-941.

[33] Zhao S, Narang A, Ding X, Eadon G (2004) Characterization and quantitative analysis of DNA adducts formed from Lower chlorinated PCB-derived quinones. Chem Res Toxicol. 17: 502–511.

[34] Ptak A, Gut P, Błachuta M, Rak A, Gregoraszczuk EŁ (2009) Direct inhibition of ERK1/2 phosphorylation as a possible mechanism for the antiproliferative action of 3,4-diOH-PCB3 in the MCF-7 cell line. Toxicol Lett. 190: 187-192.

[35] Jury HH, Zacharewski TR, Hammond GL (2000) Interactions between human plasma sex hormone-binding globulin and xenobiotic ligands. J. Steroid Biochem. Mol. Biol. 75: 167–176.

[36] Bulayeva NN, Watson CS (2004) Xenoestrogen-induced ERK-1 and ERK-2 activation via multiple membrane-initiated signaling pathways. Environ. Health Perspect. 112: 1481–1487.

[37] Radice S, Chiesara E, Fucile S, Marabini L (2008) Different effects of PCB101, PCB118, PCB138 and PCB153 alone or mixed in MCF-7 breast cancer cells. Food Chem. Toxicol. 46: 2561–2567.

[38] Dekant W, Völkel W (2008) Human exposure to bisphenol A by biomonitoring: methods, results and assessment of environmental exposures. Toxicol Appl Pharmacol. 228: 114-134.

[39] Keri RA, Ho SM, Hunt PA, Knudsen KE, Soto AM, Prins GS (2007) An evaluation of evidence for the carcinogenic activity of bisphenol A. Reprod. Toxicol. 24: 240–252.

[40] Ptak A, Wróbel A, Gregoraszczuk EL (2011) Effect of bisphenol-A on the expression of selected genes involved in cell cycle and apoptosis in the OVCAR-3 cell line. Toxicol Lett. 202: 30-35.

[41] Ricupito A, Del Pozzo G, Diano N, Grano V, Portaccio M, Marino M, Bolli A, Gzlluzzo P, Bontempo P, Mita L, Altucci L, Mita DG (2009) Effect of bisphenol A with or without enzyme treatment on the proliferation and viability of MCF-7 cells. Environ. Int. 35: 21–26.

[42] Bolli A, Galluzzo P, Ascenzi P, Del Pozzo G, Manco I, Vietri MT, Mita L, Altucci L, Mita DG, Marino M (2008) Laccase treatment impairs bisphenol A-induced cancer cell proliferation affecting estrogen receptor alpha-dependent rapid signals. IUBMB Life. 60: 843–852.

[43] Diel P, Olff S, Schmidt S, Michna H (2002) Effects of the environmental estrogens bisphenol A, o,p'-DDT, p-tert-octylphenol and coumestrol on apoptosis induction, cell proliferation and the expression of estrogen sensitive molecular parameters in the human breast cancer cell line MCF-7. J. Steroid. Biochem.Mol. Biol. 80: 61–70.

[44] Xu J, Osuga Y, Yano T, Morita Y, Tang X, Fujiwara T, Takai Y, Matsumi H, Koga K, Taketani Y, Tsutsumi O (2002) Bisphenol A induces apoptosis and G2- to-M arrest of ovarian granulosa cells. Biochem. Biophys. Res. Commun. 292: 456–462.

[45] Bredhult C, Backlin BM, Olovsson M (2007) Effects of some endocrine disruptors on the proliferation and viability ofhumanendometrial endothelial cells in vitro. Reprod. Toxicol. 23: 550–559.

[46] Ptak A, Gregoraszczuk EL (2012) Bisphenol A induces leptin receptor expression, creating more binding sites for leptin, and activates the JAK/Stat, MAPK/ERK and PI3K/Akt signalling pathways in human ovarian cancer cell. Toxicol Lett. In press

[47] Masuno H, Iwanami J, Kidani T, Sakayama K, Honda K (2005) Bisphenol a accelerates terminal differentiation of 3T3-L1 cells into adipocytes through the phosphatidylinositol 3-kinase pathway. Toxicol Sci. 84: 319-327.

[48] Dong S, Terasaka S, Kiyama R (2011) Bisphenol A induces a rapid activation of Erk1/2 through GPR30 in human breast cancer cells. Environ Pollut. 159: 212-228.

[49] Costa LG, Giordano G, Tagliaferri S, Caglieri A, Mutti A (2008) Polybrominated diphenyl ether (PBDE) flame retardants: environmental contamination, human body burden and potential adverse health effects. Acta Biomed 79: 172–183.

[50] Ptak A, Mazur K, Gregoraszczuk EL (2011) Comparison of combinatory effects of PCBs (118, 138, 153 and 180) with 17 beta-estradiol on proliferation and apoptosis in MCF-7 breast cancer cells. Toxicol Ind Health. 27: 315-321.

[51] Kwiecińska P, Wróbel A, Gregoraszczuk EŁ (2011) Combinatory effects of PBDEs and 17β-estradiol on MCF-7 cell proliferation and apoptosis. Pharmacol Rep. 63: 189-194.

Chapter 5

EPS8, an Adaptor Protein Acts as an Oncoprotein in Human Cancer

Ming-Chei Maa and Tzeng-Horng Leu

Additional information is available at the end of the chapter

http://dx.doi.org/10.5772/54906

1. Introduction

A spectrum of cellular activities including proliferation, differentiation and metabolism are controlled by growth factors and hormones. The effects of many growth factors are mediated and achieved via transmembrane receptor tyrosine kinases [1,2]. Following ligand binding, the intrinsic catalytic activity of the growth factor receptor tyrosine kinases (RTKs) is augmented. The autophosphorylated RTKs then transmit signals through their ability to recruit and/or phosphorylate intracellular substrates. Thus, identification and characterization of proteins that associate with and/or become tyrosyl phosphorylated by RTKs become critical to delineate RTKs-mediated signaling pathways. A variety of methodologies have been developed and applied to search for substrates of tyrosine kinases including RTKs [3-8]. Here, we focus on EGFR pathway substrate no. 8 (Eps8), a putative target of epidermal growth factor (EGF) receptor (EGFR), and discuss its biological function as well as its implication in human cancers. Given Eps8-elicited effects contribute to neoplasm, its potential as a therapeutic target for cancer treatment is anticipated.

1.1. The identification of Eps8

To dissect EGFR-mediated signaling, Di Fiore's laboratory took advantage of immuno-affinity purification of an entire set of proteins phosphorylated in EGF-treated EGFR-overexpressing cells, followed by generation of antisera against the purified protein pool. With these antisera, bacterial expression libraries were immunologically screened. Several murine cDNAs (*eps* clones) representing genes encoding substrates for EGFR were obtained [7,8]. One of them was designated *eps8* [9,10]. The human *eps8* locus was mapped to chromosome 12p12-p13 via fluorescence in situ hybridization (FISH) [11] and confirmed by a computer search of a genomic DNA database utilizing human *EPS8* cDNA sequence (GeneBank accession number U12535) [12]. Similarly, the murine *Eps8* genomic DNA sequences are defined on chromosome 6G1 [12]. The computer analysis also revealed three genes (designated as *Eps8R1*, *Eps8R2*, and *Eps8 R3*) that are highly homologous to both human and murine *eps8* [12]. Due to space limitation, studies on these Eps8Rs will not be described in this review.

Proteins with molecular weights of 97 kDa and 68 kDa were recognized by Eps8 antibodies and referred to as the two Eps8 isoforms ($p97^{Eps8}$ and $p68^{Eps8}$) [12,13]. The exact nature (an alternatively spliced or a proteolytic product) of $p68^{Eps8}$ was still elusive and remained to be established. By contrast, $p97^{Eps8}$ has been well characterized and is the only isoform detected in human cancer cells so far and hereinafter is called Eps8.

Eps8 contains 821 amino acids and exhibits several features of interest: a split pleckstrin homology (PH) domain, a putative nuclear targeting sequence, an Src homology 3 (SH3) domain, several proline-rich regions, and a degenerated SH2 (dSH2) domain at the N-terminus (amino acids 55-96) (Figure 1). The proline-rich Eps8 has been demonstrated to interact with the SH3 domain of Src [13] and the SH3 of Eps8 was reported to associate with Shb [14], Shc [15], RN-tre [16], and Abi1 (also known as E3b1) [17]. The SH3 domain of Eps8 binds to a consensus sequence of proline-X-X-aspartate-tyrosine (PXXDY) instead of the canonical X-proline-X-X-proline (XPXXP) consensus, implicating the existence of a novel family of SH3-containing proteins [18]. Furthermore, two Eps8 proteins were demonstrated to form an interwound dimer with their SH3 domains being located at the interface [19]. In addition to the aforementioned Eps8-interacting proteins, Eps8 was also shown to bind directly to EGFR [20], Sos1 [21], and IRSp53 [22,23].

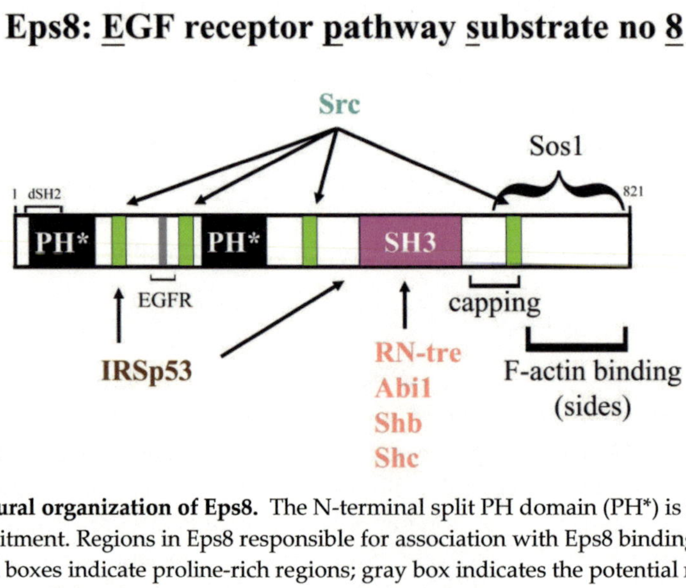

Figure 1. Structural organization of Eps8. The N-terminal split PH domain (PH*) is important for Eps8 membrane recruitment. Regions in Eps8 responsible for association with Eps8 binding partners are indicated. Green boxes indicate proline-rich regions; gray box indicates the potential nuclear localization signal. dSH2 indicates the position of a degenerated SH2.

Strikingly, Eps8 is an actin capper whose barbed-end capping activity resides in its C-terminal effector domain and is regulated by protein-protein interaction with Abi1 [24,25].

In addition to lamellipodia [26], Eps8 also localizes to other actin-rich structures such as PIP2-enriched vesicles, phagocytic cups and comet tails behind intracellular pathogens [25]. Two Abi1-containing complexes were reported to have multiple roles in regulating dynamic actin turnover [27]. One contains Nap1, Sra (PIR125), Hspc and WAVE, the other contains Eps8, Sos1, and the p85 subunit of PI3K. While the former may activate the Arp2/3 complex, the latter may regulate Rac activation and enable Eps8 to cap actin filament barbed ends. Of note, Eps8 turns out to be a novel capping protein capable of side-binding and bundling actin filaments [28]. The C-terminal Eps8 region (aa648-aa821) encompasses five helices (H1-H5). The N-terminal amphipathic helix (H1) is largely responsible for Eps8 capping activity, while a compact, globular domain composed of H2-H5 is critical for filament bundling. Thus, Eps8, as a bifunctional actin remodeller, regulates actin-based mobility and endomembrane cellular trafficking through its capping activity, whereas it contributes to proper structural organization of gut microvilli via its mediated actin filament bundling [28].

1.2. Eps8 is an oncoprotein

Known as the first identified oncoprotein, the tyrosine kinase activity of Rous sarcoma virus (RSV)-encoded v-Src is essential for its mediated transformation. Under its influence, a spectrum of proteins has their phosphotyrosine content increased and are viewed as putative v-Src substrates [3,29]. Intriguingly, some of them including Eps8 turn out to be the substrates for EGFR as well [13]. Elevated expression and tyrosyl phosphorylation of Eps8 are observed in v-Src transformed cells [13]. Overexpression of Eps8 confers the ability of fibroblasts to form foci in culture and to grow tumors in mice [30]. Consistent with its oncogenic potential [30], Eps8 attenuation retards cellular growth of fibroblasts expressing v-Src [31].

Like SH2 and SH3, PH is a common motif shared by signaling molecules, which mediates protein-protein and protein-lipid interactions. Mounting evidence indicates that via PH-mediated binding to either phospholipids [32,33] or membrane-associated proteins [34,35], the association between PH-containing molecules and plasma membrane is accelerated. The prominent examples are Akt/PKB that possesses a compact PH and PLCγ that retains a split PH. Like PLCγ, Eps8 contains a split PH (Figure 1), which does not weaken its linkage to the cell membrane. Remarkably, an intact split PH is indispensable for Eps8 membrane targeting as well as its mediated oncogenesis. In contrast, Eps8 with truncated PH fails to be recruited to plasma membrane and confers transforming ability [30].

To confirm the involvement of Eps8 in the development of cancer, the correlation between its expression and cell proliferation of various human cancer cell lines were examined [36]. In human colon cancers, there is a positive correlation between Eps8 expression and mitogenesis, implicating the importance of Eps8 in colon cancer formation. Indeed, Eps8 attenuation in high Eps8 expressing cells (i.e. SW620 and WiDr) reduces cellular growth [36]. In contrast, ectopically expressed Eps8 in low Eps8 expressing cells (i.e. SW480) or Eps8-attenuated SW620 promotes proliferation. In addition, relative to controls, there is a significant (>50%)

suppression of anchorage-independent growth in *eps8* siRNA-expressing SW620, and reintroduction of Eps8 rescues these defects. Concurrently, attenuation (or overexpression) of Eps8 significantly reduces (or promotes) the growth of tumors inoculated into nude mice [36]. In addition to fibroblasts and colon cancer cells, Eps8 also plays a pivotal role in cervical cancer formation. This can be supported by reduced proliferation and tumorigenesis in Eps8-attenuated SiHa and HeLa cells cultured in dishes or inoculated in mice [37].

1.3. Eps8-interacting proteins

As an adaptor, Eps8 intreracts with a variety of signaling proteins such as EGFR, Src, Abi1, RN-tre, Shb, and IRSp53 to exert its biological functions. The detail and implication of the interaction between Eps8 and each of its above-mentioned partners are described below.

1.3.1. EGFR

Via serial deletion mutants of Eps8 and EGFR, Castagnino et al. [20] determined the minimal region of Eps8 (aa298-aa362) and EGFR (juxtamembrane region, aa648-aa688) is required for Eps8-EGFR interaction. Obviously, this interaction is not via classical pTyr-SH2 or proline-rich region-SH3 binding manner. Interestingly, the EGFR-binding region in Eps8 is rich in basic amino acids while multiple glutamic acid residues are found in the juxtamembrane region of EGFR. Although overexpression of Eps8 enhances EGF-mediated mitogenesis, the underlying mechanisms are not yet resolved. Nevertheless, the intimately correlated transforming ability of EGFR mutants and the level of tyrosyl phosphorylated Eps8 suggested the importance of tyrosyl phosphorylation of Eps8 in cellular transformation [38].

1.3.2. Src

Oncogenic Src not only enhances Eps8 expression but also its tyrosyl phosphorylation [13]. In GST-pull down experiments, fusion proteins with Src SH3, but not SH2 domain directly interact with Eps8, presumably via its proline-rich sequences. Through *in vitro* Src kinase reactions, Eps8 was further confirmed to be directly phosphorylated by Src. Notably, simply augmenting Eps8 expression in murine C3H10T1/2 fibroblasts can not elevate its tyrosyl phosphorylation and promote cell proliferation despite these cells being tumorigenic. Given Eps8 attenuation reduced cell growth in v-Src transformed cells [31], Src-mediated Eps8 phosphorylation might be important for cell proliferation. To date, the residues on Eps8 mediated by Src are still elusive. Whether Eps8 retains the same receptor (i.e. EGFR)- and nonreceptor (i.e. Src)-mediated sites becomes an interesting issue.

1.3.3. Abi1

ABI1 (also known as E3b1) was identified as an Eps8-binding protein by screening a human embryonic fibroblast (M426) cDNA expression library with Eps8 SH3 [17]. It contains a proline-rich sequence at its C-terminus followed by an SH3 domain. The PXXDY consensus is identified at aa389-aa393 [17]. In addition to Eps8, it also interacts with Abl tyrosine kinase and is a human homologue of previously identified murine Abl-interactor 1 (Abi1) [39]. Both Abi1 and Abl contain SH3 and proline-rich sequences. These two proteins associate through the SH3 domain of Abi1 and the proline-rich region of Abl [17,39]. Overexpression of Abi1 decreased cell proliferation in NIH3T3-based EGFR overexpressors [17] while overexpression of the murine Abi1 suppressed v-Abl transforming activity [39]. Abi1/Eps8 associate with Sos1 and enable the latter protein to act as a guanine nucleotide exchange factor (GEF) of Rac to facilitate membrane ruffling in response to the activation of Ras and PI-3 kinase [21,40]. Strikingly, PI3K was also present in this multi-protein complex containing Abi1/Eps8/Sos1 to activate Rac [41]. It is noteworthy that alternatively spliced Abi1 fused with MLL has been identified in a human acute myeloid leukemia patient, suggesting the role of Abi1 in leukemogenesis [42].

1.3.4. RN-tre

RN-tre (Related to the N-terminal of *tre*) was originally identified by utilizing Eps8 SH3 as a probe to fish out its binding protein(s) in a bacterial cDNA expression library generated from NIH3T3 cells [16]. RN-tre shares a homology domain (TrH) with *tre* oncoprotein at its N-terminus and contains an extended proline-rich sequence at the C-terminus. The PXXDY consensus is present at aa725-aa729 (GeneBank database, accession number D13644; [16]). Overexpression of full-length RN-tre in NIH3T3 cells did not cause cell transformation [16]. However, NIH3T3 cells transfected with a plasmid encoding RN-tre C-terminal truncated mutant (lacking aa463-aa828) exhibited growth advantage in both soft agar and in low serum (1%) cultured medium [16]. The TrH domain in RN-tre possesses a Rab5 GTPase-activating protein (GAP) activity [43]. RN-tre overexpression suppressed EGF internalization via its Rab5 GAP activity [43]. Interactions with Grb2 [44] and/or Eps8 [43] are required for RN-tre inhibiting EGF receptor endocytosis. The association between RN-tre and Eps8 inhibits the ability of Eps8 to complex with Abi1 and Sos1 and attenuates EGF-mediated Rac activation [43].

1.3.5. Shb

Shb is an adaptor protein containing amino-terminal proline-rich sequences and a C-terminal SH2 domain [45]. Unlike Abi1 and RN-tre, there is no PXXDY consensus found in Shb sequences. Shb interacts with Eps8 SH3 domain and phosphorylated PDGFβ-receptor and FGF receptor-1 (via Shb SH2 domain) [14]. Although the role of Eps8-Shb interaction in cancer biology was not defined yet, overexpression of Shb reduced Eps8 expression [46] and induced apoptosis of NIH3T3 cells cultured in low serum [47]. Markedly, while Shb overexpression reduced tumor growth of PC3 prostate cancer cells [48], Shb attenuation sensitized SVR endothelial tumor cells to apoptotic agents such as cisplatin and staurosorine [49].

1.3.6. IRSp53

IRSp53 (Insulin/IGF-1 Receptor tyrosine kinase Substrate of 53 kDa; [50]) was also designated as brain-specific angiogenesis inhibitor 1-associated protein 2 (BAIAP2) [51,52].

Its interaction with Eps8 was originally observed from a GST-IRSp53 SH3 pull-down experiment [22] and confirmed by a yeast two-hybrid screening utilizing N-terminal Eps8 sequences as a bait to search for Eps8 binding partners [23]. IRSp53 contains an N-terminal I-BAR (inverse-Bin-Amphiphysin-Rev) domain, followed by a CRIB, an SH3, a WW-binding sequence (WWB), and a PDZ (post synaptic density 95, disc large, zonula occludens-1) domain. The I-BAR domain might form dimers and induce membrane curvature depending on the shape of I-BAR dimer (reviewed in [53,54]). In addition to the originally identified 53-kDa protein IRSp53S (designated IRSp53 from now on); three other IRSp53 isoforms (designated IRSp58M, IRSp53T, and IRSp53L) were identified in human cells. In contrast, only three murine homologues (i.e. mIRSp53S, mIRSp58M, and mIRSp53T) were detected [55]. Interaction between IRSp53 SH3 domain and Eps8 N-terminal proline-rich sequences (aa207-aa221) activates Rac and results in cell motility and invasion of cancer cells [22]. Interestingly, in addition to the SH3 domain, PPPDY (aa468-aa471; GeneBank accession number NP_001138360) within the IRSp53 C-terminal WWB domain also participates in the association with Eps8 SH3 [23]. The interplay between Eps8 and IRSp53 is important for Src-mediated STAT3 activation that leads to cell proliferation in cancer cells [23].

1.4. Eps8-mediated signal transduction

Mechanistic studies reveal that serum-induced ERK activation is involved in Eps8-mediated transformation since coexpression of dominant negative MEK1 blocks its induced oncogenesis. Consistent with the PH domain of Eps8 being critical for its oncogenic potential and membrane targeting, PH-truncated Eps8 is unable to trigger ERK activation in response to serum. These data corroborate the importance of the PH domain of Eps8 for its membrane association, ERK activation and its ability to transform cells [30].

Src becomes activated when its SH3 and/or SH2 are occupied. Given Eps8 interacts with Src SH3 *in vitro* [13] and the Src SH3-binding region of Eps8 resides in its multiple proline-rich containing sequences, Eps8 is thereby speculated to increase Src enzymatic activity. In agreement with the mechanism underlying Src activation, Eps8 does elevate Src activity. This can be verified by diminished Eps8, which reduces Src activation as reflected by decreased Src Pi-Y416, which can be restored by ectopically expressed Eps8 [36]. Remarkably, Eps8 also regulates the activity and the expression level of FAK. While activation of FAK can be achieved by Src-mediated phosphorylation [56], its elevated expression relies on Akt/mTOR/STAT3 Pi-S727 pathway, which also modulates cyclin D1 expression [36].

Expressing small interfering RNA of *eps8* in HeLa and SiHa cells impedes G1-phase progression. In addition to cyclin D1, attenuated Eps8 also reduces expression of cyclins D3 and E, elevates accumulation of p53 and $p21^{Waf1/Cip1}$, and inhibits hyperphosphorylation of Rb. Reintroduced siRNA-resistant *eps8* into Eps8-attenuated HeLa and SiHa cells reverses the described alteration, indicating that the effect of Eps8 on the mentioned cell cycle modulators is specific. Eps8 facilitates p53 degradation and decreased levels of Eps8 block this process and cause p53 accumulation. Studies of the turnover rate of p53 reveal that Eps8 attenuation significantly increases the half-life of p53 in HeLa cells from ~12 min to ~40 min [37]. It is noteworthy that via accelerated degradation of p53 as well as increased activation of Src and Akt, Eps8 enables cervical cancer cells to be resistant to chemotherapeutic agents.

With a genome-wide screen, matrix metalloproteinase 9 (MMP9) along with the forkhead transcription factor FOXM1 and a cohort of its target genes encoding the cell cycle mediators and the chemokine ligands (i.e. CXCL5 and CXCL12) are upregulated by Eps8 through a PI3K/Akt-dependent mechanism [57]. Through degradation of extracellular matrix components as well as processing of cytokine and growth factors, Eps8-elicited MMP9 plays a critical role in the migratory and invasive phenotype of squamous cell carcinoma (SCC) [58].

It is well established that Eps8 forms a complex with Sos1 and Abi1 to transmit signals to Rac from receptor tyrosine kinases [21,26,40] and PI3K [41]. By its N-terminal region, Abi1 is recruited to the tips of filopodia and lamellipodia in motile cells [59], and associates to WAVE-1 [60], the actin regulatory protein, further supporting its importance in actin remodeling. Notably, Eps8 also interacts with RN-tre (a specific Rab5 GAP) to modulate Rab5 activity, inhibit receptor internalization and prolong receptor signaling at the cell membrane [43].

IRSp53 is an adaptor protein that plays an important role in actin cytoskeleton reorganization. By pull-down assays, Eps8 is demonstrated as an IRSp53-binding protein. Through its N-terminal proline-rich sequence, Eps8 directly associates with the SH3 domain of IRSp53. This Eps8/IRSp53 complex reinforces the formation of a trimolecular Rac-GEF complex (i.e. Eps8/Abi1/Sos1) to synergistically activate Rac and contribute to cell motility [22]. Through an independent yeast two-hybrid screening, IRSp53 was identified as an Eps8-interacting protein. In addition, its C-terminal SH3/WWB-containing domain (aa376-aa521) was essential and sufficient for Eps8 association [23]. Strikingly, Eps8 modulates IRSp53 expression in cells transformed with v-Src and attenuation of IRSp53 results in reduced cell proliferation in culture and reduced tumor formation in mice, which can be partly rescued by ectopically expressed IRSp53. Src drives the formation of Eps8/IRSp53 complex, which leads to activation of Akt, ERK, STAT3 and enhancement of cyclin D1. This signaling event not only occurs in v-Src transformed cells but also in EGF-stimulated cells. Notably, Eps8/IRSp53 is important in both cell proliferation and cell mobility [23].

2. Prospective study of Eps8 as an anti-cancer drug targeting protein

As a signaling intermediate, Eps8 has been demonstrated to be critical in proliferation and control of actin dynamics that lead to increased mitogenesis and motility of various tumor cells (see below). Now, we will not only summarize the published reports regarding the role of Eps8 in human tumors, but also discuss its potential to become a novel tumor marker as well as a therapeutic target for cancer treatment.

2.1. Aberrant overexpression of Eps8 in human cancer

Eps8 overexpression confers the ability of murine fibroblasts to form foci in culture and to grow tumors in mice [30]. Its oncogenic potential invites the speculation that Eps8 might be involved and contribute to development of human cancers. Indeed, following is the published reports concerning the role of Eps8 in various human tumors.

2.1.1. *Breast cancer*

Accumulated evidence indicates that gene amplification contributes to activation of oncogenes, and is often associated with tumor progression, acquired drug resistance and poor prognosis [61]. By an integration of serial analysis of gene expression with cDNA array comparative genomic hybridization, Yao et al. [62] aimed to identify and characterize amplicons and their targets in both *in situ* and invasive breast carcinomas. Their characterization of the 12p13-p12 amplicon identified four putative oncogenes including Eps8. Compared with a panel of normal mammary epithelial cells, Eps8 was confirmed to be overexpressed in breast tumors with 12p13 amplification by quantitative RT-PCR as well as fluorescence *in situ* hybridization.

2.1.2. *Pancreatic cancer*

Pancreatic ductal adenocarcinoma (PDAC) is an extremely aggressive maliganacy and characterized by early invasion and metastasis [63]. In pancreatic ductal cells, Eps8 colocalizes to the tips of F-actin filaments, filopodia, and the leading edge of cells. Its knockdown alters actin-based cytoskeletal structures and cell shape, impairs cell-cell junctions and protrusion formation.

Studies of the expression of Eps8 in cell lines derived from various tumor stages demonstrate that the levels of Eps8 are higher in cell lines derived from metastases and ascites as compared to those from primary tumors [64]. These results suggest that Eps8 plays a critical role in the metastatic potential of PDAC.

2.1.3. *Thyroid cancer*

Papillary thyroid carcinoma (PTC) is a common thyroid maligancy whose biological behavior varies widely. By studying the expression profiles of eight matched pairs of PTC and normal throid tissues, Eps8 was identified as one of the overexpressed genes in PTC [65]. Notably, Griffith et al. [66] performed a meta-review of thyroid cancer biomarkers from a large number of published studies, identified twelve candidate diagnostic biomarkers, including Eps8. Unfortunately, no follow-up study, even at the RNA level, has confirmed Eps8 upregulation in thyroid lesions. Thus, inclusion of Eps8 as a diagnostic marker for thyroid cancer requires further investigation.

2.1.4. *Oral cancer*

Oral squamous cell carcinoma (OSCC) is a common maligancy. Its local invasion and regional lymph node metastases usually cause early death. Using expression microarrays, the *eps8* gene was identified as being overexpressed in OSCC cell lines compared with normal oral keratinocytes. Despite attenuation of Eps8 in VB6, BICR56, and CA1 OSCC cells does not inhibit cell proliferation, but it does impair the cell spreading and migration toward fibronectin. Not surprisingly, Eps8 was upregulated in a subset of OSCCs where it correlated significantly with lymph node metastasis. Knockdown of Eps8 suppressed αVβ6-, and α5β1-integrin-dependent Rac1 activation and inhibited tumor cell invasion in an organotypic model of OSCC [67].

2.1.5. *Ovarian cancer*

Among gynecologic cancers, ovarian cancer has the greatest motality rate due to its metastasis [68]. Not relying on the vasculature for metastasis as seen in solid tumors, ovarian maligancy is confined within the abdominal cavity and extends to adjacent organs and/or disseminate throughout the peritoneal cavity [69]. Lysophosphatidic acid (LPA), a growth factor-like phospholipid, retains migration-stimulating potential and is present at high levels in ascites of ovarian cancer patients. LPA-mediated cell motility is confirmed to play an important role in ovarian cancer metastasis, and the integrity of Sos1/Eps8/Abi1 tricomplex is essential for LPA-induced Rac activation, cell migration and metastatic colonization. Strikingly, only coexpression of the three members of the tricomplex correlates with advanced stages and shorter survival of ovarian cancer patients [70]. For ovarian cancer metastasis, these findings not only indicate the tricomplex is a reliable marker, but also suggest targeting the tricomplex can be developed as a therapeutic approach.

2.1.6. *Colorectal cancer*

Colorectal cancer (CRC) is the most common gastrointestinal cancer and one of the leading causes of cancer mortality worldwide. Preferentially increased Eps8 in the advanced stage of human CRC specimens is detected. Intriguingly, simultaneous up-regulation of Eps8, Src and FAK in CRC is observed and these three proteins are positively correlated as indicated by Spearman rank correlation. This is in agreement with Eps8 modulating the expression of FAK via mTOR/STAT3 pathway [35].

2.1.7. *Cervical cancer*

Cervical carcinoma evolves slowly from intraepithelial neoplasia to invasive carcinoma and is the second most common malignancy among women [68]. Through clinicopathologic examination and immunohistochemical staining, an intimate correlation between Eps8 abundance and the aggressiveness (local lymph node metastasis or parametrium invasion) of early-stage cervical cancer is established. Concurrently, Eps8 expression inversely correlates with the survival rate of cervical cancer patients [36].

2.1.8. *Esophageal cancer*

A thorough analysis of both esophageal squamous cell carcinoma and esophageal adenocarcinoma revealed 4-6 fold increase in expression of Eps8 in esophageal cancers compared to adjacent normal tissues. Notably, unlike colon cancer, higher Eps8 expression in tumors as compared to their nearby normal tissue was independent of grade of esophageal cancer [72].

2.1.9. Pituitary tumor

Comprising some of the most common intracranial neoplasms, pituitary tumors can either be detected clinically (i.e. acromegaly and amenorrhea) or become clinically silent such as those of the gonadotrope lineage [73]. By DNA microarrays, *eps8* is identified as an overexpressed transcript (5.9-fold) in pituitary tumors compared with normal controls. Xu *et al.* [74] demonstrated that overexpression of Eps8 in gonadotrope pituitary cells results in activation of ERK and Akt, which provide proliferative stimulation and antiapoptotic protection respectively. Remarkably, the above mentioned signaling components are upregulated in human pituitary tumor tissues suggesting a functional significance of Eps8 in human pituitary tumorigenesis.

2.2. The potential of Eps8 attenuation in cancer treatment

Accumulated evidence revealed the significance of Eps8 in tumor development and metastasis. According to the elucidated mechanisms underlying Eps8-mediated transformation, suppressed expression of Eps8 as well as disruption of the Eps8-containing signaling complex become two promising strategies to inhibit tumorigenesis.

2.2.1. Suppressing expression of Eps8

Considering Eps8 is an oncoprotein whose overexpression is closely linked to tumor formation, suppressing its expression might provide a means to treat and eradicate tumors. Strategies published to decrease Eps8 expression are described below.

2.2.1.1. Histone deacetylase inhibitors

Epigenetic modulation of gene expression is implicated in cancer development. Emerging evidences indicate the acetylation status of histones controls the acess of transcription factors to DNA and influences gene expression. Histone acetylation and deacetylation are mediated by histone acetyl transferases (HATs) and histone deacetylases (HDACs) respectively. HDAC inhibitors are well documented to promote differentiation, growth arrest and apoptosis of cancer cells with minimal effects on normal tissues. Notably, HDAC inhibitors not only decompact histone/DNA complex, but also influence acetylation status and function of nonhistone proteins [75]. A number of HDAC inhibitors have entered preclinical and early clinical studies. Although these compounds were chosen for their ability to inhibit histone deacetylation, they still had widely varying potency and HDAC isoenzyme specificity as well as different effects on acetylation of nonhistone proteins. To date, the prominent targets of HDAC inhibitors include HDACs, $p21^{WAF1/CIP1}$, p53, death receptor proteins (i.e. TNF-α, Fas and TRAIL receptors), HIF-1α, and VEGFR [75].

Trichostatin A (TSA), an antifungal agent, is a HDAC inhibitor. The reversal of v-Src-mediated transformation by TSA is attributable to its suppression of Eps8 expression. RT-

PCR and Northern analyses reveal the significant decrease of *eps8* transcripts in TSA-treated v-Src-expressing cells relative to control cells [31]. Similar reduction of Eps8 is also obtained when butyrate, another well known HDAC inhibitor is applied (unpublished result). These data indicate Eps8 can be added to the growing list of HDAC inhibitor targets and its downregulation contributes to the antineoplastic effects of HDAC inhibitors.

2.2.1.2. Mithramycin

Mithramycin (MIT, also known as mithracin, aureolic acid and plicamycin), a polyketide produced by various soil bacteria of the genus *streptomyces*, is an inhibitor that blocks the binding of the Sp-family transcription factors to the GC box [76]. To date, expression of several proto-oncoproteins such as Met, Myb, Myc, Ras and Src can be suppressed by MIT. Interestingly, in several cancer cell lines, MIT also reduces the protein and mRNA levels of Eps8 in dose- and time-dependent manners [77]. Considering the mechanistic action exerted by MIT, the promoter composition and the transcriptional regulation of *eps8* gene warrant further investigation.

2.2.1.3. Small interference RNA or short hairpin RNA methodology

Expressing either small interference RNA (siRNA) [31,36,37] or short hairpin RNA (shRNA) of *eps8* [58] in tumor cells efficiently inhibits the expression of Eps8. Decreased levels of Eps8 alters the behavior of cancer cells such as (1) suppressed v-Src-mediated transformation in fibroblasts [31], (2) reduced colonocyte proliferation and motility in colon cancer cells [36], (3) retarded cell cycle and decreased chemoresistance in cervical cancer cells [37], (4) impaired tumorigenicity of HNSCC cells in xenograft assays [58]. Hence, using siRNA (or shRNA) methodology to suppress Eps8 expression in tumor cells might block their progression, invasion and increase their chemosensitivity to anti-cancer drugs.

2.2.2. Disruption of the formation of Eps8-containing complexes

Eps8 exerts its effects through the formation of various complexes. The well-studied ones are Sos1/Eps8/Abi1 and Eps8/IRSp53. Formation of both complexes results in Rac activation and promotes cell proliferation and cell motility.

2.2.2.1. Disruption of Sos1/Eps8/Abi1 complex formation

Sos1/Eps8/Abi1 tricomplex is well established to mediate Rac activation and whose integrity is required for LPA-stimulated cell motility and metastatic colonization in ovarian cancer cells. Given coexpression of Sos1, Eps8 and Abi1, but not any one alone, correlates with advanced stages as well as shorter survival of ovarian cancer patients [70], silencing any member of Sos1/Eps8/Abi1 tricomplex and/or targeting this tricomplex can be developed as a therapeutic approach for tumor metastasis.

2.2.2.2. Disruption of Eps8/IRSp53 complex formation

Eps8/IRSp53 complex, occurs at the leading edge of motile cells, augments Sos1/Eps8/Abi1 trimolecular complex formation, and synergistically activates Rac. Inhibiting its formation reduces the mobility and invasiveness of fibrosarcoma cells [22]. Strikingly, elevated activity of Akt, ERK, STAT3, and augmented expression of cyclin D1 are also dictated by Eps8/IRSp53 that can be reduced by SU6656, an inhibitor of Src family kinases [23]. Of note, through activation of Src, EGF induces the formation of Eps8/IRSp53 and activation of STAT3 in HeLa cells [23]. Since the association between Eps8 and IRSp53 is Src-dependent and might be a physiological event in relaying EGF signaling, strategies that interrupt the interaction between Eps8 and IRSp53 can be developed and applied for cancer treatment. Specifically designed peptides, naturally occurring or artificially synthesized chemicals that block the association between Eps8 and IRSp53 might fulfill the purpose and become novel cancer therapeutics.

3. Concluding remarks

Considering a spectrum of proteins bind to Eps8 and play important roles in cell proliferation and migration (Figure 2), Eps8 upregulation is thus expected to cause human carcinogenesis. Indeed, aberrant overexpression of Eps8 is closely linked to many types of human cancer. Although Eps8-mediated signal transduction is gradually being resolved, several important questions still remain unanswered. For instance, tyrosyl phosphorylation of Eps8 mediated by either Src or EGFR is not addressed yet. Where are these tyrosine residues located? How does their phosphorylation contribute to abnormal cell proliferation and motility in cancer cells? In addition, Eps8 possesses a nuclear localization signal (Figure 1). However, to date there are no reports regarding the role of nuclear Eps8 and how the nuclear localization of Eps8 is regulated? Tremendous work needs to be done before these questions get answers.

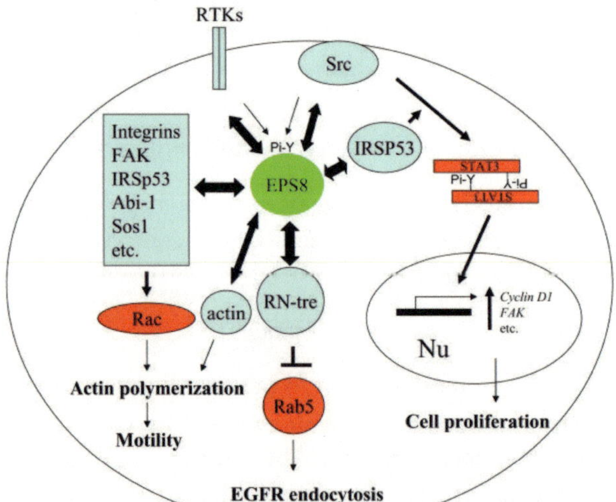

Figure 2. The signals transmitted by Eps8. Active EGFR and Src phosphorylate Eps8 and induce Eps8-IRSp53 interaction that facilitates Src-mediated STAT3 Pi-Y705 and dimerization, resulting in the increased transcription of *Cyclin D1* and *FAK* and in cell cycle progression. By binding to RN-tre, Eps8 reduces Rab5 activity and hinders EGFR endocytosis. In addition to its actin-capping activity, Eps8 interacts with proteins listed in the square box, activates Rac, promotes membrane actin polymerization, and increases motility. Nu: nucleus.

Author details

Ming-Chei Maa
Graduate Institute of Basic Medical Science, China Medical University, Taichung, Taiwan

Tzeng-Horng Leu*
Department of Pharmacology, Institute of Basic Medical Sciences and Center of Infectious Disease and Signaling Research, College of Medicine, National Cheng Kung University, Tainan, Taiwan

Acknowledgement

This study is supported in part by grants from National Health Research Institute (NHRI-EX101-1013BI to T.-H.L.), National Science Council (NSC101-2325-B-006-010 to T.-H.L; NSC98-2311-B-039-002-MY3 to M.-C. M), Comprehensive Cancer Center in Southern Taiwan (DOH100-TD-C-111-003 to T.-H. L.), Taiwan Department of Health Clinical Trial and Research Center of Excellence (DOH101-TD-B-111-004 to M.-C.M.) and China Medical University (CMU97-193 to M.-C.M.).

4. References

[1] Schlessinger J, Ullrich A (1992) Growth factor signaling by receptor tyrosine kinases. Neuron 9: 383-391.

[2] Van der Geer P, Hunter T, Lindberg RA (1994) Receptor protein-tyrosine kinases and their signal transduction pathways. Annu. Rev. Cell Biol. 10: 251-337.

[3] Kanner SB, Reynolds AB, Vines RR, Parsons JT (1990) Monoclonal antibodies to individual tyrosine-phosphorylated proteins substrates of oncogene-encoded tyrosine kinases. Proc. Natl. Acad. Sci. U.S.A. 87: 3328-3332.

[4] Glenney JR (1991) Isolation of tyrosine-phosphorylated proteins and generation of monoclonal antibodies. Methods Enzymol. 201: 92-100.

[5] Skolnik EY, Margolis B, Mohammadi M, Lowenstein E, Fischer R, Drepps A, Ullrich A, Schlessinger J (1991) Cloning of PI3 kinase-associated p85 utilizing a novel method for expression/cloning of target proteins for receptor tyrosine kinases. Cell 65: 83-90.

[6] Lowenstein EJ, Daly RJ, Batzer AG, Li W, Margolis B, Lammers R, Ullrich A, Skolnik EY, Bar-Sagi D, Schlessinger J (1992) The SH2 and SH3 domain-containing protein GRB2 links receptor tyrosine kinases to ras signaling. Cell 70: 431-442.

[7] Fazioli F, Bottaro DP, Minichiello L, Auricchio A, Wong WT, Segatto O, Di Fiore PP (1992) Identification and biochemical characterization of novel putative substrates for the epidermal growth factor receptor kinase. J. Biol. Chem. 267: 5155-5161.

[8] Fazioli F, Wong WT, Ullrich SJ, Sakaguchi K, Appella E, Di Fiore PP (1993) The ezrin-like family of tyrosine kinase substrates: receptor-specific pattern of tyrosine phosphorylation and relationship to malignant transformation. Oncogene 8: 1335-1345.

* Corresponding Author

[9] Fazioli F, Minichiello L, Matoska V, Castagnino P, Miki T, Wong WT, Di Fiore PP (1993) Eps8, a substrate for the epidermal growth factor receptor kinase, enhances EGF-dependent mitogenic signals. EMBO J. 12: 3799-3808.

[10] Wong WT, Carlomagno F, Druck T, Barletta C, Croce CM, Huebner K. Kraus MH, Di Fiore PP (1994) Evolutionary conservation of the EPS8 gene and its mapping to human chromosome 12q23-q24. Oncogene 9: 3057-3061.

[11] Ion A, Crosby AH, Kremer H, Kenmochi N, Van Reen M, Fenske C, Van Der Burgt I, Brunner HG, Montgomery K, Kucherlapati RS, Patton MA, Page C, Marima E, Jeffery S (2000) Detailed mapping, mutation analysis, and intragenic polymorphism identification in candidate Noonan syndrome genes MYL2, DCN, EPS8, and RPL6. J. Med. Genet. 37: 884-886.

[12] Tocchetti A, Confalonieri S, Scita G, Di Fiore PP, Betsholtz C (2003) In silico analysis of the EPS8 gene family: genomic organization, expression profile, and protein structure. Genomics 81: 234-244.

[13] Maa MC, Lai JR, Lin RW, Leu TH (1999) Enhancement of tyrosyl phosphorylation and protein expression of eps8 by v-Src. Biochim. Biophys. Acta 1450: 341-351.

[14] Karlsson T, Songyang Z, Landgren E, Lavergne C, Di Fiore PP, Anafi M, Pawson T, Cantley LC, Claesson-Welsh L, Welsh M (1995) Molecular interactions of the Src homology 2 domain protein Shb with phosphotyrosine residues, tyrosine kinase receptors and Src homology 3 domain proteins. Oncogene 10: 1475-1483.

[15] Matòsková B, Wong WT, Salcini AE, Pelicci PG, Di Fiore PP (1995) Constitutive phosphorylation of eps8 in tumor cell lines: relevance to malignant transformation. Mol. Cell. Biol. 15: 3805-3812.

[16] Matòsková B, Wong WT, Nomura N, Robbins KC, Di Fiore PP. (1996) RN-tre specifically binds to the SH3 domain of eps8 with high affinity and confers growth advantage to NIH3T3 upon carboxy-terminal truncation. Oncogene 12: 2679-2688.

[17] Biesova Z, Piccoli C, Wong WT (1997) Isolation and characterization of e3B1, an eps8 binding protein that regulates cell growth. Oncogene 14: 233-241.

[18] Mongioví AM, Romano PR, Panni S, Mendoza M, Wong WT, Musacchio A, Cesareni G, Di Fiore PP (1999) A novel peptide-SH3 interaction. EMBO J. 18: 5300-5309.

[19] Kishan KV, Scita G, Wong WT, Di Fiore PP, Newcomer ME (1997) The SH3 domain of Eps8 exists as a novel interwined dimmer. Nat. Struct. Biol. 4: 739-743.

[20] Castagnino P, Biesova Z, Wong WT, Fazioli F, Gill GN, Di Fiore PP (1995) Direct binding of eps8 to the juxtamembrane domain of EGFR is phosphotyrosine- and SH2-independent. Oncogene 10: 723-729.

[21] Scita G, Nordstrom J, Carbone R, Tenca P, Glardina G, Gutkind S, Bjarnegard M, Betsholtz C, Di Fiore PP (1999) EPS8 and E3B1 transduce signals from Ras to Rac. Nature 401: 290-293.

[22] Funato Y, Terabayashi T, Suenaga N, Seiki M, Takenawa T, Miki H (2004) IRSp53/Eps8 complex is important for positive regulation of Rac and cancer cell motility/invasiveness. Cancer Res. 64: 5237-5244.

[23] Liu PS, Jong TH, Maa MC, Leu TH (2010) The interplay between Eps8 and IRSp53 contributes to Src-mediated transformation. Oncogene 29: 3977-3989.

[24] Di Fiore PP, Scita G (2002) Eps8 in the midst of GTPases. Int. J. Biochem. Cell Biol. 34: 1178-1183.

[25] Disanza A, Carlier MF, Stradal T, Didry D, Frittoli E, Confalonieri S, Croce A, Wehland J, Di Fiore PP, Scita G (2004) Eps8 controls actin-based motility by capping the barbed ends of actin filaments. Nat. Cell Biol. 6: 1180-1188.

[26] Scita G, Tenca P, Areces LB, Tocchetti A, Frittoli E, Giardina G, Ponzanelli I, Sini P, Innocenti M, Di Fiore PP (2001) An effector region in Eps8 is responsible for the activation of the Rac-specific GEF activity of Sos-1 and for the proper localization of the Rac-based actin-polymerizing machine. J. Cell Biol. 154: 1031-1044.

[27] Higgs HN (2004) There goes the neighbourhood: Eps8 joins the barbed-end crowd. Nat. Cell Biol. 6: 1147-1149.

[28] Hertzog M, Milanesi F, Hazelwood L, Disanza A, Liu H, Perlade E, Malabarba MG, Pasqualato S, Maiolica A, Confalonieri S, Le Clainche C, Offenhauser N, Block J, Rottner K, Di Fiore PP, Carlier MF, Volkmann N, Hanein D, Scita G (2010) Molecular basis for the dual function of Eps8 on actin dynamics: bundling and capping. PLos Biol. 8: e1000387.

[29] Brown MT, Cooper JA (1996) Regulation, substrates and functions of src. Biochim. Biophys. Acta 1287: 121-149.

[30] Maa MC, Hsieh CY, Leu TH (2001) Overexpression of $p97^{Eps8}$ leads to cellular transformation: implication of pleckstrin homology domain in $p97^{Eps8}$-mediated ERK activation. Oncogene 20: 106-112.

[31] Leu TH, Yeh HH, Huang CC, Chuang YC, Su SL, Maa MC (2004) Participation of $p97^{Eps8}$ in Src-mediated transformation. J. Biol. Chem. 279: 9875-9881.

[32] Harlan JE, Hajduk PJ, Yoon HS, Fesik SW (1994) Pleckstrin homology domains bind to phosphatidylinositol-4,5-bisphosphate. Nature 371: 168-170.

[33] Ferguson KM, Lemmon MA, Schlessinger J, Sigler PB (1995) Structure of the high affinity complex of inositol trisphosphate with a phospholipase C pleckstrin homology domain. Cell 83: 1037-1046.

[34] Touhara K, Inglese J, Pitcher JA, Shaw G, Lefkowitz RJ (1994) Binding of G protein beta gamma-subunits to pleckstrin homology domains. J. Biol. Chem. 269: 10217-10220.

[35] Tsukada S, Simon MI, Witte ON, Katz A (1994) Binding of beta gamma subunits of heterotrimeric G proteins to the PH domain of Bruton tyrosine kinase. Proc. Natl. Acad. Sci. U.S.A. 91: 11256-11260.

[36] Maa MC, Lee JC, Chen YJ, Chen YJ, Lee YC, Wang ST, Huang CC, Chow NH, Leu TH (2007) Eps8 facilitates cellular growth and motility of colon cancer cells by increasing the expression and activity of focal adhesion kinase. J. Biol. Chem. 282: 19399-19409.

[37] Chen YJ, Shen MR, Chen YJ, Maa MC, Leu TH (2008) Eps8 decreases chemosensitivity and affects survival of cervical cancer patients. Mol. Cancer Ther. 7: 1376-1385.

[38] Alvarez CV, Shon KJ, Miloso M, Beguinot L (1995) Structural requirements of the Epidermal growth factor receptor for tyrosine phosphorylation of eps8 and eps15, substrates lacking Src SH2 homology domains. J. Biol. Chem. 270: 16271-16272.

[39] Shi Y, Alin K, Goff SP (1995) Abl-interactor-1, a novel SH3 protein binding to the carboxy-terminal portion of the Abl protein, suppresses v-abl transforming activity. Gene Dev. 9: 2583-2597.

[40] Innocenti M, Tenca P, Frittoli E, Faretta M, Tocchetti A, Di Fiore PP, Scita G (2002) Mechanisms through which Sos-1 coordinates the activation of Ras and Rac. J. Cell Biol. 156: 125-136.

[41] Innocenti M, Frittoli E, Ponzanelli I, Falck JR, Brachmann SM, Di Fiore PP, Scita G (2003) Phosphoinositide 3-kinase activates Rac by entering in a complex with Eps8, Abi1, and Sos-1. J. Cell Biol. 160: 17-23.

[42] Taki T, Shibuya N, Taniwaki M, Handa R, Morishita K, Bessho F, Yanagisawa M, Hayahi Y (2012) *ABI-1*, a human homolog to mouse Abl-interactor 1, fuses the *MLL* gene in acute myeloid leukemia with t(10;11)(p11.2;q23). Blood 92: 1125-1130

[43] Lanzetti L, Rybin V, Malabarba MG, Christoforidis S, Scita G, Zerial M, Di Fiore PP (2000) The Eps8 protein coordinates EGF receptor signalling through Rac and trafficking through Rab5. Nature 408: 374-377.

[44] Martinu L, Santiago-Walker A, Qi H, Chou MM (2002) Endocytosis of Epidermal Growth Factor Receptor regulated by Grb2-mediated recruitment of the Rab5 GTPase-activating protein RN-tre. J. Biol. Chem. 277: 50996-51002.

[45] Welsh M, Mares J, Karsson T, Lavergne C, Breant B, Claesson-Welsh L (1994) Shb is a ubiquitously expressed Src homology 2 protein. Oncogene 9: 19-27.

[46] Karlsson T, Welsh M (1997) Modulation of Src homology 3 proteins by the proline-rich adaptor protein Shb. Exp. Cell Res. 231: 269-275.

[47] Karlsson T, Welsh M (1996) Apoptosis of NIH3T3 cells overexpressing the Src homology 2 domain protein Shb. Oncogene 13: 955-961.

[48] Davoodpour P, Landstrom M, Welsh M (2007) Reduced tumor growth in vivo and increased c-Abl activity in PC3 prostate cancer cells overexpressing the Shb adaptor protein. BMC Cancer 7: 161.

[49] Funa NS, Reddy K, Bhandarkar S, Kurenova EV, Yang L, Cance WG, Welsh M, Arbiser JL (2008) Shb gene knockdown increases the susceptibility of SVR endothelial tumor cells to apoptotic stimuli in vitro and in vivo. J. Investig. Dermatol. 128: 710-716.

[50] Yeh TC, Ogawa W, Danielsen AG, Roth RA (1996) Characterization and cloning of a 58/53-kDa substrate of the insulin receptor tyrosine kinase. J. Biol. Chem. 271: 2921-2928.

[51] Abbott MA, Wells DG, Fallon JR (1999) The insulin receptor tyrosine kinase substrate p58/53 and the insulin receptor are components of CNS synapses. J. Neurosci. 19: 7300-7308.

[52] Oda K, Shiratsuchi T, Nishimori H, Inazawa J, Yoshikawa H, Taketani Y, Nakamura Y, Tokino T (1999) Identification of BAIAP2 (BAI-associated protein 2), a novel human homologue of hamster IRSp53, whose SH3 interacts with the cytoplasmic domain of BAI1. *Cytogenet Cell Genet* **84**: 75-82.

[53] Scita G, Confalonieri S, Lappalainen P, Suetsugu S (2008) IRSp53: crossing the road of membrane and actin dynamics in the formation of membrane protrusions. Trends Cell Biol. 18: 52-60.

[54] Ahmed S, Goh WI, Bu W (2010) I-BAR domains, IRSp53 and filopodium formation. Semin. Cell Dev. Biol. 21: 350-356.

[55] Leu TH, Maa MC (2002) Tyr-863 phosphorylation enhances focal adhesion kinase autophosphorylation at Tyr-397. Oncogene 21: 6992-7000.

[56] Miyahara, A, Okamura-Oho, Y, Miyahita, T, Hoshika, A, Yamada, M (2003) Genomic structure and alternative splicing of the insulin receptor tyrosine kinase substrate of 53-kDa protein. *J. Hum. Genet.* 48: 410-414.

[57] Wang H, Teh MT, Ji Y, Patel V, Firouzabadian S, Patel AA, Gutkind JS, Yeudall WA (2010) Eps8 upregulates FOXM1 expression, enhancing cell growth and motility. Carcinogenesis 31: 1132-1141.

[58] Wang H, Patel V, Miyazaki H, Gutkind JS, Yeudall WA (2009) Role for Eps8 in squamous carcinogenesis. Carcinogenesis 30: 165-174.

[59] Stradal T, Courtney KD, Rottner K, Hahne P, Small JV, Pendergast AM (2001) The Abl interactor proteins localize to sites of actin polymerization at the tips of lamellipodia and filopodia. Curr. Biol. 11: 891-895.

[60] Echarri A, Lai MJ, Robinson MR, Pendergast AM (2004) Abl interactor 1 (Abi-1) wave-binding and SNARE domains regulate its nucleocytoplasmic shuttling, lamellipodium localization, and wave-1 levels. Mol. Cell. Biol. 24: 4979-4993.

[61] Savelyeva L, Schwab M (2001) Amplification of oncogenes revisited: from expression profiling to clinical application. Cancer Lett. 167: 115-123.

[62] Yao J, Weremowicz S, Feng B, Gentleman RC, Marks JR, Gelman R, Brennan C, Polyak K (2006) Combined cDNA array comparative genomic hybridization and serial analysis of gene expression analysis of breast tumor progression. Cancer Res. 66: 4065-4078.

[63] Kleeff J, Michalski C, Friess H, Büchler MW (2006) Pancreatic cancer: from bench to 5-year survival. Pancreas 33: 111-118.

[64] Welsch T, Endlich K, Giese T, Büchler MW, Schmidt J (2007) Eps8 is increased in pancreatic cancer and required for dynamic actin-based cell protrusions and intercellular cytoskeletal organization. Cancer Lett. 255: 205-218.

[65] Huang Y, Prasad M, Lemon WJ, Hampel H, Wright FA, Kornacker K, LiVolsi V, Frankel W, Kloos RT, Eng C, Pellegata NS, de la Chapelle A (2001) Gene expression in papillary thyroid carcinoma reveals highly consistent profiles. Proc. Natl. Acad. Sci. U. S. A. 98: 15044-15049.

[66] Griffith OL, Melck A, Jones SJ, Wiseman SM (2008) Meta-analysis and meta-review of thyroid cancer gene expression profiling studies identifies important diagnostic biomarkers. J. Clin. Oncol. 24: 5043-5051.

[67] Yap LF, Jenei V, Robinson CM, Moutasim K, Benn TM, Threadgold SP, Lopes V, Wei W, Thomas GJ, Paterson IC (2009) Upregulation of Eps8 in oral squamous cell carcinoma promotes cell migration and invasion through integrin-dependent Rac1 activation. Oncogene 28: 2524-2534.

[68] Cannistra SA (2004) Cancer of the ovary. N. Engl. J. Med. 351: 2519-2529.

[69] Naora H, Montell DJ (2005) Ovarian cancer metastasis: integrating insights from disparate model organisms. Nat. Rev. Cancer 5: 355-366.

[70] Chen H, Wu X, Pan ZK, Huang S (2010) Integrity of SOS1/EPS8/ABI1 tri-complex determines ovarian cancer metastasis. Cancer Res. 70: 9979-9990.
[71] Pisani P, Bray F, Parkin DM (2002) Estimates of the world-wide prevalence of cancer for 25 sites in the adult population. Int. J. Cancer 97: 72-81.
[72] Bashir M, Kirmani D, Bhat HF, Baba RA, Hamza R, Naqash S, Wani NA, Andrabi KI, Zargar MA, Khanday FA (2010) P66shc and its downstream Eps8 and Rac1 proteins are upregulated in esophageal cancers. Cell Commun. Signal. 8: 13.
[73] Ezzat S, Asa SL, Couldwell WT, Barr CE, Dodge WE, Vance ML, McCutcheon IE (2004) The prevalence of pituitary adenomas: a systematic review. Cancer 101: 613-619.
[74] Xu M, Shorts-Cary L, Knox AJ, Kleinsmidt-DeMasters B, Lillehei K, Wierman ME (2009) Epidermal growth factor receptor pathway substrate 8 is overexpressed in human pituitary tumors: role in proliferation and survival. Endocrinology 150: 2064-2071.
[75] Lane AA, Chabner BA (2009) Histone deacetylase inhibitors in cancer therapy. J. Clin. Oncol. 27: 5459-5468.
[76] Jia Z, Gao Y, Wang L, Li Q, Zhang J, Le X, Wei D, Yao JC, Chang DZ, Huang S, Xie K (2010) Combined treatment of pancreatic cancer with mithramycin A and tolfenamic acid promotes Sp1 degradation and synergistic antitumor activity. Cancer Res. 70: 1111-1119.
[77] Yang TP, Chiou HL, Maa MC, Wang CJ (2010) Mithramycin inhibits human epithelial carcinoma cell proliferation and migration involving downregulation of Eps8 expression. Chem. Biol. Interact. 183: 181-186.

Chapter 6

FJ194940.1 Gene and Its Protein Product ACJ04040.1 – Potential Tumor Marker – From Protein to cDNA and Chromosomal Localization

Ewa Balcerczak, Aleksandra Sałagacka,
Malwina Bartczak-Tomczyk and Marek Mirowski

Additional information is available at the end of the chapter

http://dx.doi.org/10.5772/54972

1. Introduction

1.1. Investigations connected with a 65 kDa tumor associated protein

1.1.1. Purification and characterization of a 65 kDa tumor associated protein

Tumorigenesis is a multistep process during which appearance of tumor-specific antigens can occur. A wide variety of transformed rodent cells secrete transformation-related proteins. In 1992, a tumor-associated phosphoprotein with molecular weight (MW) of about 65 kDa (p65) was isolated from cell culture medium containing rat transplantable hepatocellular carcinoma 1682C cell line and purified to homogeneity [1]. For purification, in the first step ammonium-sulfate precipitation and high-performance liquid chromatography on molecular-sieving and phenyl hydrophobic interaction columns were used. Next, the protein was concentrated in a Rotofor isoelectrofocusing cell and finally separated by isoelectrofocusing followed by SDS-polyacrylamide gel electrophoresis. Purification fold after the Rotofor concentration step was about 11 000. This protein had a pI of 5.8 in isoelectrofocusing gels and in SDS-PAGE migrated as a single band. The tumor origin of this 65 kDa protein was confirmed by *in vivo* labeling of hepatocellular carcinoma cells in culture with [^{32}P]orthophosphate or [^{35}S]methionine followed by immunoprecipitation of the p65 from cell culture medium, SDS-PAGE and autoradiography. Thin-layer chromatography (TLC) showed that the p65 molecule contains phosphotyrosine, phosphothreonine, and phosphoserine. The carbohydrate content of the purified p65 protein was confirmed by Western blot analysis with the use of biotinylated lectins. Positive reaction with concanavalin A, wheat-germ agglutinin, and *Ricinus communis* agglutinin I was observed, which suggested the presence of D-mannose or N-acetyl-D-glucosamine, D-galactose and N-acetylglucosamine respectively [1].

In our further purification procedure of P65 protein from tissue culture of human breast carcinoma MCF-7 cells the extensive rotofor concentration step was successfully replaced with TCA precipitation. Having in hand purified p65 rat / P65 human, a comparison of both proteins isolated from different sources was performed [2]. Analysis of the amino acid compositions revealed a high degree of relatedness between the human and rat proteins. Also, N-terminal amino acid sequences of p65/P65 proteins were identical for the first 9 residues and no homology with other proteins was indicated. Amino acid sequence established for the N-terminal end of the p65 molecule was as follow: DPENVVRADT. Furthermore, peptide maps of the rat and human p65/P65 were generated by cyanogen bromide (CNBr) treatment. The cleavage of p65/P65 with CNBr resulted in four major peptides identifiable by silver staining of the Tricine SDS-PAGE prepared according to Schagger and Von Jagow 1987 [3]. The peptide patterns for p65/P65 were identical. The peptides have molecular weights of about 51, 39, 30, 19 kDa. Identical cleavage maps were obtained for rat and mouse p65. N-terminal sequence analysis of four peptides generated by CNBr treatment, resulted in short amino-acids residues 1-6, 1-10, 1-14 and 1-10, respectively, were almost identical, therefore the most probable sequences were established and their sequences were as follows: 51 kDa – TGPPWT, 39 kDa – FSLQLNSRGG, 30 kDa – REKVRLSSARQRLR and 19 kDa - TTHNRNPKKW. High degree of homology between human and rat proteins resulted in cross-reaction of both antigens with antibodies raised in rabbits against p65 isolated from the rat cell line THC 1682C. Similar cross reactivity to polyclonal anti-rat p65 antibodies was observed for p65 from mice bearing chemically induced papillomas. On the basis of collected data it was suggested the p65 is highly conserved in different species [4].

1.2. P65 Protein in experimental models of carcinogenesis

Polyclonal antibodies raised against p65 antigen isolated from cell culture medium of transplantable hepatocellular carcinoma (THC 1682C) have been employed to monitor the carcinogenic process in multistage rodent models of liver, skin and mammary gland carcinogenesis. In the first experimental model female Sprague-Dawley rats were initiated by the single dose of 10 mg/kg body weight of N-diethylnitrosamine (DEN) in physiological saline by gastric intubation. Twenty four hours later a 2/3 of liver was removed by surgery (partial hepatectomy). Six weeks after DEN administration a part of the animals were sacrificed at one -week intervals and their livers were used for immunohistochemical analysis and their blood was analyzed for the presence of p65 by ELISA (Enzyme Linked Immunosorbent Assay). In the liver the detectable number of p65 positive minifoci were observed one week after promotion by partial hepatectomy (PH). The number of p65 positive hepatocytes increased steadily during the first three weeks after DEN/PH. Positive p65 immunoreaction was observed in the nuclei of the hepatocytes, more precisely, within the nuclear envelopes and also in the cytoplasm. Also, three weeks after DEN/PH the p65 rapidly accumulated in the blood plasma, reached a plateau by the 3rd week and then markedly dropped by the 6th week, probably due to immune clearance. Later it increased again in parallel with the growth of p65 positive foci [4].

The second model was based on seven week old male SENCAR mice. Skin tumors were induced on the back by a single dose of 10 mmol of 7,12-dimethylbenz[a]antracene (DMBA) and repetitive application of 1 μg of 12-0-tetradecanoylphorbol-13-acetate (TPA, carcinogenesis promoter) twice a week for 20 weeks on the shaved dorsal skin. Blood samples were randomly obtained from four mice at monthly intervals to detect p65 antigen by the use of ELISA. The p65 was detected in this system as early as 4 weeks after the 1st TPA application, with slow increases in its activity for up to 24 weeks [4].

The third model was also based on chemically {N-methyl-N-nitrosourea (NMU)}-induced mammary adenocarcinoma in rats. The presence of p65 in urine and serum of rats bearing N-methyl-N-nitrosourea-induced mammary gland adenocarcinomas were analyzed by ELISA developed on the basis of polyclonal antibodies raised against rat p65 antigen. The correlation coefficient between tumor burden and p65 concentration in urine and serum was 0.65 and 0.77, respectively. The average levels of p65 in normal urine and normal serum were 37 + 32 and 48 + 38 ng/ml, respectively. In the case of urine obtained from rats bearing mammary adenocarcinoma, the mean p65 level was 119.0 + 35.9 ng/ml and its serum level was 225.4 + 67.5 ng/ml. Sensitivity, specificity and predictive value for serum and urine marker elevation were 78.5, 70.0 and 78.5% respectively. Concentrated urinary proteins were phosphorylated *in vitro* and separated by IEF or SDS-PAGE. IEF analysis of phosphorylated proteins followed by autoradiography barely showed any radioactive bands in the urine of control rats but three major radioactive bands with pI of 5.8, 5.5 and 5.0 in the urine of adenocarcinomas-bearing animals were observed. The strongest of these bands corresponded to pI ~ 5.8 in IEF was further analyzed by SDS-PAGE and showed a MW of 65 kDa. Two lighter bands corresponded to pI 5.5 and 5.0 and MW of 50 and 41 kDa apparently representing degradation products of the p65. The 65 kDa protein with a pI of 5.8 identified in the urine of tumor-bearing rats bound to an antiphosphotyrosine monoclonal and an anti-p65 polyclonal antibody as determined by Western blot analysis [5].

Also *in vivo* phosphorylation of urinary proteins was performed by i.p. injection of [^{32}P]orotophosphate into control- and mammary adenocarcinoma-bearing animals, which was followed by immunoprecipitation and subsequent separation of the in vivo-labeled urinary proteins by SDS-PAGE. No radioactive bands were observed in the case of immunoprecipitation of control urinary proteins with the preimmune or anti-p65 IgG, as well as in experimental urinary proteins treated with preimmune serum. By using anti-p65 antibodies for immunoprecipitation of *in vivo* phosphorylated urinary proteins we were able to detect the p65 antigen only in urine of rats bearing adenocarcinomas [5].

1.3. Anti-p65 antibodies as a tool in cancer detection

Described data strongly suggest that p65 is highly conserved in various species and this phenomenon could explain why human, rat, and mouse p65 antigens cross-reacted with polyclonal antibodies raised in rabbits against p65 isolated from the rat cell line THC 1682C.

On the basis of such antibodies the ELISA procedure was developed in order to analyze the presence of p65 in blood plasma, serum and urine of rats bearing adenocarcinoma [5]. The ELISA was also tested on a limited panel of cancer patients' sera as well as sera from non-cancer patients. It was proven that serum samples obtained from patients with advanced leukemia and lung adenocarcinoma contain significantly higher levels of P65 antigen than those present in control serum [4]. Anti-p65 rabbit polyclonal antibodies were also useful in immunohistochemical studies on p65 detection in either frozen or paraffin-embedded liver sections taken from experimental animals [4].

Having in hand purified p65/P65 antigens from rat transplantable hepatocellular carcinoma THC 1682C cell line and the human breast carcinoma MCF-7 cell line the possibility to produce monoclonal antibodies (MABs) against human and rat antigen was opened [6]. A few hybridomas secreting monoclonal antibodies against p65/P65 protein were established. MAbs expanded in culture medium were isolated with the use of affinity chromatography on Protein A-Sepharose, and their subclass was determined as IgG_1 by isotyping using immunodiffusion assay on 1.5% agarose gel containing goat anti-mouse subclasses of IgG and IgM. A rapid and sensitive sandwich type ELISA, with the use of purified MAbs was established to measure markedly elevated amounts of p65/P65 in sera obtained from tumor-bearing animals and from cancer patients. The average level of p65 in normal rat sera was 38 ng/ml (SD 13 ng/ml), and in sera from rats bearing mammary adenocarcinomas, the average value was 1005 $\pm$ 140 ng/ml, ranging from 200 to 3400 ng/ml. In control human sera, the mean P65 level was 34 + 35 ng/ml, while sera of patients with a variety of cancers had a 10-fold higher average P65 value of 344 + 57 ng/ml, ranging from 50 to 2230 ng/ml. More than 80% of tested sera from adenocarcinoma-bearing rats as well as from cancer patients had p65/P65 levels elevated. Overall the assay had a sensitivity of 80.9% and specificity of 85%. Different categories of cancer such as breast, ovary and endometrium, head and neck, lung and leukemia had increased P65 levels: 83.5%, 95.0%, 81.2%, 55.5% and 88.9%, respectively [6]. The purified IgG_1 MAbs with high titers and strong anti-P65 specificities were also suitable for visualization of the P65 antigen expression in tumor tissue sections [6]. Human P65 antigen has been isolated from culture medium of the breast cancer cell line (MCF-7). That is why detailed analysis of sera as well as paraffin slides from breast cancer patients was performed [7]. ELISA showed that 90.2% of cancer patients' sera were positive for P65. The average level of P65 was 446.5 ±243.8 ng/ml and the range was from 135.2 to 958.9 ng/ml. The average P65 level in control sera was 37 $\pm$ 29.5 ng/ml. Furthermore, in the group of patients with benign breast disease P65 levels were slightly elevated above the mean, with the average P65 value of 74.0 $\pm$ 41.2 ng/ml. It was also noticed that serum P65 level correlated with the pathological state of the disease. Elevation of P65 was not obvious in patients with pathological stages 0 and 1, but in stages IIA, IIB, IIIB and IV showed a marked increase above the cut-off point 2$\pm$SD (96ng/ml). In case of immunohistochemical analysis with the use of monoclonal antibodies against P65 80% of analyzed tissue slides were positive showing nucleocytoplasmic reaction [7].

Preliminary screening study based on P65 level determination in sera taken from patients with different categories of cancer showed increased P65 levels in the case of leukemias

(88.9%) [6]. It was the reason of P65 examination in patients with lymphocytic and granulocytic leukemia [8]. Using the anti-P65 monoclonal antibodies (MB2 and MF11) in a double-antibody sandwich ELISA the expression of the protein in sera of healthy controls, in patients with benign, non-neoplastic disease as well as in sera of patients with leukemia in different stages of development were established. The upper limit of normal P65 concentration was 115 U/ml (mean plus two standard deviations above the mean in the control group) [8]. The level of P65 was above normal in 95% of acute lymphocytic leukemia (ALL), 83% of acute myeloblastic leukemia (AML), 37% of chronic lymphocytic leukemia (CLL), and 30% of chronic myelogenous leukemia (CML). Monoclonal antibody was also used for immunocytochemical staining of isolated lymphocytes from normal peripheral blood and from blood of leukemic patients. The P65 positivity was 83% in CLL, 100% in ALL and 75% in AML patients [8]. Distribution of P65 in noncancer and cancer human sera samples base on already published results: [6-8] are presented in Table 1.

Diagnosis		**Average concentration of P65 (ng/ml) in human sera ± SD**	**P65-positive cases (%)**
Leukemia (n=71)	ALL – acute lymphoblastic leukemia	570.6 + 86.0	95
	AML – acute myelocytic leukemia	429,5 + 71.3	83
	CLL – chronic lymphocytic leukemia	252.2 +80.6	37
	CML – chronic myelocytic leukemia	196.3 + 87.6	30
Normal (n=80)		34.8 + 34	0
Benign (n=61)		124 + 149.4	8
Breast cancer (n=132)		466.5 + 243.8	90.2
Benign (n=68)		74.0 = 41.2	20
Normal (n=112)		37.4 +29.5	10.8
Ovary/Endometrium		232 + 74	95
Head /Neck		328 + 121	81.2
Lung		328 +158	55.5

Table 1. The medium concentrations of P65 (ng/ml) in sera from normal donors and from patients with benign diseases and different malignant cancers as well as leukemias

1.4. P65-like protein

The presence of a protein antigenically related to P65 (p65-like) was also shown in fetal serum [9]. Isoelectrofocusing followed by polyacrylamide gel electrophoresis in the presence of SDS was used for its isolation. Fractionated serum proteins after transfer onto nitrocellulose sheets were further analyzed by Western blot technique with the use of anti-P65 monoclonal antibody. Such analysis revealed that P65 protein has four isoforms. The isoforms, after isolation from polyacrylamide gels were used together for polyclonal antibody production [9]. Additional analysis of fetal serum fractions separated by electrophoresis on cellulose acetate membrane followed by immunostaining with anti-P65 monoclonal antibody revealed that the p65-like protein had a similar location to one of γ-globulin [9].

1.5. Anti-p65-like protein antibodies as a tool in cancer detection

Polyclonal antibody raised in rabbits against p65-like protein was tested by immunohistochemistry technique in breast cancer patients (frozen sections) and compared with that of anti-human-P65 monoclonal antibodies [10]. Comparison of the percentage of tumor cells showing positive immunoreaction with mono- and polyclonal antibodies showed a weak reactivity in significantly higher percentage of investigated cases 27% for MAb and 7% for PAb. On the other hand, medium and strong reactions were observed in a larger amount of cases after probing of the tumor tissue with a polyclonal antibody – 91% in comparison to 73% stained by a monoclonal antibody. In all cases positive for P65, immunohistochemical reaction was observed in the cytoplasm and in the area surrounding the nuclei [10].

Further comparative studies connected with clinical evaluation of the usefulness of polyclonal and monoclonal antibodies raised against P65/p65 protein were done by immunohistochemistry on paraffin-embedded tissue slides from breast cancer patients [11]. More than one hundred cases including infiltrating ductal breast carcinomas, fibrocystic disease and fibroadenoma were assessed immunohistochemically using monoclonal antibodies against human P65 antigen, and polyclonal antibodies against p65-like protein present in fetal serum. There were no evident differences in P65 detection between polyclonal and monoclonal antibodies, but monoclonal antibody causes more specific immunohistochemical reactions. Fibrocystic disease with large epithelioplasia that had precancerous status, gave a positive response when anti-P65 antibodies were utilized. This observation correlated with our previous data showing unique properties of anti-p65 antibodies of staining premalignant foci in the early stages of chemical carcinogenesis. In the most cases of breast cancer, a positive immunoreaction occurred with poly- and monoclonal anti-p65/P65 antibodies in the cytoplasm and/or nuclei.

The p65-like protein was also analyzed in B-chronic lymphocytic leukemia (CLL) cells as well as in normal lymphocytes, followed by their separation to nuclear, mitochondrial, and microsomal fractions by differential centrifugation. The cellular fraction of CLL and normal lymphocytes were separated by SDS-PAGE electrophoresis followed by Western blot analysis with the use of anti-p65 like polyclonal antibody [12]. P65 antigen was recognized as a predominant polypeptide in the leukemic nuclear fraction. No cross reactivity was observed with normal lymphocyte nuclear proteins in the region of 65 kDa [12].

To get a better idea about the role of the P65 protein in cancer formation and growth a more advanced study was undertaken on paraffin-embedded infiltrating ductal breast cancer tissue slides [13]. It was noticed that the percentage of positive cells with cytoplasmic expression of P65 was significantly higher in histologically more differentiated cancers (grade I and II according to Bloom & Richardson) than in grade III. The percentage of immunopositive nuclei grew with the advance of the disease and was the highest in poorly-differentiated (grade III) tumors. The tumors with P65 cytoplasmic reaction were mainly small (T1, T2), without lymph nodes (N0) and distant (M0) metastases. The straight dependence existed between P65 nucleic reaction and tumor size, metastases to lymph nodes and distant metastases. The obtained results suggested that transfer of P65 protein from cytoplasm to nuclei of the breast cancer cells is connected with more clinically advanced stages and worse prognosis for patients [13].

1.6. P65 and selected factors employed in clinical diagnosis and prognosis in breast cancer

Steroid hormone receptors (estrogen and progesterone), proliferating cell nuclear antigen (PCNA), Ki67, epidermal growth factor receptor (EGFR), oncogene c-ErbB2, tumor suppressor gene P53, anti-apoptotic gene Bcl-2 are among factors often used in clinical diagnosis and monitoring breast cancer, among other types of cancer. A computer search of Protein Sequence Database (PSD) revealed that the N-terminal peptide of human and rat P65/p65, which have been sequenced for the first 10 residues, is unique. Analysis of the amino-acid sequences of several internal peptides, generated by CNBr treatment, as described above, showed 100% identity in 6 amino-acids to c-erbA upstream of the DNA-binding domain, and 87.5% of identity in 10 amino-acids to human prostate specific antigen among other proteins [2]. On the basis of partial amino acid sequence analysis it could be suggested that P65/p65 is like the thyroid hormone receptor (THRA) or c-erbA1 and belongs to a family of nuclear receptors for various hydrophobic ligands such as steroids, vitamin D, retinoic acid and thyroid hormones. These hormones are composed of several domains important in hormone binding, DNA-binding dimerization and activation of transcription. It was shown that P65/p65 is located in nuclei of malignant cells of different cancers and this observation may support such hypothesis. It is well known that cytoplasmic receptors bind hormone and rapidly translocate it to the nucleus. This fact may explain immunostaining showing the presence of p65/P65 not only in nuclei, but also in the cytoplasm in breast cancer tissues. The presence of P65 in the cytoplasm as well as in nuclei of cancer cell may also suggest that P65 may function as a transcriptional factor.

Taking into consideration above mentioned data P65 expression was investigated in paraffin-embedded tissue slides from infiltrating ductal breast cancer specimens by immunohistochemistry using monoclonal antibodies recognizing human P65 antigen and polyclonal antibodies recognizing p65-like protein present in fetal serum in parallel with estrogen and progesterone receptors, which are very important prognostic factors in mammary gland tumors [14]. The P65/p65 expression was correlated with estrogen receptor (ER) and progesterone receptor (PR) levels. Statistically significant correlation was found between ER or PR level and P65/p65 cytoplasmic reaction and inverse correlation with nucleic localization of P65/p65 protein [13,14]. It should be underlined that patients with high levels of ER and PR are more sensitive to antiestrogen therapy. Usually a high ER level is accompanied by a high PR level. When only one type of receptor is present, the percentage of patients sensitive to such therapy significantly decreases.

PCNA and Ki67 belong to prognostic factors for clinical evaluation of breast cancer; especially their proliferating indexes (PI-PCNA, PI-Ki67) are very useful prognostic factors. A strong correlation between PI-PCNA and PI-Ki67 was established in our studies in the group of patients suffering from infiltrating ductal breast carcinoma. High PI-PCNA was accompanied by loss of steroid receptors (ER/PR) and low level of P65/p65 antigen. Those data confirmed that appearance of P65 protein is connected to carcinogenic or tumorigenic processes and that this factor is not induced by cellular proliferation associated with non-neoplastic diseases [15]. It was also established that there is no correlation between P65 and c-ErbB2, EGFR or P53 expression. In low differentiated tumors (grade III) high P53 index and high EGFR and c-ErbB2 expression was connected with low P65 expression [16].

2. Studies of *P65/p65* gene expression at the mRNA level

2.1. Development of PCR studies of *P65/p65* gene expression in different cancers and comparison with prognostic factors

Having in hand short N-terminal amino acid sequence for whole P65/p65 molecule as well as for four peptides generated by CNBr treatment, the most probable nucleotide sequences were generated. To establish RT-PCR conditions, a forward primer was designed on the basis of N-terminal domain of whole P65 molecule and reverse primers designed on the basis of its four internal peptides. As a source of RNA for RT-PCR method optimization human promyelocytic leukemic cell line (HL-60), which secretes P65 antigen was chosen. The best primers and the best condition for the PCR were established in preliminary experiments. The best results were achieved for primers based on N-terminal sequence of whole P65 molecule and N-terminal sequence established for 51 kDa peptide. The size of the product of PCR reaction was about 150 bp long [17].

On the basis of this technique P65 gene expression was analyzed in various types of leukemia: acute myeloblastic leukemia (AML), acute lymphoblastic leukemia (ALL) and chronic lymphocytic leukemia (CLL). No relationship between the expression of *P65* gene and clinical stage of leukemia was observed. The highest frequency of *P65* gene expression was found in the group of patients with CLL (average 66%). This percentage was lower in patients with acute leukemia and took out 42% in ALL and 46% in AML [17]. When *P65* gene expression was analyzed in limited groups of ALL and AML patients, where both peripheral blood and bone marrow were collected, the percentage of *P65* positivity increased to 83 and 75, respectively. Predominant presence of *P65* gene transcript in bone marrow cells may be explained by the hypothesis that investigated gene is expressed preferentially in some type of white blood cells, which do not pass through the bone marrow-blood barrier [17].

P65 gene expression was also investigated in the cases of follicular thyroid cancer and follicular adenomas and in the contrary to our earlier studies this gene was not observed in any of the analyzed follicular cancers but it was observed in 65% of follicular adenoma cases [18].

P65 gene expression was also analyzed in frozen tissue slides taken from patients diagnosed as ductal and lobular breast cancer, classified as G3, and in a limited panel of proliferative breast disease cases [19]. It was shown that *P65* gene expression is connected with small tumor size and with absence of metastases to regional lymph nodes. In contrast to *P65, c-ErbB2* expression was observed in patients with large tumors and with metastases to regional lymph nodes. Thus, an inverse relationship was found between these two genes (*P65 and c-ErbB2*). Notably, the P65 gene expression occurred in the group of proliferating breast disease cases, which were correlated with higher risk of breast cancer. In contrast, lack of P65 was evident in cases classified as fibroadenomas [19].

Because of the biological similarity between breast and prostate adenocarcinomas and some evidence suggested that the *P65* gene may be a novel member of the superfamily of genes that encode nuclear receptors for hydrophobic ligands, *P65* gene expression was also evaluated in prostate cancer. Similarly to the investigated breast cancer cases, the expression of *P65* was observed in a significant percentage of well- and moderately-differentiated tumors [20]. *P65* gene expression was also compared to expression of other factors connected with prostate cancer like well-known oncogene *c-ErbB2* (poor prognostic factor) and prostate specific gene *DD3,* highly overexpressed in prostate cancer tissue. In all investigated stages of disease straight dependence between *P65* and *DD3* gene expression and opposite dependence between *P65* and *c-ErbB2* expression were observed [20]. *P65* gene expression was also observed in some cases diagnosed as benign prostatic hyperplasia (BPH) (Balcerczak et al., unpublished data), which may suggest that its appearance may follow transition from benign to adenocarcinoma state. It is already well documented that *H. pylori* causes critical alterations in gastric mucin structure. Long-term bacterial infection is associated with development of gastritis and peptic ulcer and is presumed to be a risk factor for gastric cancer development. The presence of *H. pylori* infection was determined by urease test. Additionally, we had been looking for the presence of *P65* gene transcript in the group of gastric cancers and adjacent normal gastric mucosa. There was no correlation between P65 gene expression and *H. pylori* infection, which suggests that *H. pylori* is not involved in the process of P65 gene activation. In the case of gastric cancers *P65* gene expression was connected with poor prognosis for the patients because its expression was detectable in cases with lymph nodes and distant metastases [21]. Taking into consideration that *H. pylori* has been suggested to be a tumor-promoter in gastric carcinogenesis, our earlier results confirmed such hypothesis because anti-P65 antibodies detected only preneoplastic foci that were tumor-promoter independent [4].

2.2. Qualitative and quantitative analysis of *P65* gene expression in colorectal cancer - comparison with bad prognostic factors

When we analyzed gastric cancer cases, it was first time the positive dependence between *P65* gene expression and poor prognosis for the patients was observed. That is why our further work was focused on colorectal cancer. Patients with colorectal cancer have the highest mortality among those with cancer. We examined 109 couples of colorectal cancer tissue and adjacent, healthy colorectal mucosa from the same patients and a few samples of colorectal mucosa from patients without colorectal neoplastic disease. For 19 of them the *P65* expression was observed both in cancer tissue and in adjacent colorectal mucosa. In 58 remaining pairs *P65* gene expression was not detected. None of a few cases of healthy mucosa revealed the expression of *P65* gene. Analysis was performed by qualitative technique based on reverse transcription followed by PCR [22] and quantitative analysis by real-time PCR based on fluorescence dye SYBR Green [23]. *P65* gene expression was detected in nearly 50% (n=51) of investigated colorectal cancer cases. There was no statistically significant correlation between age, gender and expression of the *P65* gene. The investigated group consisted of 37 cases of rectal and 72 cases of colon cancers. *P65* gene expression levels determined by quantitative analysis were statistically lower in cancers originating in the rectum as compared to those originating in the colon (p=0.0099, Mann-Whitney U test). The analyzed carcinomas were histologically classified as tubular and mucinous adenocarcinomas. There was no statistical correlation between histological type of tumor and *P65* gene expression. There was no statistically significant dependence between *P65* gene expression and histological grade. *P65* gene expression was compared with several clinicopathological parameters (TNM classification) such as depth of tumor invasion (T), lymph node metastases (N), and distant metastases (M). Expression of *P65* was also correlated with vessel invasion and the presence of lymphocytes in tumor tissue. *P65* gene expression was higher in more advanced tumors (T3 and T4, deep wall penetration), while in the T1-T2 group lower levels were recorded. There was statistical dependence between the expression of *P65* and the depth of tumor penetration. Another parameter analyzed was the expression of *P65* gene in cases with (N1-N2) and without (N0) lymph-node metastasis. This analysis also revealed significant statistical correlation between them and, in cases classified as N0, the P65 expression level was lower than in the N1-N2 cases. Statistically significant correlation was also found between *P65* gene expression and distant metastases. In carcinomas with distant metastases (M1) the levels of *P65* were two times higher than in the group of cancers without distant metastases (M0). The cases without lymphocytes in tumor tissue showed higher levels of *P65* then those with the presence of lymphocytes. Furthermore, in the group of tumors without vessel invasion, *P65* gene expression was lower than in tumors with the vessel invasion, but these differences were not statistically significant [22, 23].

2.3. Influence of anticancer drugs on *P65*/*p65* expression

In our further studies, we aimed to get information about the possible stimulation of apoptosis and *P65* expression by different compounds in HL-60 cells. For this reason, we have tested the expression of different genes connected with apoptosis like *Bcl-2, c-Myc, ICE, P53* and *Bax* as well as *P65* expression after treatment of human acute promyelocytic leukemia cell line HL-60 by carboplatin alone and in combination with cytoprotective agent amifostine. *Bcl-2, c-Myc, ICE* and *P53* gene expression was estimated semi-quantitatively using a human apoptosis set 1 detection kit (hAPO1-MPCR) based on multiplex PCR reaction. *Bax* and *P65* gene expression was also estimated semi-quantitatively with the use of multiplex PCR method where cDNA was generated from total RNA isolated from HL-60 cells with the use of reverse transcriptase. Expression of the investigated genes was determined by normalization to the expression of reference (housekeeping) GAPDH or β-actin genes. HL-60 cells exposed to carboplatin alone showed about 120-fold increase in caspase 3 activity. Combination of carboplatin with amifostine induced the enzyme activity up to 280 times. The level of *Bcl-2* gene expression was diminished, whereas *Bax* gene showed tendency to grow in HL-60 cells treated with carboplatin in combination with amifostine as compared to the cells treated with carboplatin only. Protein product of *Bcl-2* has been shown to block apoptosis in experimental systems and also genetic evidence has indicated that *Bcl-2* suppresses apoptosis. It is known that *Bax* expression is usually connected with induction of programmed cell death. Similarly, to the *Bax* gene, an increasing tendency was also noticed for the *P65*, but its biological role in this process is still unknown [24].

In the same model (HL-60 cells in culture), the influence of amifostine alone and in combination with doxorubicin, cytarabine, or etoposite on *Bcl-2*, *Bax*, and *P65* genes expression was investigated. It was shown that amifostine potentiated cytotoxic action of doxorubicin but not cytarabine and etoposide. HL-60 cells treated with doxorubicin alone showed about 35-fold increase in caspase 3 activity. The enzyme activity was stimulated by combination of doxorubicin with amifostin up to 94 times. Semi-quantitative reverse transcriptase-polymerase chain reaction showed a decrease in *Bcl-2* and an increase in *Bax* and *P65* expression in HL-60 cells treated with doxorubicin in combination with amifostine when compared with the cells treated only with doxorubicin [25].

Expression of the *p65* gene was also analyzed in experimental colon cancer under the influence of 5-fluorouracil (5-FU) given alone and in combination with hormonal modulation. It was found that in the control group (mice bearing colon 38 cancer without treatment) the expression of *p65* gene was present in 57% of investigated samples. In the groups treated with tamoxifen (TAM) or lanreotide (LAN) *p65* expression was detected in 87.5% and 83.3% of analyzed cases, respectively. Both these substances increased apoptotic index in colon 38 cancer as determined by TUNEL method, and a tumor mass. After combined treatment with TAM and LAN a percentage of *p65* positive cases in the cancer group was similar to that of the control group and equal to approximately 60%. This treatment did not increase proapoptotic effects of these drugs used individually. In the group treated with 5-FU and LAN *p65* gene expression was also close to the control value (about 66%). Similarly in this group the combined treatment with these two drugs did not cause any favorable effect on apoptosis. In the group treated with 5-FU alone the expression of *p65* was present in about 80% of samples and increased apoptotic index was observed. In the group treated with a combination of 5-FU and TAM, all analyzed cases exhibited *p65* gene expression [26].

On the basis of these studies, we can conclude that different types of *in vitro* treatment of HL-60 cells, as well as mice bearing colon 38 cancer treated *in vivo*, which leads to apoptosis, is connected with stimulation of *p65*/*P65* gene expression.

2.4. Cloning, sequencing and chromosomal localization of *P65* gene

Our next goal was to clone and sequence human *P65* cDNA and analyze its expression in malignant tissues. The 5'-RACE and 3'-RACE with previously designed primers [17] were carried out to obtain the 5' and 3' missing portions of the cDNA, respectively. Amplification product of about 900 bp was obtained in 5'-RACE only and cloned in pCR 2.1. Fourteen clones were obtained and gene inserts in seven of them sequenced. The complete cDNA of the human *P65* gene was compiled by overlapping the sequences of cloned 5'-RACE PCR products. The human P65 transcript consisting of 921 bp was deposited in GenBank Acc No *FJ194940.1.* and, from that time, the P65 name was replaced by *FJ194940.1.* [27]

BLAT (BLAST-Like **A**lignment **T**ool) located the cloned cDNA sequence on human chromosome 1. The cloned sequence spans 2150 bp genomic DNA and consists of five exons. The sequence of intron 1 and intron 4 does not match human genomic sequence. The best matches for intron 1 covered only 37% of sequence in length. Better results were obtained in the BLAT search against the Human Endogenous Retrovirus Database HERVd [28]. Intron 1 sequence was similar to rv_001141. This is a complete typical provirus (soloLTR) with TSD belonging to family HERVL66. Provirus rv_001141 is located on chromosome 1. The most probable explanation is that an integration of additional copy of rv_001141 took place. Part of intron 4 sequence shows similarity (52% coverage, 83% identity) to the second intron of MLLT3 (NW_001839149).

Integration of an additional copy of rv_001141 changed transcription in this chromosome region. In normal human tissues, this chromosome region (224789942 – 224797092) corresponds to an uncharacterized transcript (GenBank Acc No AK055856) and three EST: DA627076, DA625438, and DA627327. All of them were found in kidney [27].

Chromosomal localization of cDNA of the human *FJ194940.1.* gene was experimentally determined with the use of CHORI-17 (Hydatidiform Mole) Homo sapiens BAC Library from BACPAC Resource Center (http://bacpac.chori.org) and was shown to be located on chromosome 1: 224792167-224794166. On the basis of established sequence 40 bp long synthetic probe for *FJ194940.1.* was designed to target a conserved sequence ~900 bp upstream of exon 1. Hybridizations with a ^{32}P-labeled probe were performed with high-density colony filters containing clones from chromosome 1 segments. The library was hybridized using radioactive probes. Clones from probe-positive well positions were recovered from freezer archives and grown in liquid culture (Balcerczak, Mirowski unpublished data).

2.5. Possible splice variants for *FJ194940.1* gene transcript

To confirm the exon-intron structure of *FJ194940.1* gene generated by the bioinformatics program, eight pairs of primers were designed (Table 2). Four of these primers corresponded to the interior sequences of potential exons. They were denoted as II, III, IV and V. The other corresponded respectively to 3′ end and 5′ end of adjacent exons. They were denoted as I/II, II/III, III/IV and IV/V [29].

Exon	Primer sequence		Expected amplicon length
	Forward primer	Reverse primer	
I/II	TGGTGTCCTATGGAATGCAG	CAGTTCTTCTGGCCCATCCT	153
II	CACTAGAAAACCCTATGACTTTCACA	GGACAGTTACTTGCAGTTCTTCTG	103
II/III	TGTGAAACAAGCAGTGCAAC	GCTTGTTGGTCAGCCTTCTG	155
III	TTTTCCATGTTGATGCTCA	CGCCTGAGTCTGCAGTAAT	101
III/IV	TGCTCATGCATCTCTGCTTT	TTTGAAATGGGAGCCACTGT	218
IV	CAGTGGCTCCCATTTCAAAG	TCAAACAGGTGATCGTTCCA	189
IV/V	CAGCTGGCCTAATCGAAAGA	TCCAGCATTTCAGCAAGAGA	155
V	CTCTCTTGCTGAAATGCTGG	GGCCCAGGCTTTAAACTATA	94

Table 2. Primer sequence specific for potential exons and exon junctions of *FJ194940.1* gene and expected product size

The preliminary study has indicated that *FJ194940.1.* gene transcript probably has different splice variants. The mRNA expression of *FJ194940.1* was determined in various types of cancers (breast n =25, colon n=30, thyroid n=25, and acute and chronic leukemias n=50) by semi-quantitative RT-PCR. Amplification conditions were established by gradient PCR. Messenger RNAs for exon III as well as for junction of III/IV and IV/V were found in all investigated samples. PCR product with primers set for exon V was observed in all types of cancers, but it occurred irregularly. Also irregularly, but only in some types of cancer (breast cancer, colon cancer and acute leukemia) products appeared from exon II and IV and junction of II/III. Additionally, it was proven that there is no statistically significant correlation between the presence of exon V and clinical stage and/or cancer grade.

2.6. Detailed investigation of *FJ194940.1* gene alternative splicing in colon cancer

A detailed analysis of 102 colon cancer cases was conducted to confirm an initial observation that pre-mRNA of *FJ194940.1.* gene has undergone alternative splicing. Using the method developed earlier and the above mentioned sets of primers, a total of 18 forms of mRNA *FJ194940.1* splice variants were identified. They have appeared with differential prevalence. Those isoforms arise from different combinations of 4 interior parts of exons (II, III, IV, V) and 4 different exon-exon junctions (created by 3′ and 5′ ends of particular, adjacent exons I/II, II/III, III/IV and IV/V). The full-length transcript, which was defined as exons I-V and all exon-exon junctions, was seen as the most prevalent in colon cancer samples, being identified in 40 of 102 (39.2%) cases. On the other hand, taking all detected variants (rest of the 17 types of isoforms) into account, they were found in 62 of 102 (60.8%) of patients. Some variants were not observed more frequently than full-length transcripts [29].

The variants of *FJ194940.1* gene are characterized by the lack at least one, as well as the lack of two, three or four investigated elements simultaneously in this gene transcript.

- 5 of the 18 *FJ194940.1* isoforms represented the lack of only one investigated component. Those types of isoforms were detected in 33 of the 102 colon cancer cases (32.4%). The most frequent single omitted element was the junction of II/III exons (16.7%), whereas the most infrequently isolated omitted element was the junction of III/IV as well as IV/V exons (1.9% and 1.9% respectively).
- Two elements were missing in 6 out of 18 *FJ194940.1* isoforms. Those types of isoforms were detected in 18 of the 102 colon cancer cases (17.6%). All but 2 of these variants had omissions of interior sequence of exon with the deleted region of exon-exon junction, i.e. a) II and II/III, b) III and III/IV, c) IV, IV/V, d) II/III, III.
- Three elements were missing in 4/18 *FJ194940.1* isoforms. Those types of isoforms were detected in 7 of the 102 colon cancer cases (6.9%).
- Four elements were missing in 2/18 *FJ194940.1* isoforms. Those types of isoforms were detected in 4 of the 102 colon cancer cases (3.9%). One of these isoforms was missing the entire exon IV.

To sum up the results mentioned above, the splice variant with one element deleted is the most prevalent isoform of *FJ194940.1*. The most frequently omitted element of *FJ194940.1* gene transcript was the junction of II/III exons (36/102, 35.3%). This junction of exons was missing less frequently than in combination with other elements of *FJ194940.1* cDNA. The most infrequently skipped element was the junction of IV/V exons (5.9%). This was incidental to the lack of an interior sequence in exon IV. All samples contained amplification products for the junction of I/II exons and exon V. All possible splice variants of *FJ194940.1* gene are presented on Figure 1 and number of cases with the presence and absence of analyzed splice variants are presented in Table 3.

Additionally, to assess applicability of *FJ194940.1* splice variants elements as prognostic factors in colon cancer, their expression with established prognostic features and survival time of patients suffering from this disease were also compared. Statistical analysis was carried out with reference to whole *FJ194940.1* transcript and to particular exons and exon-exon junctions, but no significant correlations were found. The whole transcript was divided into two parts A and B. The part A consists of exons II and III as well as I/II, II/III exon-exon junctions, while part B is composed of exons IV, V, III/IV, and IV/V exon-exon junctions. Part A contains the most frequently skipped element of the examined transcript, while part B contains its longest component.

No associations were found between gender, familial history and expression of both examined parts of *FJ194940.1* gene transcript. Expressions of both parts A and B were not connected with tumor localization. There was not a statistically significant association between part A and B of *FJ194940.1* gene expression and histological type of tumor. There was link between part B of *FJ194940.1* gene transcript expression and tumor grading. Expression of part B is connected with well (G1) and moderately (G2) differentiated cases. Expression of both parts of investigated gene transcript and some clinical staging features, including depth of tumor invasion, lymph nodes metastases, distant metastases, and stage, according to pTNM classification, were compared. No statistically significant associations were noted between mentioned parameters and expression of part A as well as part B of

FJ194940.1 gene transcript. The expression levels of analyzed parts of *FJ19940.1* gene transcript were also compared to the presence of lymphocytes in tumor and vascular invasion. Venous invasion was significantly related to presence of all elements in part A of the *FJ194940.1* gene transcript (p=0.0477). There was no statistical significance connection between the presence of lymphocytes in tumor and expression of part A or B of *FJ194940.1* gene transcript. There was no statistically significant difference in survival time comparing patient with presence and absence of whole transcript in spite of the visible tendency for shorter survival of those without at least one element in whole transcript (*p=0.0690*).

	I/II	II	II/III	III	III/IV	IV	IV/V	V
40	------	------	------	------	------	------	------	------
17	------	------		------	------	------	------	------
8	------	------	------		------	------	------	------
7	------			------	------	------	------	------
6	------	------	------	------			------	------
4	------		------	------	------	------	------	------
2	------	------	------	------		------	------	------
2	------	------	------	------	------	------		------
2	------	------	------	------	------			------
2	------				------	------	------	------
2	------	------		------				------
2	------	------		------			------	------
2	------			------			------	------
2	------			------	------		------	------
1	------	------			------	------	------	------
1	------	------	------				------	------
1	------	------		------		------	------	------
1	------		------	------	------		------	------

Figure 1. 18 possible splice variants of *FJ194940.1* gene in colorectal cancer cases (n=102). From the left - the number of cases where splice variants were detected. Amplified exons II, III, IV and V and their junctions I/II, II/III, III/IV, IV/V.

	Number of cases with the presence of investigated amplicon	Number of cases with the absence of investigated amplicon
I/II	102 (100,0%)	0 (0,0%)
II	84 (82,4%)	18 (17,6%)
II/III	66 (64,7%)	36 (35,3%)
III	90 (88,2%)	12 (11,8%)
III/IV	86 (84,3%)	16 (15,7%)
IV	84 (82,4%)	18 (17,6%)
IV/V	96 (94,1%)	6 (5,9%)
V	102 (100,0%)	0 (0,0%)

Table 3. The expression frequency of investigated exons and their junctions in investigated transcript of *FJ194940* gene.

2.7. From cDNA to amino acid sequence

ORF (Open Reading Frame) Finder found several open reading frames on cDNA, which could code protein(s). Sequences of generated peptides were compared by BLAST with sequences of proteins available in GenBank and SwissProt databases. The best results were obtained for ORF number 2 in reading frame 2 on the direct strand extending from base 374 to base 790 (Balcerczak and Mirowski unpublished data).

The peptide amino acids sequences were found to be significantly similar to the integrase core domain in the Conserved Domain Database, and to the human protein EAW69787 referred as similar to Pro-Pol-dUTPase polyprotein, RNaseH, dUTPase, integrase, protease and reverse transcriptase (LOC768966) in the GenBank database. The deduced peptide has a molecular weight of 15.74 kDa and is probably one of possible *FJ194940.1.* gene protein products. This hypothesis is in agreement with results that confirmed alternative splicing of the investigated gene. It is also possible that the TAA stop codon at the 790 position is skipped and protein synthesis further continued.

2.8. Anti-peptide antibodies

The deduced protein (15.74 kDa) is substantially smaller than P65. For experimental evidence of this protein sequence potential antigenic region(s) were searched for future experimental analysis. The EMBOSS (European Molecular Biology Open Software Suite) ANTIGENIC program, Kolaskar and Tongaonkar and Peptide Select Program were used. Sequences predicted as antigenic by all the software were used for induction of antibody production. Three peptides (IC14, CL14 and CR14) were chosen for further experiments. Peptides were modified by adding cysteine to the C-terminus or N-terminus and conjugated with KLH. Obtained antibodies were used in Western-blotting analysis of two cell lines: promyelocytic HL-60 and lymphoblastic NALM-6. Positive results were obtained for antibodies IC14 and CR 14 and, in Western blot analysis, two immunoactive bands were detected. The first one had a molecular weight of about 65 kDa and the second about 15 kDa (Mirowski, Balcerczak unpublished data).

2.9. Possible mechanism of transcription in human neoplasm

Sequence of *FJ194940.1* fragment determined in this study had the length of 921 bp. An insertion of an additional copy of HERV provirus rv_001141 probably occurs during the carcinogenic process, which changes transcription of chromosome 1 224792176 - 222794166 region. In normal human tissues this chromosome region encodes transcript AK055856 expressed in kidney. Integration of rv_001141 leads to alteration of transcription [27].

It is already well known that the retrovirus family is an etiological agent of human cancer, mainly leukemia and lymphomas. The presence of endogenous retroviruses (HERV) sequences in the human genome is well documented. In contrast to the normal tissues, HERV sequences are transcriptionally-active in embryonic cells, such as placenta and theratocarcinoma [30] as well as in tumor cells [31]. Several factors regulate HERV expression. In tumor cells, HERV expression can be stimulated by INF-α [32], TNF-α, IL-1α and IL-1β [33]. Other factors, which can stimulate their transcription, are steroid hormones, including glucocorticoids. HERV-K10 (in breast cancer cells) belongs to the family of sequences that are activated in placenta by steroids. On the other hand, HERV-E expression is hindered during therapy with the use of steroids [34]. Another group of factors, which can influence activity of endogenous retroviruses, are products of exogenous viruses e.g., Epstein-Barr, which upregulate transcription of *env* gene of HERV-K18, which is located in the intron of the *CD48* gene [30]. Endogenous retroviruses have influence on genomic DNA organization and deregulate genes expression, creating additional transcription initiation sites, incorrect splicing, inserting stop codons or or polyadenylation signal [30,32,35]. As a consequence of interruption of gene function, many diseases can develop e.g., cancer, if HERV insertion is present in a proto-oncogene or suppressor gene or their vicinity. Such situation is observed in rats with N-methyl–N nitrosurea induced mammary gland carcinoma, where defective sequence of HERV in *c-H-ras* gene intron leads this gene to overexpression [36]. In our previous study P65 antigen was found in the serum and urine of rats with N-methyl-N-nitrosourea-induced mammary adenocarcinomas [5].

3. Conclusion

FJ194940.1 and its protein product seem to be a potential new molecular marker, which may be used for monitoring of oncological patients, especially with colon cancer. Its chromosomal localization and exon-intron structure was predicted by BLAT, confirmed by RT-PCR and also with the use of CHORI-17 (Hydatidiform Mole) Homo sapiens BAC Library from BACPAC Resource Center analysis. The best matches in cloned sequence of *FJ194940.1* gene were found for the Human Endogenous Retrovirus Database HERVd, especially with the family of HERVL66. RT-PCR analysis with sets of primers designed for different exons and junctions of exons, showed alternative splicing of mRNA *FJ194940.1* in different tumors. It leads to production of different *FJ194940.1* isoforms that are expressed with differential prevalence in colon cancer cases. Established nucleotide sequence of *FJ194940.1* gene opens the possibility for further studies with the use of labeled probes or polyclonal / monoclonal antibodies raised against recombinant proteins and such investigations are in progress.

Author details

Ewa Balcerczak, Aleksandra Sałagacka, Malwina Bartczak-Tomczyk and Marek Mirowski
Laboratory of Molecular Diagnostic and Pharmacogenomics,
Department of Pharmaceutical Biochemistry, Medical University of Lodz Muszyńskiego 1, PL Łódź, Poland

Acknowledgement

Supported by grant NN405 341 633 from the MNiSW and NCN, Poland.

4. References

[1] Mirowski M, Sherman U, Hanausek M (1992) Purification and Characterization of a 65 kDa Tumor-associated Phosphoprotein from Rat Transplantable Hepatocellular Carcinoma 1682C Cell Line. Protein Expr. Purif. 3: 196-203.
[2] Mirowski M, Walaszek Z, Sherman U, Hanausek M (1993) Comparative Structural Analysis of Human and Rat 65 kDa Tumor-associated Phosphoproteins. Int. J. Biochem. 25: 1865-1871.
[3] Schagger H, Von Jagow G (1987) Tricine-sodium Dodecyl Sulfate-polyacrylamide Gel Electrophoresis for the Separation of Proteins in the Range from 1 to 100 kDa. Anal. Biochem. 166: 368-379.
[4] Mirowski M, Hanausek M, Sherman U, Adams AK, Walaszek Z, Slaga TJ (1992) An Enzyme-linked Immunosorbent Assay for P65 Oncofetal Protein its Potential as a New Marker for Cancer Risk Assessment in Rodents and Humans. In: Relevance of Animal Studies to the Evaluation of Human Cancer Risk, Ed. D`Amato R, Slaga TJ, Farland WH, Henry C. pages 281-294.
[5] Mirowski M, Walaszek Z, Sherman U, Adams AK, Hanausek M (1993) Demonstration of a 65 kDa Tumor-specific Phosphoprotein in Urine and Serum of Rats with N-methyl-N-nitrosourea-induced Mammary Adenocarcinomas. Carcinogenesis 14: 1659-1664.
[6] Wang S, Mirowski M, Sherman U, Walaszek Z, Hanausek M (1993) Monoclonal Antibodies Against a 65 kDa Tumor-Associated Phosphoprotein: Development and Use in Cancer Detection. Hybridoma 12: 167-176.
[7] Mirowski M, Klijanienko J, Wang S, Vielh P, Walaszek Z, Hanausek M (1994) Serological and Immunohistochemical Detection of a 65 kDa Oncofetal Protein in Breast Cancer. Eur. J. Cancer 30A: 1108-1113.
[8] Hanausek M, Wang SC, Blonski JZ, Polkowska-Kulesza E, Walaszek Z, Mirowski M (1996) Expression of an Oncofetal 65-kDa Phosphoprotein in Lymphocytic and Granulocytic Leukemias. Int. J. Hematol. 63: 193-203.
[9] Mirowski M, Walaszek Z, Hanausek M (1996) Presence in Bovine Fetal Serum of the Protein Antigenically Related to p65-tumor Associated Antigen: Its Isolation and Polyclonal Antibody Production. Neoplasma 43: 83-88.

[10] Mirowski M, Błoński JZ, Niewiadomska H, Olborski B, Walaszek Z, Hanausek M, Wozniak L (1997) Immunohistochemical Study of 65-kDa Oncofetal Protein Expression in Breast Cancer. The Breast 6: 284-290.

[11] Niewiadomska H, Mirowski M, Stempien M, Blonski JZ, Hanausek M (1996) Clinical Evaluation of the Usefulness of Polyclonal and Monoclonal Antibodies Raised Against p65 Protein in Immunohistochemical Diagnosis of Breast Cancer: a Comparative Study. Biomed. Lett. 54: 223-231.

[12] Chrusciel J, Blonski JZ, Krykowski E, Mirowski M, Hanausek M, Kilianska ZM (1996) Characterization of Proteins from Chronić Lymphocytic Leukemic Cells: Electrophoretic and Immunological Approach. Cytobios 85: 39-49.

[13] Niewiadomska H, Mirowski M, Świtalska J, Balcerczak E, Kubiak R, Wierzbicki R (2004) Polyclonal Antibodies Raised Against P65 Protein in Immunohistochemical Diagnosis of Breast Cancer. J. Exp. Clin. Cancer Res. 23: 113-119.

[14] Niewiadomska H, Mirowski M, Barkowiak J, Stempien M, Blonski JZ, Walaszek Z, Hanausek M, Wierzbicki R (1997) Oestrogen/Progesterone Receptors and 65 kD Tumor-associated Phosphoprotein (p65) Expression in Breast Cancer Patients. Biomed. Lett. 56: 91-99.

[15] Niewiadomska H, Mirowski M, Stempien M, Olborski B, Blonski JZ, Hanausek M, Wierzbicki R (1998) A 65 kDa Oncofetal Protein (p65), Proliferating Cell Nuclear Antigen (PCNA) and Ki67 Expression in Breast Cancer Patients. Neoplasma 1998, 45, 216-222.

[16] Niewiadomska H, Mirowski M, Stempien M, Blonski JZ, Czyz W, Switalska J, Matyga E, Hanausek M, Wierzbicki R (2000) Immunohistochemical Analysis of Expression of a 65 kDa Oncofetal Protein (p65), Epidermal Growth Factor Receptor (EGFR), Oncogene c-erb B2 and Tumor Suppressor Gene p53 Protein Products in Breast Cancer Patients. Neoplasma 47: 8-14.

[17] Balcerczak E, Bartkowiak J, Błoński JZ, Robak T, Mirowski M (2002) Expression of Gene Encoding P65 Oncofetal Protein in Acute and Chronic Leukemias. Neoplasma 49: 295-299.

[18] Czyz W, Balcerczak E, Rudowicz M, Niewiadomska H, Pasieka Z, Kuzdak K, Mirowski M (2003) Expression of C-ERBB2 and P65 Genes and Their Protein Products in Follicular Neoplasms of Thyroid Gland. Fol. Histochem. Cytobiol. 41: 91-95.

[19] Balcerczak E, Mirowski M, Jesionek-Kupnicka D, Bartkowiak J, Kubiak R, Wierzbicki R (2003) P65 and c-erbB2 Genes Expression in Breast Tumors: Comparison with Some Histological Typing, Grading and Clinical Staging. J. Exp. Clin. Cancer Res. 22: 421-427.

[20] Balcerczak E, Mirowski M, Sasor A, Wierzbicki R (2003) Expression of p65, DD3 and c-erbB2 Genes in Prostate Cancer. Neoplasma 50: 97-101.

[21] Balcerczak E, Jankowski T, Becht A, Balcerczak M, Janiuk R, Jesionek-Kupnicka D, Sztompka J, Mirowski M (2005) Expression of the P65 Gene in Gastric Cancer and in Tissues with or without Helicobacter pylori Infection. Neoplasma 52: 464-468.

[22] Balcerczak M, Balcerczak E, Pasz-Walczak G, Kordek R, Mirowski M (2004) Expression of the p65 Gene in Patients with Colorectal Cancer: Comparison with some Histological Typing, Grading and Clinical Staging. Eur. J. Surg. Oncol. 30: 266-270.

[23] Balcerczak E, Balcerczak M, Mirowski M (2007) Quantitative Analysis of the P65 Gene Expression in Patients with Coloroctal Cancer. Int. J. Biomed. Sci. 3: 287-291.

[24] Mirowski M, Różalski M, Krajewska U, Balcerczak E, Młynarski W, Wierzbicki R (2003) Induction of Caspase 3 and Modulation of some Apoptotic Genes in Human Acute Promyelocytic Leukemia HL-60 Cells by Carboplatin with Amifostine. Pol. J. Pharmacol. 55: 227-234.

[25] Rózalski M, Mirowski M, Balcerczak E, Krajewska U, Młynarski W, Wierzbicki R (2005) Induction of Caspase 3 Activity, bcl-2 bax and p65 Gene Expression Modulation in Human Acute Promyelocytic Leukemia HL-60 Cells by Doxorubicin with Amifostine. Pharmacol. Rep. 57: 360-366.

[26] Mełeń-Mucha G, Balcerczak E, Mucha S, Panczyk M, Lipa S, Mirowski M (2004) Expression of p65 Gene in Experimental Colon Cancer under the Influence of 5-fluorouracil Given Alone and in Combination with Hormonal Modulation. Neoplasma 51: 319-324.

[27] Balcerczak E, Malewski T, Bartczak M, Mirowski M (2011) Alteration of FJ194940.1 Transcript Expression after Retrovirus Integration in Human Neoplasms. Int. J. Integ. Biol. 11: 58-63.

[28] Paces J, Pavlícek A, Zika R, Kapitonov VV, Jurka J, Paces V (2004) HERVd: the Human Endogenous Retroviruses Database: update. Nucleic Acids Res. 32: D50.

[29] Bartczak-Tomczyk M, Sałagacka A, Mirowski M, Balcerczak E (2011) Investigation of FJ194940.1 Gene Alternative Splicing in Colon Cancer and its Association with Clinicopathological Parameters. Exp. Therap. Med. DOI: 10.3892/etm.2011.378

[30] Löwer R, Löwer J, Kurth R (1996) The Viruses in All of Us: Characteristics and Biological Significance of Human Endogenous Retrovirus Sequences. Proc. Natl. Acad. Si. USA, 93: 5177–5184.

[31] Stauffer Y, Theiler G, Sperisen P, Lebedev Y, Jongeneel CV (2004) Digital Expression Profiles of Human Endogenous Retroviral Families in Normal and Cancerous Tissues. Cancer Immunity 4: 2-20.

[32] Villesen P, Aagaard L, Wiufl C, Pedersen FS (2004) Identification of Endogenous Retroviral Reading Frames in the Human Genome. Retrovirology 1: 1-13.

[33] Portis JL (2002) Perspectives on the Role of Endogenous Human Retroviruses in Autoimmune Diseases. Virology 296: 1-5.

[34] Ono M, Kawakami M, Ushikubo H (1987) Stimulation of Expression of the Human Endogenous Retrovirus Genome by Female Steroid Hormones in Human Breast Cancer Cell Line T47D. J Virol. 61: 2059-2062.

[35] Patience C, Wilkinson DA, Weiss RA (1997) Our retroviral heritage. Trends. Genet. 13: 116-120.

[36] Nelson PN, Carnegie PR, Martin J, Davari Ejtehadi H, Hooley P, Roden D, Rowland-Jones S, Warren P, Astley J, Murray PG (2003) Demystified . . . Human endogenous retroviruses. Mol. Path. 56: 11-18.

Chapter 7

The Interaction Between Redox and Hypoxic Signalling Pathways in the Dynamic Oxygen Environment of Cancer Cells

Maneet Bhatia, Therese C. Karlenius, Giovanna Di Trapani and Kathryn F. Tonissen

Additional information is available at the end of the chapter

http://dx.doi.org/10.5772/55185

1. Introduction

Oxygen is essential for the survival of all living beings. A balanced oxygen environment is required since both lower and higher than the required oxygen levels can be detrimental to the cells (Figure 1). The oxygen state of a tissue results from the relative contributions of oxygen consumption and delivery. Different organs in the body exist under different oxygen environments, depending on the location and function of the cells in an organ. Most healthy organs reside in 3-6% oxygen [1] while conditions lower than 3% oxygen are described as hypoxia. Cells also survive in hypoxic environments during normal development [2]. However, hypoxia is mostly detrimental to the cells by disrupting the oxygen homeostasis.

Cancer cells are capable of surviving under hypoxic conditions by inducing the expression of metabolic enzymes required for anaerobic metabolism. To fulfill their oxygen and nutritional requirements, cancer cells can also induce the formation of blood vessels by a process called angiogenesis. A transcription factor called hypoxia inducible factor-1 (HIF-1) is responsible for induction of specific gene expression by binding to hypoxic response elements (HRE) present in the promoters of these target genes, which are essential for cells to survive under a low oxygen environment, as reviewed recently in [3]. When hypoxic tumor cells are reoxygenated due to angiogenesis, oxidative stress may occur. However, angiogenesis in tumors is aberrant due to sparse arteriolar supply [4], low vascular density [5], and inefficient orientation of microvessels [6]. This creates a scenario where cancer cells are in flux, where they cycle between hypoxia and the reoxygenated state. There are two dominant timescales that contribute to the cycling kinetics. One is of a faster frequency with a few cycles per hour and primarily arises from fluctuations in red blood cell flux [7]. The slower timescale varies from hours to days and is due to vascular remodeling [8]. This makes angiogenesis irregular with respect to both space and time, thereby leading to an unstable cancer environment that oscillates between low and high oxygen conditions. This cycling phenomenon is termed intermittent hypoxia or cycling hypoxia [9]. The involvement of reoxygenation phases in intermittent hypoxia suggests the possibility that redox enzymes, such as thioredoxin, may be upregulated in addition to the hypoxic enzymes.

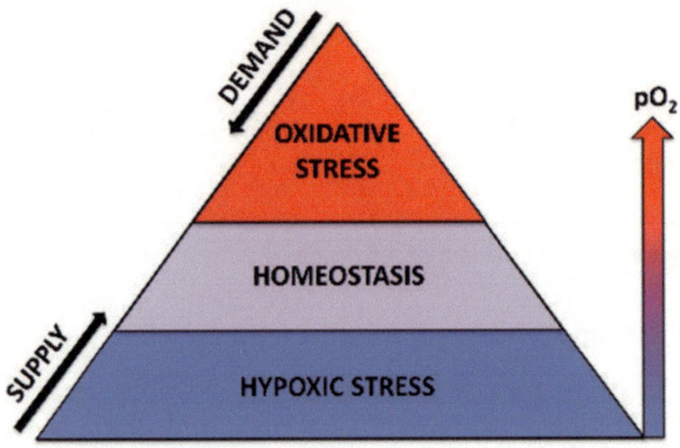

Figure 1. Oxygen homeostasis. Low cellular oxygen results in hypoxic stress causing cells to upregulate pathways involved in increasing the oxygen supply. On the other hand, higher oxygen levels result in oxidative stress and many antioxidants are induced in response, in order to reduce the available oxygen and prevent subsequent cellular damage.

2. The thioredoxin system

Cellular oxygen status is a key regulator of several important biological functions. To maintain the oxygen homeostasis, cells utilize antioxidant systems. An important antioxidant system that is present in all species and is conserved through evolution is the thioredoxin system. It comprises thioredoxin and thioredoxin reductase and catalyses oxidoreductase reactions through a dithiol-disulfide exchange mechanism [10]. Thioredoxin is a small 12kDa protein containing an active site motif of Cys-Gly-Pro-Cys. Reduced thioredoxin catalyses the reduction of disulphide bonds in other oxidised proteins and in the process itself becomes oxidised such that a disulphide bond forms between the two cysteine residues in its active site. Thioredoxin is then restored to a reduced state by thioredoxin reductase with the use of NADPH [10].

2.1. Subcellular localisation and functions of thioredoxin

Thioredoxin is found in the cytoplasm, in the nucleus and also in the extracellular environment and it has distinct functions in each location (Figure 2). The key function of the thioredoxin system is to maintain the redox balance of cells by either directly scavenging highly unstable and reactive molecules known as reactive oxygen species (ROS) [11] or by regulating the activity of several other important enzymes, such as peroxiredoxins [12] and methionine sulfoxide reductase (MSR) [13] that also maintain the cellular oxygen balance. Peroxiredoxins are a family of small (22-27 kDa) peroxidases comprised of 6 isoforms. They use their -SH groups as reducing equivalents and act to reduce peroxides such as H_2O_2, organic hydroperoxides and peroxynitrite [12]. The oxidised form of peroxiredoxins can then be recycled back to their active reduced form through the action of an electron donor, which for peroxiredoxins 1-5 is thioredoxin. The MSR family consists of MSRA and MSRB antioxidant proteins and provides an indirect defense against ROS. Methionine residues in several proteins become oxidised by ROS to Met-S-O and Met-R-O, epimers of methionine sulfoxide (Met-O). This can render the proteins non-functional. MSRA and MSRB can restore the functionality of proteins by reducing the Met-S-O and Met-R-O bound proteins respectively [14]. During this process the MSR proteins become oxidised, but are reduced to their active form by thioredoxin. Thioredoxin also directly interacts with the apoptotic pathway by binding to apoptosis signal-regulating kinase-1 (ASK-1), a member of the MAPKKK family. The reduced form of thioredoxin binds to ASK-1 but in the presence of ROS, thioredoxin becomes oxidised and dissociates. This allows the free ASK-1 to promote apoptosis [15].

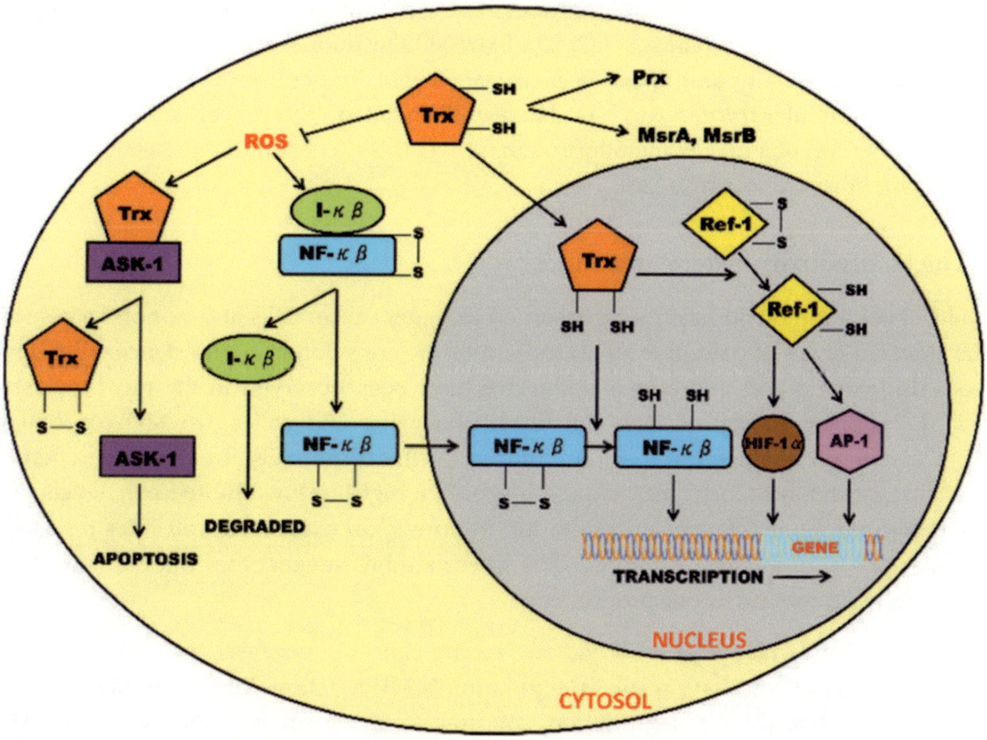

Figure 2. Localisation of thioredoxin with some of its functions and regulatory pathways.

In the nucleus, thioredoxin is responsible for regulating the activity of several transcription factors. Nuclear factor-κB (NF-κB) is a transcription factor involved in the regulation of apoptosis and is activated in response to ROS [16]. Under normal conditions, NF-κB is inhibited by I-κβ, which keeps NF-κB sequestered in the cytosol. In response to oxidative stress, I-κβ is degraded and releases NF-κβ, which is translocated to the nucleus. In the nucleus, thioredoxin directly reduces Cys62 in the p50 subunit of NF-κB, which allows NF-κB to bind to the specific recognition sequence in the promoter of its target genes, such as those involved in cell survival, to induce their expression [16]. Thus, thioredoxin contributes to the upregulation of anti-apoptotic proteins. Thioredoxin can also regulate transcription factors via indirect mechanisms through redox factor-1 (Ref-1), which is an intermediate protein that reduces several other transcription factors to enhance their binding to the promoters of their target genes [17]. Activator protein-1 (AP-1) is a heterodimeric complex of Fos and Jun proteins that binds to the DNA regulatory element known as the AP-1 binding site [18]. AP-1 mediates growth of cells in response to external stimuli. Thioredoxin acts on Ref-1, which in turn activates AP-1 by reducing the highly conserved cysteine residues in the DNA-binding domains of Fos (Cys154) and Jun (Cys272) [17]. Therefore, thioredoxin is also involved in cell growth. Furthermore, under hypoxic conditions, thioredoxin activates HIF-1 through Ref-1.

Thioredoxin is also secreted by a variety of normal and neoplastic cells through an as yet unknown pathway [19]. Secreted thioredoxin has been implicated in immune responses [20, 21] and in cell survival mechanisms [22, 23]. Extracellular thioredoxin has been suggested to have chemotactic activity and to act as chemo-attractant for neutrophils, monocytes and T-cells [24]. Extracellular thioredoxin has also been associated with cancer cell metastasis [25] and the promotion of a matrix metalloproteinase-9 (MMP-9) dependent invasive phenotype in malignant breast cancer cells [26].

2.2. The thioredoxin system and cancer

High levels of thioredoxin have been observed in many cancer cells and tumors in response to the elevated levels of oxidative stress these cells are considered to experience. High levels of both thioredoxin and thioredoxin reductase have been observed in the most metastatic tumors [27]. Using prostate cancer cell lines, Chaiswing and colleagues showed that the more invasive cell line displayed a more reduced cellular state [28]. In addition, when two human lung carcinoma cell lines expressing either high or low thioredoxin levels were injected into immuno-deficient mice, the high thioredoxin expressing cell lines resulted in more aggressive tumors being formed [29]. These studies suggest that thioredoxin plays a critical role in promoting tumor progression.

While the specific roles that thioredoxin has in cancer metastasis are yet to be fully identified, it is known to have a role in regulating MMP function. MMPs are involved with extracellular matrix (ECM) degradation, an important aspect of metastasis [30]. MMP activity is regulated by tissue inhibitor of matrix metalloproteinases (TIMPs) [31]. In normal cells, MMP levels are maintained by TIMPs and ECM degradation is inhibited. In tumor cells, the MMP/TIMP balance is disturbed, leading to ECM degradation and subsequent tumor invasion. Addition of extracellular thioredoxin was shown to preferentially inhibit TIMPs, leading to an increase in overall MMP activity and thus, stimulating neuroblastoma cell invasion [25]. Recently, it was shown that over-expression of thioredoxin in MDA-MB-231 breast cancer cells stimulated MMP-9 expression by upregulating NF-κB, Sp1 and AP-1 activity and enhancing binding of these transcription factors to the MMP-9 gene promoter. Transfection of a construct expressing a dominant negative redox inactive thioredoxin protein inhibited MMP-9 promoter activity and subsequent NF-κB, SP1 and AP-1 binding [26].

2.3. Induction of the thioredoxin system by oxidative stress

The induction of thioredoxin expression during oxidative stress in both normal and cancer cells has been well documented and occurs primarily through an antioxidant response element (ARE) in the thioredoxin gene promoter. ARE elements are short cis-acting elements found in the promoter regions of many genes encoding antioxidant enzymes and they regulate gene expression during oxidative stress [32]. A redox-sensitive transcription factor, nuclear factor (erythroid-derived 2)-like 2 (Nrf2) plays a critical role in mediating the antioxidant gene expression via the ARE element [33]. Nrf2 is ubiquitously expressed in most tissues and is continuously degraded in the cytosol under normal oxygen conditions via its inhibitor "kelch-like erythroid cell-derived protein-1" (Keap1) [34]. Keap1 contains several cysteine residues that act as redox sensors. Upon changes in the cellular oxygen environment, these cysteine residues are oxidised [35]. As a result, Keap1 undergoes a conformational change and releases Nrf2, which is translocated into the nucleus [32]. In the nucleus, Nrf2 forms a heterodimer with small maf proteins and binds to the ARE of the target antioxidant genes [36], including thioredoxin [37] and thioredoxin reductase [38] (Figure 3).

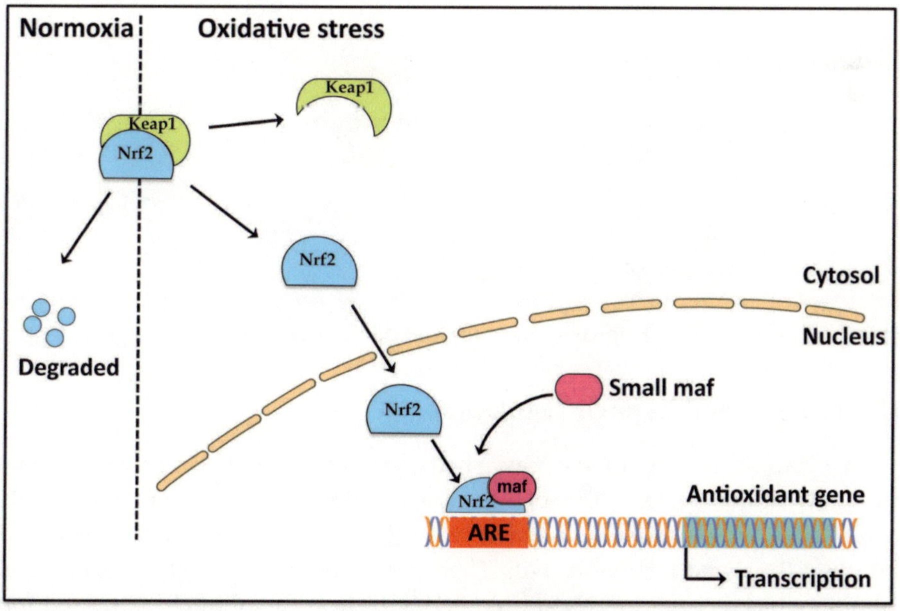

Figure 3. Antioxidant gene expression via the ARE/Nrf2 pathway.

3. The HIF-1 signaling pathway

Hypoxia-inducible factor-1 (HIF-1) is an important transcription factor that regulates the expression of several vital genes in response to oxygen deficient conditions [3]. These include genes encoding metabolic enzymes to allow growth under hypoxia and proteins that assist hypoxic tissues to re-establish oxygen supply. Of particular relevance to tumors, HIF-1 induces the expression of vascular endothelial growth factor (VEGF), which is required for angiogenesis. HIF-1 transcription factor is a complex of two subunits: aryl hydrocarbon receptor nuclear translocator (ARNT), also known as HIF-1β, which is constitutively expressed in all cells, and HIF-α, which is stabilised under hypoxia. Normally, HIF-α is synthesized and continuously degraded in the cytosol, but in response to a low oxygen environment it starts accumulating rapidly [39]. HIF-α is then translocated into the nucleus, where it dimerises with HIF-1β to form the HIF-1 complex, which then binds to the hypoxia responsive element (HRE) in the promoters of target genes to activate their expression [3] (Figure 4).

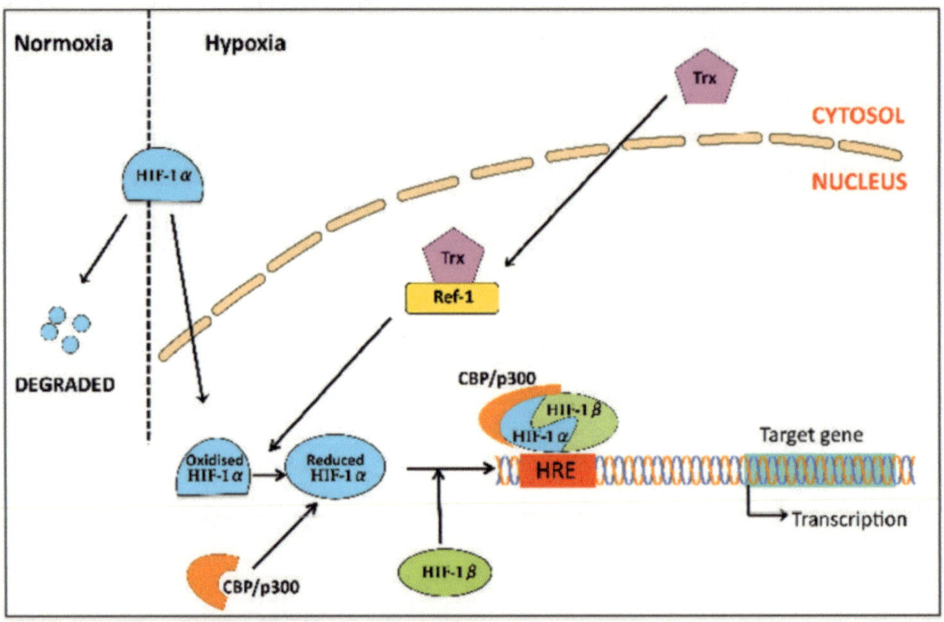

Figure 4. Regulation of the HIF-1 signaling pathway and the expression of its target genes.

3.1. HIF-1 proteins and hypoxic regulation

Both HIF-1 subunits belong to the basic helix-loop-helix (bHLH)/Per-ARNT-Sim (PAS) family of transcription factors. The bHLH domain aids in DNA-binding while the PAS domain mediates protein-protein interaction. Both domains also act as an interface for dimerisation of the α and β subunits [40]. There are three identified HIF-α subunits [3] and one β subunit, which is alternatively spliced [41]. HIF-1α is the most characterised form and will be discussed in this chapter. HIF-1α and HIF-2α have structurally similar DNA binding and dimerisation domains, but they differ in their transactivation domains. This may explain why a genome wide screen detected both HIF-1α and HIF-2α bound to the same HRE consensus sites, but without initiating the same transcriptional response [42]. Moreover, HIF-2α is only expressed in certain tissues [43], while HIF-1α is ubiquitously expressed. Overall their biological actions in response to hypoxia are distinct, as reviewed by Loboda and colleagues [44]. For example, HIF-1α, but not HIF-2α regulates the transcription of genes encoding enzymes involved in glycolysis [45], while HIF-2α has been associated with adaptation to high altitude exposure [46]. Furthermore, Bracken and co-workers showed in PC12 rat cells that HIF-1α required a shorter duration (4h) under hypoxia to be stabilized, whereas a longer hypoxic exposure (16h) was required for HIF-2α stabilization. However, this difference was cell-line specific [47]. In human colon cancer, advanced tumors displayed strong HIF-1α staining and weak HIF-2α staining, while in early stage tumors, strong HIF-2α and weak HIF-1α staining was observed. This implies that HIF-1α and HIF-2α have different roles in colon cancer [48]. In contrast, HIF-3α has inhibitory function since it lacks the transactivation domain, but binds to HIF-1α and prevents it from activating transcription. Therefore, HIF-3α is also called 'inhibitory PAS domain' (IPAS) and arises as an alternatively spliced product of the HIF-1α gene [49].

There are two transactivation domains in HIF-1α: the amino-terminal transactivation domain (NAD) and the carboxy-terminal transactivation domain (CAD) [50, 51]. These domains are involved in the transcriptional activation of HIF-1α under hypoxia. The NAD overlaps the oxygen-dependent degradation domain (ODD), linking the transcriptional activity of HIF-1 with the stabilisation of the protein [50]. On the other hand, the transcriptional activity of the CAD is associated with the binding of transcriptional co-activators, including CREB-binding protein (CBP)/p300 [52]. The recruitment of the co-activators is redox-regulated and requires Ref-1, which reduces the cysteine residue at position 800 of HIF-1α within the CAD region [53]. The co-activators are then able to bind HIF-1 and subsequently initiate transcription. It should be noted that Ref-1 is an intermediate protein that is regulated by thioredoxin.

3.2. Regulation of HIF-1 under normoxia

Although the HIF-1α proteins are activated in response to hypoxia, they do not sense the changes in the oxygen environment themselves. Sensors to such changes have been identified as oxygen-dependent hydroxylases. The hydroxylases responsible for modifying HIF-1α are the 'prolyl hydroxylase domain-containing proteins' (PHDs) and an asparaginyl hydroxylase called 'Factor Inhibiting HIF-1' (FIH-1) [54]. These hydroxylases continuously modify HIF-1α in presence of oxygen. When there is a negative change in oxygen availability, PHDs and FIH-1 can no longer hydroxylate HIF-1α, which is stabilised and translocated to the nucleus [55] (Figure 5).

Under higher oxygen conditions, PHDs modify distinct proline residues (Pro 402 and Pro 564) in the ODD domain of HIF-1α [56], leading to the recruitment of von Hippel-Lindau (VHL) proteins [57] and subsequent degradation of HIF-1α [58]. The PHD family has three members: PHD1, PHD2 and PHD3, with PHD2 being the most abundant and highly active towards HIF-1α [59]. PHDs require only a short stretch of HIF-1α amino acids (as short as 20 residues) for the selective recognition of proline hydroxylation sites and subsequent VHL-binding. These sites reside within an LXXLAP motif, which is highly conserved between the HIF-α isoforms as well as across species [58]. The hydroxylation enables the VHL protein to bind HIF-1α, which initiates degradation via the ubiquitination pathway [58, 60]. VHL-deficient cells have the HIF-1α subunit constitutively stabilised and thus, HIF-1 is constantly activated in these cells [57].

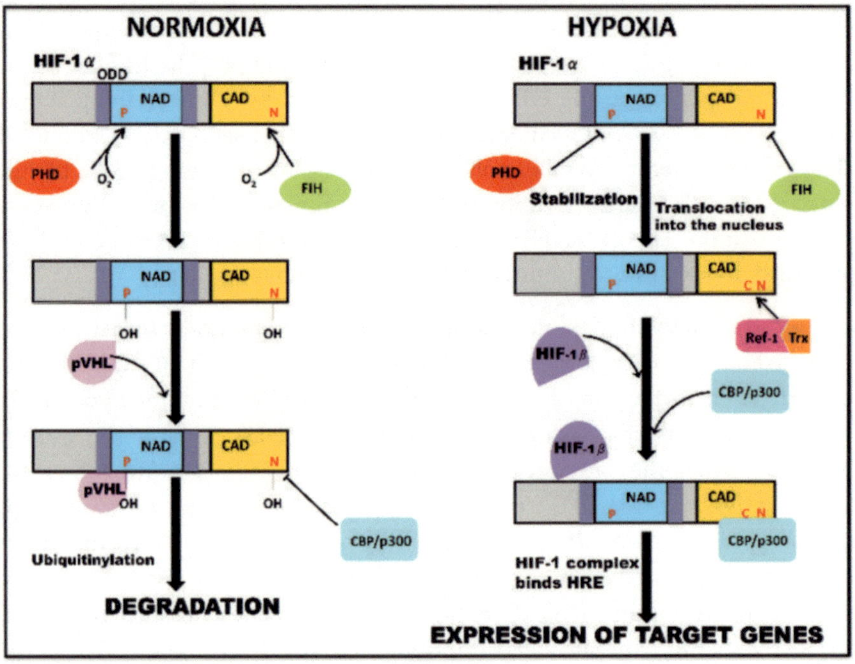

Figure 5. Regulation of HIF-1α during normoxia and hypoxia.

An additional hydroxylation event in the CAD domain ensures that any HIF-1α that escapes degradation is rendered inactive. This process involves the hydroxylation of an asparagine residue instead of a proline and suppresses the recruitment of CBP/p300 co-activators [54]. This asparaginyl hydroxylase is the FIH-1, and uses both HIF-1α and HIF-2α as substrates. In HIF-1α, FIH-1 hydroxylates an asparagine residue at position 803. FIH-1 is an Fe(II)-dependent enzyme and plays the role of a second oxygen sensor within the hypoxic response pathway [61].

Thus, under normoxia, prolyl and asparaginyl hydroxylases prevent the activation of HIF-1α by acting on the NAD and CAD domains respectively. However, when oxygen levels decrease, these hydroxylases become inactive, HIF-1α proteins are stabilised and translocated to the nucleus where they dimerise with HIF-1β. The reduction of a key cysteine residue in the CAD by Ref-1, through the action of thioredoxin, results in the recruitment of transcriptional co-activators and subsequent expression of the target genes.

3.3. Regulation of the HIF-1 system by ROS

While HIF-1 is stabilised and active under conditions of low oxygen, paradoxically ROS can also stabilise HIF-1. Under normoxia, the addition of H_2O_2 caused HIF-1α stabilisation and enhanced expression from HRE-reporter constructs [62]. In addition, Hep3B ρ^0 cells, which do not have mitochondrial electron transport function, can exhibit HRE-luciferase reporter activity under normoxia upon addition of H_2O_2 [62]. The molecular basis for ROS stabilising HIF-1 was shown by exposing murine breast tumor cells to nitric oxide (NO). Addition of NO caused nitrosylation of a specific cysteine residue in the ODD domain of HIF-1α under normoxia. The VHL protein was therefore unable to bind to HIF-1α, thereby preventing its degradation [63]. This represents a control mechanism that bypasses the function of the PHD enzymes under normoxia, since the nitrosylation did not prevent or change the level of proline hydroxylation detected in the NAD domain.

ROS is also believed to play a role in the HIF-1 signaling pathway during hypoxia. Cells with non-functional mitochondria, and therefore, reduced ROS levels, were unable to stabilise HIF-1α in response to hypoxia [62, 64]. When H_2O_2 was inhibited by catalase over-expression in human 293 cells under hypoxia, there was reduced HRE-luciferase reporter activity, suggesting lower HIF-1α activity, which was restored by the addition of H_2O_2 [62]. These observations suggest that the presence of H_2O_2 in the cytosol is necessary for HIF-1α stabilisation under hypoxia. One possible role of ROS may be to inhibit the PHD enzymes. Addition of 10 μM H_2O_2 showed more than 50% inhibition of PHD enzyme function *in vitro* but did not increase HIF-1α transcriptional activity in Hep3B cells [65]. This is implies that HIF-1α activation by ROS can occur through multiple pathways including both stabilisation and recruitment of co-activators.

While ROS appears to exert some regulatory function on HIF-1, there is still debate as to whether ROS levels are increased [62, 66, 67] or decreased [68-70] during hypoxia. Contradictory results may occur due to differences in cell type, mode of generating hypoxia, oxygen levels and assays used to measure ROS. Work from our laboratory demonstrated that MDA-MB-231 breast cancer cells grown under hypoxia have reduced ROS levels [68]. However, we found that how the cells were processed was extremely important. If cells were processed under normoxic conditions following the hypoxic growth then increased ROS levels were observed. When cells were maintained under hypoxia throughout the processing steps, then a decrease was evident [68]. This indicates that cells grown in hypoxia must be maintained in hypoxia during processing to avoid introduction of an inadvertent reoxygenation step (however brief), thus, mimicking the intermittent hypoxia observed in tumors.

3.4. Redox regulation of the HIF-1 system

The activity of the HIF-1 system is regulated by the thioredoxin redox system, via Ref-1. Thioredoxin provides the reducing potential for Ref-1 to reduce a cysteine residue in the CAD domain of HIF-1α that enhances the ability of HIF-1 to recruit co-activators [53].

Consequently, cell lines engineered to over-express thioredoxin also displayed increased HIF-1α levels, enhanced HIF-1 DNA binding and increased activation of HIF-1 regulated gene promoters. This results in increased levels of hypoxia regulated proteins such as VEGF [71, 72] and cyclooxygenase-2 (COX-2) [73]. In contrast, when cells were transfected with the dominant negative redox inactive thioredoxin protein, VEGF and COX-2 levels were decreased. Other small molecule inhibitors of the thioredoxin system, such as quinols, also led to down regulation of HIF-1 activity [72] and subsequently to a decrease in VEGF and inducible nitric oxide synthase (iNOS) expression in MCF-7 breast cancer cells [74].

A recent study showed that thioredoxin reductase levels were decreased during hypoxia and as a consequence higher ROS levels were observed [75]. They concluded that hypoxia does not increase mitochondrial ROS production, but that lower thioredoxin reductase levels are responsible for higher ROS levels. Since HIF-1 is also regulated by ROS, this study demonstrated that the thioredoxin redox system could modulate HIF-1 signalling by indirectly affecting ROS levels, in addition to the direct interaction described above.

4. Redox and hypoxic systems: the intermittent hypoxia link

The tumor environment is in flux between hypoxia and reoxygenation. Hypoxia induces the formation of new blood vessels, which are often poorly formed, causing an inconsistent oxygen supply [7]. Therefore, cells can experience a cycling between hypoxia and reoxygenation. Hypoxic pathways are induced during periods of low oxygen while the reoxygenation results in induction of antioxidant proteins, including the redox enzymes. Thus, the interplay between the two systems is important to study in tumors. Interestingly, the cycling between hypoxia and reoxygenation enhances HIF-1 activity. Many of the studies undertaken to assess the role of HIF-1 and redox signaling in cancer are performed using cancer cell lines. Therefore, each cancer cell line should be evaluated for its suitability as a model system for intermittent hypoxia.

4.1. Use of an *in vitro* model system for intermittent hypoxia

The MDA-MB-231 breast cancer cell line is often used as an *in vitro* model system for metastatic cancer. However, most researchers grow these cells under what is usually regarded as normoxia, that is 20% oxygen, despite this not being physiologically relevant. We wanted to assess the suitability of this cell line for hypoxic cycling studies. Our first aim was to determine the most appropriate level of oxygen to use to ensure a strong hypoxic response is generated. We assayed the lactate dehydrogenase (LDH) activity present in MDA-MB-231 cells grown in either 1% oxygen or 0.1% oxygen. LDH is a glycolytic enzyme, which is upregulated in response to hypoxia through the binding of HIF-1 to an HRE element in its gene's promoter [76]. Cells were cultured in 5% CO_2 with either 1% oxygen or 0.1% oxygen for 24 hours in a hypoxic C-chamber (Biospherix, New York, USA), and then lysed within a C-shuttle glovebox (Biospherix) using a buffer comprised of 150 mM NaCl, 50 mM Tris-HCl pH 8.0, 0.5 % (v/v) Nonidet P-40, 0.5 mM EDTA, 2 mM PMSF, 1 μl/ml proteinase inhibitor cocktail VI (AG-Scientific, California, USA). Protein estimation was performed using the DC protein assay kit (BioRad, NSW, Australia) and equal amounts of cell lysate were used to measure LDH activity. The assay buffer contained 50 mM Tris-HCl pH 7.5, 1 mg/ml NADH, 1 mg/ml pyruvate and the LDH activity was measured at 340 nm using a Spectromax Plate reader. The results are presented in Figure 6. The data is expressed as a change in percentage of LDH activity relative to normoxic treated cells, with normoxia represented as 100%. While cells grown at both 1% and 0.1% oxygen levels showed an increase in LDH activity, only cells grown in 0.1% oxygen had a statistical significance compared to cells grown under normoxia.

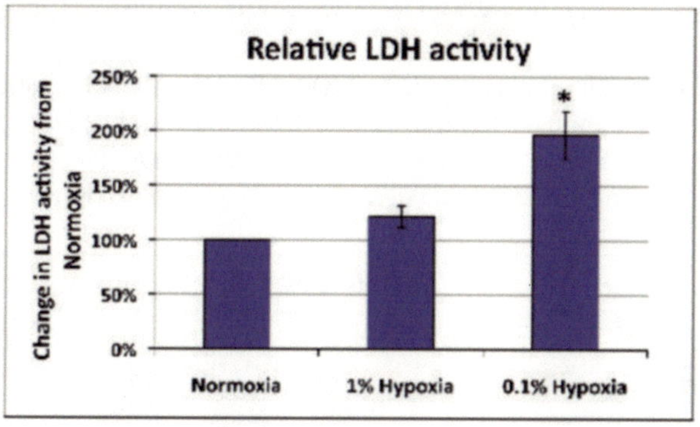

Figure 6. Relative LDH activities in MDA-MB-231 cells after 24 hours of 1% O_2 or 0.1 % O_2 growth. Normoxia and 0.1% hypoxia treated cells showed significant difference using a one-way ANOVA employing Tukey's Post-Hoc test, as indicated by * ($p < 0.05$). Data presented as mean ± SEM from three independent experiments conducted in triplicate.

We then wanted to assess the morphology and viability of the MDA-MB-231 cells grown under various oxygen growth conditions. We selected 0.1% oxygen as the hypoxic condition to culture these cells in, to ensure a strong hypoxic response. The MDA-MB-231 cells were grown under prolonged hypoxia (16 hours) followed by different lengths of reoxygenation by transferring cells to 20% oxygen (referred to as normoxia). To assess the effect of cycling hypoxia, cells were also subjected to 4 pre-conditioning (PC) cycles (comprising 10 minutes hypoxia and 20 minutes reoxygenation) prior to the hypoxic growth phase. These different conditions are illustrated in Figure 7. The cycling between hypoxia and normoxia was repeated four times within a 2 hour period before cells were transferred into prolonged hypoxia for 16 hours. Since 20% oxygen is much higher than 0.1% oxygen switching to normoxia results in a reoxygenation step. After cells were grown in 0.1% hypoxia for 16 hours they were either processed using the hypoxic C-Shuttle glovebox to maintain hypoxic conditions or re-oxygenated by being transferred to normoxic conditions for 2, 4 or 6 hours. These cells were processed under normoxia.

To confirm that cells were viable under these oxygen growth conditions, a fluorescence activated cell sorting (FACS) based assay was used. Cells were harvested and detached using cell dissociation buffer (Life Technologies), washed in phosphate buffered saline (PBS) pH 7.4, and then resuspended at a concentration of 1×10^6 cells/ml containing an appropriate dilution of 7-aminoactinomycin D. The cells were then stored on ice until they were

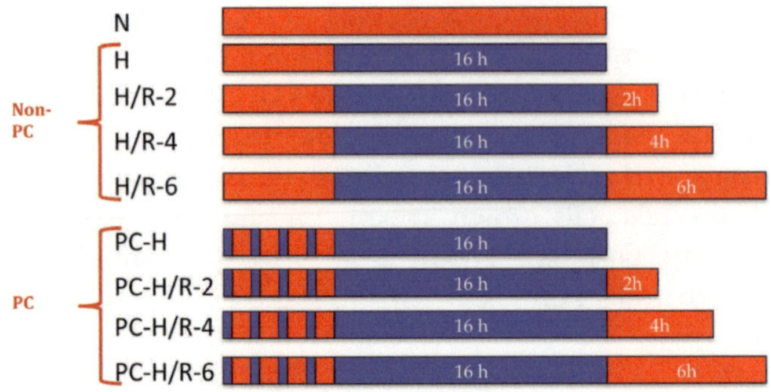

Figure 7. Oxygen growth conditions used to grow MDA-MB-231 cells. Schematic representation outlining the different combinations of hypoxia and reoxygenation and their respective length of exposure used to grow MDA-MB-231 cells. Red indicates growth under 20% oxygen. Blue indicates growth in 0.1% oxygen. N: normoxia (20% oxygen); R: reoxygenation; H: hypoxia; PC: pre-conditioning.

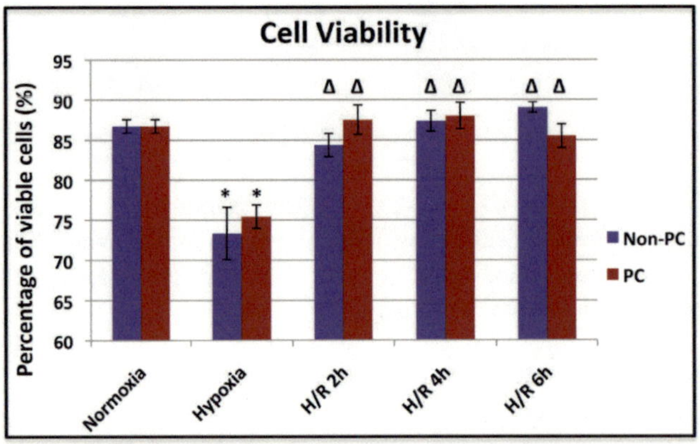

Figure 8. Viability of MDA-MB-231 cells in response to different oxygen growth conditions. Non-PC treated samples and PC treated samples were analysed separately using a one-way ANOVA employing Tukey's Post-Hoc test. A statistical difference was observed compared to normoxia, as indicated by * ($P < 0.01$). A statistical difference was observed for all reoxygenation samples compared to hypoxic cells, as indicated by Δ ($p < 0.01$). Data is presented as mean ± SEM from at least two independent experiments.

analysed for viability using the BD FACSAria flow cytometer (BD Biosciences). The results are shown in Figure 8. Upon growth in hypoxia cellular viability decreases, while after reoxygenation cell viability returns to levels consistent with those of cells grown in normoxia. A decrease in cell viability following hypoxic growth has also been observed by other researchers using different cell lines [77, 78].

The morphology of the cells grown in each oxygen growth condition was assessed by microscopy. Cells were also grown in media containing 100μM H_2O_2 for 30 minutes as a control for oxidative stressed cells. After exposing MDA-MB-231 cells to different oxygen growth conditions, cell morphology was examined under an Olympus CK30 microscope (Olympus Co., Japan) at 100X magnification. Experiments were performed multiple times with representative images shown in Figure 9. Cells exposed to 100μM H_2O_2 for 30 minutes

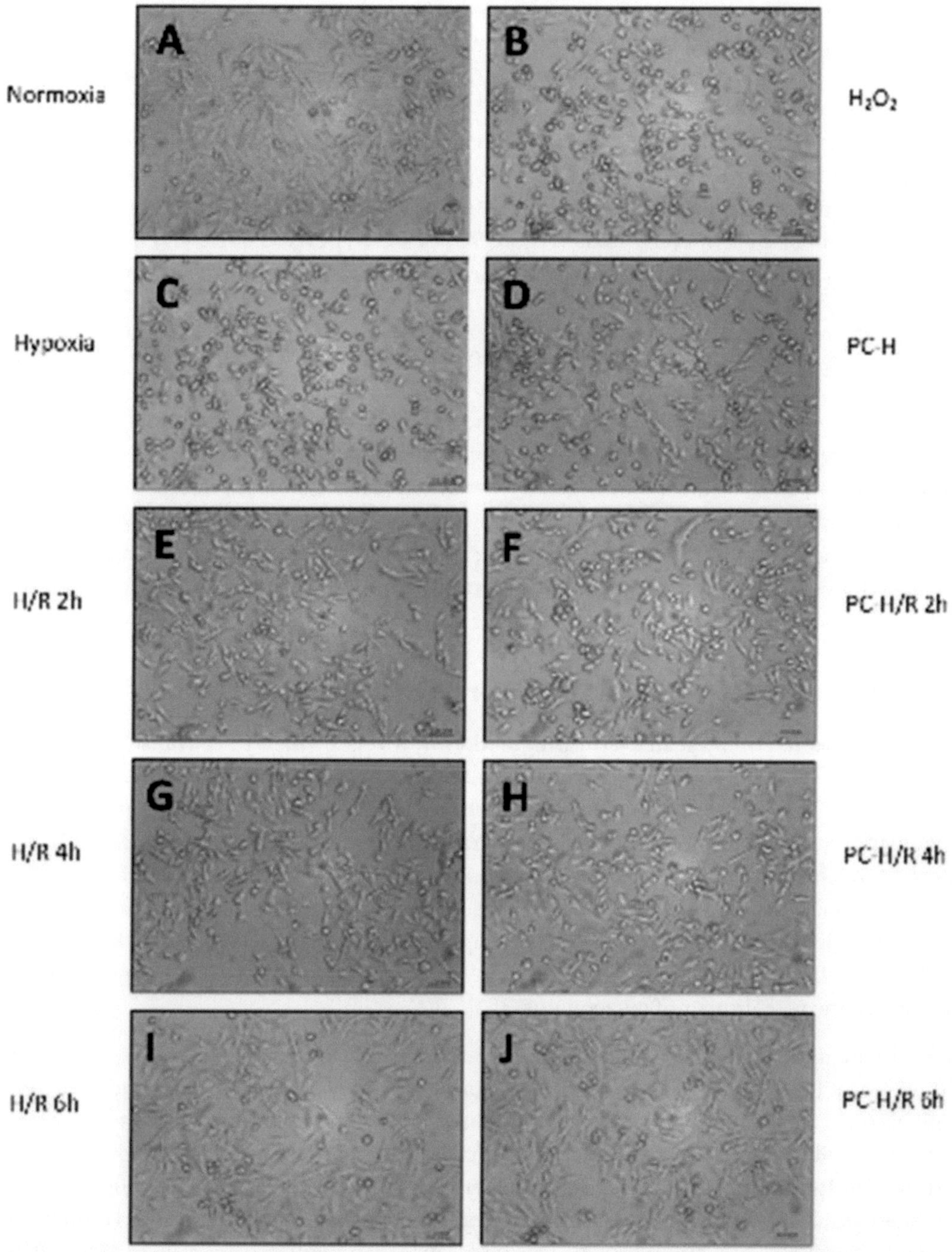

Figure 9. Morphology of MDA-MB-231 cells after different oxygen growth treatments. A): Normoxia treated cells, B): 100μM H_2O_2 treated cells, C): 0.1% hypoxia treated cells, D): PC-H treated cells, E): H/R 2h treated cells, F): PC-H/R 2h treated cells, G): H/R 4h treated cells, H): PC-H/R 4h treated cells, I): H/R 6h treated cells, J): PC-H/R 6h treated cells. Images were taken using an Olympus CK30 microscope at 100X magnification. Scale bar = 0.05mm.

(Figure 9B) exhibited altered cell morphology compared to normoxia treated cells (Figure 9A). These cells appeared to be less elongated and more rounded in shape. The cells exposed to hypoxia (Figure 9C) or PC-hypoxia (Figure 9D) showed a similar morphology to H_2O_2 treated cells. When hypoxia or PC-hypoxia treated cells were exposed to a longer period of reoxygenation (Figure 9I and J) their morphology becomes very similar to that of the normoxia treated cells. This trend suggests that the cells become stressed when exposed to hypoxia but recover during the reoxygenation phase. No difference was observed in overall morphology between hypoxia (Figure 9C) or PC-hypoxia (Figure 9D) treated cells or their respective reoxygenation exposures (Figure 9E, G and I compared to Figure 9F, H and J, respectively).

Since various methodologies are used to generate hypoxia it is important to establish the appropriate conditions for each cell line. MDA-MB-231 cells grown at 0.1% oxygen elicited a hypoxic response, whereas 1% oxygen did not induce a significant hypoxic response. A decrease in cellular viability in response to hypoxia was observed compared to normoxia, but returned to normal levels during reoxygenation. Cells also exhibited a more rounded morphology during hypoxia, consistent with a stress response. The recovery of the cells during reoxygenation suggests that signaling pathways are involved that enable cells to adapt to these changing oxygen conditions, with the most likely candidates being the HIF-1 and redox-dependent pathways.

4.2. Expression of the HIF-1 system under intermittent hypoxia

Several studies have implicated an upregulation in levels of the HIF-1 transcription factor under intermittent hypoxia. This increase supersedes the HIF-1 levels found in acute hypoxia [79, 80]. Yuan and co-workers found this to be Ca^{+2} dependent [80]. They demonstrated the involvement of calcium-calmodium dependent kinase II (CaMK II) under intermittent hypoxia. CaMK II phosphorylates p300, a co-activator required for the transcriptional activity of HIF-1, thereby increasing the HIF-1 transactivation [80]. In contrast, under acute hypoxia, HIF-1 transcriptional activity is increased as a result of a decrease in the O_2 dependent asparaginyl hydroxylation in the CAD region of HIF-1α, assisting in the recruitment of co-activators [54].

Intermittent hypoxia has been linked to increased tumor invasion and resistance against radiotherapy [81, 82] and to enhanced metastasis in rodent lungs [83]. Liu and colleagues demonstrated that intermittent hypoxia treated H446 lung cancer cells had a greater metastatic ability and radio-resistance. They found HIF-1α was involved in both processes [84]. Intermittent hypoxia exposed endothelial cells also showed enhanced migration and exhibited an increased resistance against irradiation as compared to their counterparts grown in normoxia or acute hypoxia. This effect was also mediated by HIF-1α since siRNA targeting HIF-1α abolished the radiation resistance [82]. Therefore, HIF-1α may be expected to have a role in tumor invasion observed under intermittent hypoxia.

Differences in expression of HIF-1α and HIF-2α under acute and intermittent hypoxia have been shown in sleep-disordered breathing. While intermittent hypoxia caused an upregulation in HIF-1α levels, the HIF-2α levels were down-regulated in intermittent hypoxia treated rat PC12 cells and also in *in vivo* rat models. In contrast, acute hypoxia upregulated both HIF-1α and HIF-2α [85]. It was proposed that down-regulation of HIF-2α contributes to oxidative stress, at least in part via transcriptional down-regulation of a HIF-2 target gene, an antioxidant called superoxide dismutase (SOD). Intermittent hypoxia also increased ROS by decreasing the mitochondrial complex I activity. The increase in ROS levels was linked to the upregulated HIF-1α levels under intermittent hypoxia [86]. Therefore, the differential regulation of HIF-1α and HIF-2α is believed to cause oxidative stress resulting from an imbalance between ROS and antioxidants [85]. Similar mechanisms may contribute to higher levels of ROS in cancer cells. However, as antioxidants are proteins that scavenge ROS, one may expect that antioxidant levels would be augmented in such a scenario. Interestingly, a number of studies implicate an upregulation of antioxidants in cancer cells cultured under intermittent hypoxia.

4.3. Expression of redox enzymes under hypoxia and intermittent hypoxia

Since intermittent hypoxia involves phases of reoxygenation, it is reasonable to expect that redox enzymes would be induced during these reoxygenation phases. The expression of thioredoxin during the hypoxic phase has been less clear. In hypoxic regions of tumors, thioredoxin expression has been reported as high [87], but intermittent hypoxia may contribute to this high expression. In cells cultured *in vitro* there has been conflicting reports regarding thioredoxin expression levels under hypoxia.

Thioredoxin protein levels were increased in A549 human lung cancer cells during growth in 0.05% oxygen [88] and in both human endothelial progenitor cells and human umbilical vein endothelial cells cultured in 1% oxygen [78], as assessed by Western blotting. Our work [68] showed a visible increase (by Western blotting) in thioredoxin levels in MDA-MB-231 cells cultured in 0.1% hypoxia, but this increase was not statistically significant. In addition, neither thioredoxin nor thioredoxin reductase promoter activity was increased under hypoxia [68]. Ref-1 protein levels were also not increased [68] while other studies reported that peroxiredoxin protein levels were not increased in A549 cells cultured in hypoxia [89]. A recent study showed a decrease in thioredoxin reductase protein levels under hypoxia [75]. Previously, it was reported that thioredoxin reductase was increased in human endothelial progenitor cells but not in human umbilical vein endothelial cells under hypoxia [78]. This conflicting data suggests that as with the variable ROS levels reported under hypoxia, expression of the thioredoxin system under hypoxia may depend on the specific cell line, oxygen levels or how samples are processed. For example, Jewell and co-workers observed that thioredoxin levels in the nucleus were increased after as little as 30 seconds of oxygen exposure following hypoxic growth [90]. Thus, in some reported cases, cells may have received an inadvertent reoxygenation stimulus during processing of cells after hypoxic growth, which was sufficient to induce antioxidant gene expression.

Since reoxygenation stimulates the production of ROS, one might expect that high levels of thioredoxin would be detected in cells reoxygenated after hypoxia. However, this appears not to be the case. In our studies [68] MDA-MB-231 cells cultured in 0.1% oxygen followed by reoxygenation had increased thioredoxin levels as assessed visually on Western blots, but this was statistically non-significant when quantitated by densitometry. In addition, after 6 hours of reoxygenation, the levels were visually decreasing. This correlates with other studies that reported a visible decrease in thioredoxin protein levels in A549 cells grown in 0.2% oxygen followed by 6 hours or more of reoxygenation [91]. Their work showed that thioredoxin was oxidised during the reoxygenation phase [91], probably by the increased ROS levels [68]. After 6 hours of reoxygenation, ROS levels start to decrease and it is possible that the cells no longer require thioredoxin. No change in Ref-1 was observed during reoxygenation [68], but peroxiredoxin 1 expression was increased [89].

When conditions mimicking intermittent hypoxia are utilized, the involvement of thioredoxin is quite apparent. Malec and co-workers utilized several different schemes to grow A549 cells alternating between hypoxia and reoxygenation [92]. While a maximum of three 2-hour cycles were used for either hypoxia or reoxygenation, the schemes with the greatest number of cycles of hypoxia and reoxygenation resulted in the highest thioredoxin levels. Nrf2 was also increased under these conditions and may be responsible for the increased thioredoxin expression [92]. Our work [68] used a scheme that mimicked an ischemia/reperfusion study performed in the heart [93]. In that study, 4 short cycles of ischemia and reperfusion (of 10 and 20 minutes respectively) prior to longer-term growth in ischemia and subsequent reperfusion led to very high levels of thioredoxin. These pre-conditioning conditions also provided the heart protection from damage otherwise caused by the longer-term ischemia and reperfusion. We applied these oxygen growth conditions (Figure 7) to cancer cells and also detected high levels of thioredoxin in cells pre-conditioned with short cycles of hypoxia and reoxygenation followed by a longer exposure to hypoxia and reoxygenation [68]. Maximum thioredoxin protein levels were obtained after 4 hours of reoxygenation, which was confirmed to be statistically significant. These short cycles may also represent what happens in tumors due to red blood cell flux [7] and may provide the tumor with protection against subsequent oxidative insult. Without the pre-conditioning cycling, thioredoxin levels were not increased by as much during reoxygenation, indicating that the cycling may provide an advantage to the cells. Of interest is that Ref-1 levels were also higher in MDA-MB-231 cells subjected to the pre-conditioning, but not in cells grown without this step [68]. Since Ref-1 and thioredoxin regulate HIF-1 activity, the short pulses of hypoxia may be responsible for their induction. We found that the promoter activity of both thioredoxin and thioredoxin reductase were dependent on Nrf2 in the reoxygenation phase, and that cells cultured with the pre-conditioning cycles did not exhibit higher promoter activity [68]. Therefore, the mechanism for inducing higher thioredoxin protein levels in cells subjected to cycling may not be at the transcriptional level.

4.4. The Interaction of redox and hypoxic pathways under intermittent hypoxia

Cancer cells can reside in conditions of hypoxic as well as oxidative stress. HIF-1 and Nrf2 are two important transcription factors that play a crucial role in each of these conditions. While HIF-1 is important for cell survival under low oxygen conditions, Nrf2 provides cytoprotection against oxidative stress by upregulating antioxidants such as thioredoxin. Both HIF-1 and Nrf2 are induced in cells under intermittent hypoxia. This presents a possible link between the oxygen- and redox-dependent regulatory pathways. As described in 4.2, the increase in HIF-1 levels under intermittent hypoxia supersedes the HIF-1 levels observed in acute hypoxia. Similarly, higher thioredoxin levels were observed under intermittent hypoxia in comparison to acute hypoxia [68, 92]. Higher levels of other antioxidants have also been observed under intermittent hypoxia. For example, Prx1 was upregulated in response to hypoxia/reoxygenation, through the action of Nrf2, which binds to the ARE in the Prx1 promoter. In cells lacking Nrf2, Prx1 expression was compromised [89]. ROS levels are also higher under intermittent hypoxia [68] and are involved in both HIF-1 regulation and induction of antioxidant expression through the action of Nrf2. This may induce higher thioredoxin levels, which in turn results in the higher HIF-1 levels observed under intermittent hypoxia.

The high levels of both thioredoxin and HIF-1 in cancer cells cultured under intermittent hypoxia also have implications for tumor metastasis [79, 92]. Thioredoxin enhances the invasive behavior of tumor cells by regulating MMP activity, which is required for ECM degradation [25, 26]. HIF-1 over-expression during hypoxia has also been associated with ECM degradation by upregulating MMP-2 [94] and MMP-9 gene expression [95]. In a separate study, intermittent hypoxia treated A549 and H446 lung cancer cells exhibited increased invasion in comparison to normoxic cells. Down-regulation of the HIF-1α gene decreased the cellular migration in these cells, thereby linking HIF-1 to cancer cell invasion under intermittent hypoxia [84]. Moreover, both thioredoxin and HIF-1 have been linked to the development of resistance against anticancer therapeutics [82, 96, 97]. These common outcomes suggest an interplay of redox and hypoxic systems under intermittent hypoxia, with possible consequences for the design and testing of therapeutics.

5. Consequences for drug development

Development of resistance in cancer cells against chemotherapies presents a major setback in the prevention and cure of the disease that kills millions of people every year. Many chemotherapeutics are based on heavy metals, such as gold and platinum that generate ROS in cells, causing damage to DNA, proteins and lipids, and ultimately leading to apoptosis [98]. However, cells upregulate their antioxidant defenses in order to scavenge ROS, and as a result cancer cells become resistant to these drugs. High levels of thioredoxin and other antioxidant proteins in tumors are correlated with resistance to various chemotherapeutic agents, including cisplatin [97], docetaxel [96] and tamoxifen [99]. Furthermore, breast tumors with high levels of thioredoxin and other antioxidants prior to treatment with docetaxel were correlated with a high likelihood of developing resistance during therapy [100]. Therefore, anti-cancer therapies could be designed to inhibit the thioredoxin system in combination with radiation or chemotherapy.

Radiation treatment has been shown to cause reoxygenation of hypoxic tumors by increasing perfusion. As the better oxygenated cells die due to irradiation, the oxygen consumption decreases [101]. This has been linked with accumulation of ROS. Moeller and colleagues observed an elevation in levels of HIF-1 regulated proteins after 72 hours of radiation exposure [102]. Inhibition of ROS by a SOD mimetic prevented the stabilisation of HIF-1α and sensitized the tumor to the damage caused by radiation [103]. In a separate study, they observed a delay in tumor growth following radiation when HIF-1 was inhibited using an antisense knockdown technique [104]. HIF-1β null tumor lines were also found to be sensitive to radiotherapy as they prevent the HIF-1 response [105]. All these studies suggest that radiation treatment causes an increase in ROS levels that stabilise HIF-1α and leads to the subsequent increase in levels of HIF-1 mediated proteins.

The formation of stress granules has been observed in hypoxic tumors, which were found to disaggregate upon radiation exposure [102]. Stress granules contain mRNA transcripts and are formed in cells under stress. To save energy during stress, these transcripts are not translated into proteins [106]. Upon reoxygenation of hypoxic cells (during irradiation), the HIF-1 regulated transcripts are released and are translated, leading to an increase in VEGF and erythropoietin levels. This promotes angiogenesis, cell survival and proliferation, ultimately making the cells resistant to radiotherapy [102].

Cancer cells are often resistant not only to a single drug but develop cross-resistance against a range of drugs. Multidrug resistance (MDR) in cancer cells induces resistance against the efficacy of structurally and mechanistically different anticancer drugs, significantly decreasing their effectiveness. Higher drug doses in MDR cells not only produce toxic effects but also further stimulate the resistance, making tumors hard to treat [107]. MDR may arise due to alterations in targets, evasion of apoptosis, alteration in drug-uptake and transport of drugs out of cells [108]. The efflux of drugs from cells is mediated by transmembrane transporters belonging to the ATP-binding cassette (ABC) protein superfamily. These proteins use ATP to transport drugs out of cells [109]. One highly studied ABC transporter protein is P-glycoprotein (Pgp) (an MDR1 gene product) that has been linked to MDR in cancer cells [110]. High levels of Pgp are found in MDR cells and coincide with higher expression of HIF-1 [111-113]. Doublier and co-workers found MCF7 breast cancer cells grown under hypoxia to be resistant to doxorubicin. This resistance was associated with an increased Pgp expression via increased HIF-1 activation since transfection with siRNA specific to HIF-1 abolished this increase. They also observed that the binding of HIF-1 to the MDR1 gene promoter was higher in hypoxic cells. These cells accumulated lower levels of doxorubicin compared to normoxic cells [112]. Therefore, these roles of HIF-1 should be assessed during optimization of treatment strategies.

6. Conclusion

The oxygenation state of the cells has immense importance in cancer biology and both oxygen- and redox-dependent regulatory pathways are crucial for the process of carcinogenesis. While HIF-1 is important for tumor cells to adapt to hypoxia, thioredoxin protects cells from damage due to high oxygen levels. Since cancer cells have the ability to survive under conditions of both hypoxic and oxidative stress, one may expect a cross talk between the oxygen- and redox-dependent systems in tumors. This idea is further potentiated by the role of ROS in regulating the HIF-1 activity under both normoxia and hypoxia, and in inducing the thioredoxin system under oxidative stress.

The *in vivo* tumor environment is dynamic and cycles between low and high oxygen conditions. Surprisingly, these conditions are not taken into account while designing anticancer drugs. Most anticancer drugs are evaluated under normoxia (20% oxygen), which is not physiologically relevant and does not reflect the actual *in vivo* tumor environment. Therefore, drugs tested under normoxic laboratory conditions may not respond similarly in the patient's body. Hence, it is important to evaluate the effectiveness of various chemotherapeutics under a wide range of oxygen conditions, particularly under intermittent hypoxia. Furthermore, both HIF-1 and thioredoxin levels are higher in cells grown under intermittent hypoxia. The higher levels of both these proteins have also been linked to enhanced invasion and resistance to treatment in cancer cells (Figure 10).

Therefore, the pathological implications of an upregulation of these important systems in cancer demonstrate the vital need to increase our understanding of the molecular mechanisms involved in the hypoxic and reoxygenation conditions encountered by the cancer cells *in vivo,* in order to design and test more effective therapeutics.

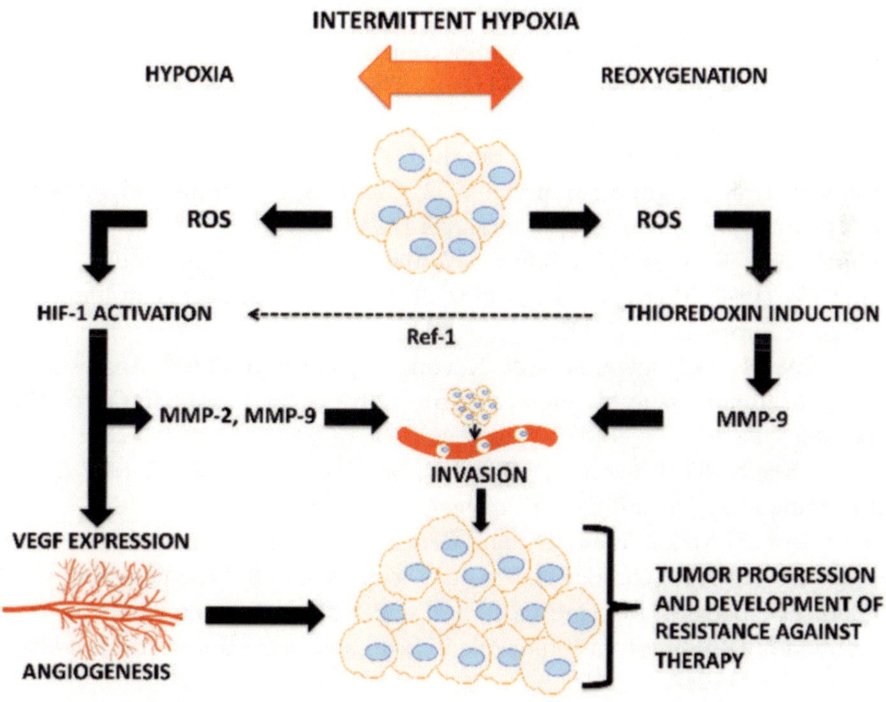

Figure 10. Overview of Trx and HIF-1 interaction under intermittent hypoxia and consequences for cancer progression.

Author details

Maneet Bhatia, Therese C. Karlenius and Kathryn F. Tonissen*
School of Biomolecular and Physical Sciences, Griffith University, Nathan, Qld, Australia
Eskitis Institute for Cell and Molecular Therapies, Griffith University, Nathan, Qld, Australia

Giovanna Di Trapani
School of Biomolecular and Physical Sciences, Griffith University, Nathan, Qld, Australia

Acknowledgement

This research was supported by Griffith University Postgraduate Research Scholarships (to M.B. and T.K.), a Griffith University International Postgraduate Research Scholarship (to M.B.) and an Endeavour International Postgraduate Research Scholarship (to T.K.).

7. References

[1] Roy S, Khanna S, Bickerstaff AA, Subramanian SV, Atalay M, Bierl M, Pendyala S, Levy D, Sharma N, Venojarvi M, Strauch A, Orosz CG, Sen CK (2003) Oxygen sensing by primary cardiac fibroblasts: a key role of p21(Waf1/Cip1/Sdi1). Circ Res. 92: 264-271.

[2] Muniyappa H, Song S, Mathews CK, Das KC (2009) Reactive oxygen species-independent oxidation of thioredoxin in hypoxia: inactivation of ribonucleotide reductase and redox-mediated checkpoint control. J Biol Chem. 284: 17069-17081.

[3] Greer SN, Metcalf JL, Wang Y, Ohh M (2012) The updated biology of hypoxia-inducible factor. EMBO J. 31: 2448-2460.

[4] Dewhirst MW, Ong ET, Braun RD, Smith B, Klitzman B, Evans SM, Wilson D (1999) Quantification of longitudinal tissue pO2 gradients in window chamber tumours: impact on tumour hypoxia. Br. J. Cancer. 79: 1717-1722.

[5] Dewhirst MW, Kimura H, Rehmus SW, Braun RD, Papahadjopoulos D, Hong K, Secomb TW (1996) Microvascular studies on the origins of perfusion-limited hypoxia. Br. J. Cancer Suppl. 27: S247-251.

[6] Secomb TW, Hsu R, Dewhirst MW, Klitzman B, Gross JF (1993) Analysis of oxygen transport to tumor tissue by microvascular networks. Int. J. Radiat. Oncol. Biol. Phys. 25: 481-489.

[7] Lanzen J, Braun RD, Klitzman B, Brizel D, Secomb TW, Dewhirst MW (2006) Direct demonstration of instabilities in oxygen concentrations within the extravascular compartment of an experimental tumor. Cancer Res. 66: 2219-2223.

[8] Nehmeh SA, Lee NY, Schroder H, Squire O, Zanzonico PB, Erdi YE, Greco C, Mageras G, Pham HS, Larson SM, Ling CC, Humm JL (2008) Reproducibility of intratumor distribution of (18)F-fluoromisonidazole in head and neck cancer. Int. J. Radiat. Oncol. Biol. Phys. 70: 235-242.

* Corresponding Author

[9] Dewhirst MW (2007) Intermittent hypoxia furthers the rationale for hypoxia-inducible factor-1 targeting. Cancer Res. 67: 854-855.

[10] Holmgren A (1985) Thioredoxin. Annu. Rev. Biochem. 54: 237-271.

[11] Das KC,Das CK (2000) Thioredoxin, a singlet oxygen quencher and hydroxyl radical scavenger: redox independent functions. Biochem Biophys Res Commun. 277: 443-447.

[12] Rhee SG, Chae HZ, Kim K (2005) Peroxiredoxins: a historical overview and speculative preview of novel mechanisms and emerging concepts in cell signaling. Free Radic. Biol. Med. 38: 1543-1552.

[13] Kim HY,Kim JR (2008) Thioredoxin as a reducing agent for mammalian methionine sulfoxide reductases B lacking resolving cysteine. Biochem Biophys Res Commun. 371: 490-494.

[14] Zhang C, Jia P, Jia Y, Weissbach H, Webster KA, Huang X, Lemanski SL, Achary M, Lemanski LF (2010) Methionine sulfoxide reductase A (MsrA) protects cultured mouse embryonic stem cells from H2O2-mediated oxidative stress. J Cell Biochem. 111: 94-103.

[15] Saitoh M, Nishitoh H, Fujii M, Takeda K, Tobiume K, Sawada Y, Kawabata M, Miyazono K, Ichijo H (1998) Mammalian thioredoxin is a direct inhibitor of apoptosis signal-regulating kinase (ASK) 1. EMBO J. 17: 2596-2606.

[16] Hirota K, Murata M, Sachi Y, Nakamura H, Takeuchi J, Mori K, Yodoi J (1999) Distinct roles of thioredoxin in the cytoplasm and in the nucleus. A two-step mechanism of redox regulation of transcription factor NF-kappaB. J. Biol. Chem. 274: 27891-27897.

[17] Xanthoudakis S,Curran T (1992) Identification and characterization of Ref-1, a nuclear protein that facilitates AP-1 DNA-binding activity. EMBO J. 11: 653-665.

[18] Abate C, Patel L, Rauscher FJ, 3rd, Curran T (1990) Redox regulation of fos and jun DNA-binding activity in vitro. Science. 249: 1157-1161.

[19] Rubartelli A, Bajetto A, Allavena G, Wollman E, Sitia R (1992) Secretion of thioredoxin by normal and neoplastic cells through a leaderless secretory pathway. J Biol Chem. 267: 24161-24164.

[20] Schwertassek U, Balmer Y, Gutscher M, Weingarten L, Preuss M, Engelhard J, Winkler M, Dick TP (2007) Selective redox regulation of cytokine receptor signaling by extracellular thioredoxin-1. EMBO J. 26: 3086-3097.

[21] Angelini G, Gardella S, Ardy M, Ciriolo MR, Filomeni G, Di Trapani G, Clarke F, Sitia R, Rubartelli A (2002) Antigen-presenting dendritic cells provide the reducing extracellular microenvironment required for T lymphocyte activation. Proceedings of the National Academy of Sciences of the United States of America. 99: 1491-1496.

[22] Backman E, Bergh AC, Lagerdahl I, Rydberg B, Sundstrom C, Tobin G, Rosenquist R, Linderholm M, Rosen A (2007) Thioredoxin, produced by stromal cells retrieved from the lymph node microenvironment, rescues chronic lymphocytic leukemia cells from apoptosis in vitro. Haematologica. 92: 1495-1504.

[23] Mougiakakos D, Johansson CC, Jitschin R, Bottcher M, Kiessling R (2011) Increased thioredoxin-1 production in human naturally occurring regulatory T cells confers enhanced tolerance to oxidative stress. Blood. 117: 857-861.

[24] Bertini R, Howard OM, Dong HF, Oppenheim JJ, Bizzarri C, Sergi R, Caselli G, Pagliei S, Romines B, Wilshire JA, Mengozzi M, Nakamura H, Yodoi J, Pekkari K, Gurunath R,

Holmgren A, Herzenberg LA, Ghezzi P (1999) Thioredoxin, a redox enzyme released in infection and inflammation, is a unique chemoattractant for neutrophils, monocytes, and T cells. J. Exp. Med. 189: 1783-1789.
[25] Farina AR, Tacconelli A, Cappabianca L, Masciulli MP, Holmgren A, Beckett GJ, Gulino A, Mackay AR (2001) Thioredoxin alters the matrix metalloproteinase/tissue inhibitors of metalloproteinase balance and stimulates human SK-N-SH neuroblastoma cell invasion. Eur. J. Biochem. 268: 405-413.
[26] Farina AR, Cappabianca L, DeSantis G, Di Ianni N, Ruggeri P, Ragone M, Merolle S, Tonissen KF, Gulino A, Mackay AR (2011) Thioredoxin stimulates MMP-9 expression, de-regulates the MMP-9/TIMP-1 equilibrium and promotes MMP-9 dependent invasion in human MDA-MB-231 breast cancer cells. FEBS Lett. 585: 3328-3336.
[27] Lincoln DT, Ali Emadi EM, Tonissen KF, Clarke FM (2003) The thioredoxin-thioredoxin reductase system: over-expression in human cancer. Anticancer Res 23:2425-33
[28] Chaiswing L, Bourdeau-Heller JM, Zhong W, Oberley TD (2007) Characterization of redox state of two human prostate carcinoma cell lines with different degrees of aggressiveness. Free Radic Biol Med. 43: 202-215.
[29] Ceccarelli J, Delfino L, Zappia E, Castellani P, Borghi M, Ferrini S, Tosetti F, Rubartelli A (2008) The redox state of the lung cancer microenvironment depends on the levels of thioredoxin expressed by tumor cells and affects tumor progression and response to prooxidants. Int J Cancer. 123: 1770-1778.
[30] Sato H, Takino T, Okada Y, Cao J, Shinagawa A, Yamamoto E, Seiki M (1994) A matrix metalloproteinase expressed on the surface of invasive tumour cells. Nature. 370: 61-65.
[31] Nagase H (1997) Activation mechanisms of matrix metalloproteinases. Biol Chem. 378: 151-160.
[32] Rushmore TH, Morton MR, Pickett CB (1991) The antioxidant responsive element. Activation by oxidative stress and identification of the DNA consensus sequence required for functional activity. J Biol Chem. 266: 11632-11639.
[33] Ishii T, Itoh K, Takahashi S, Sato H, Yanagawa T, Katoh Y, Bannai S, Yamamoto M (2000) Transcription factor Nrf2 coordinately regulates a group of oxidative stress-inducible genes in macrophages. J. Biol. Chem. 275: 16023-16029.
[34] Itoh K, Wakabayashi N, Katoh Y, Ishii T, Igarashi K, Engel JD, Yamamoto M (1999) Keap1 represses nuclear activation of antioxidant responsive elements by Nrf2 through binding to the amino-terminal Neh2 domain. Genes Dev. 13: 76-86.
[35] Zhang DD,Hannink M (2003) Distinct cysteine residues in Keap1 are required for Keap1-dependent ubiquitination of Nrf2 and for stabilization of Nrf2 by chemopreventive agents and oxidative stress. Mol Cell Biol. 23: 8137-8151.
[36] Itoh K, Chiba T, Takahashi S, Ishii T, Igarashi K, Katoh Y, Oyake T, Hayashi N, Satoh K, Hatayama I, Yamamoto M, Nabeshima Y (1997) An Nrf2/small Maf heterodimer mediates the induction of phase II detoxifying enzyme genes through antioxidant response elements. Biochem Biophys Res Commun. 236: 313-322.
[37] Kim YC, Masutani H, Yamaguchi Y, Itoh K, Yamamoto M, Yodoi J (2001) Hemin-induced activation of the thioredoxin gene by Nrf2. A differential regulation of the

antioxidant responsive element by a switch of its binding factors. J. Biol. Chem. 276: 18399-18406.

[38] Hintze KJ, Wald KA, Zeng H, Jeffery EH, Finley JW (2003) Thioredoxin reductase in human hepatoma cells is transcriptionally regulated by sulforaphane and other electrophiles via an antioxidant response element. J. Nutr. 133: 2721-2727.

[39] Salceda S,Caro J (1997) Hypoxia-inducible factor 1alpha (HIF-1alpha) protein is rapidly degraded by the ubiquitin-proteasome system under normoxic conditions. Its stabilization by hypoxia depends on redox-induced changes. J Biol Chem. 272: 22642-47.

[40] Huang ZJ, Edery I, Rosbash M (1993) PAS is a dimerization domain common to Drosophila period and several transcription factors. Nature. 364: 259-262.

[41] Qin C, Wilson C, Blancher C, Taylor M, Safe S, Harris AL (2001) Association of ARNT splice variants with estrogen receptor-negative breast cancer, poor induction of vascular endothelial growth factor under hypoxia, and poor prognosis. Clin Cancer Res. 7: 818-823.

[42] Mole DR, Blancher C, Copley RR, Pollard PJ, Gleadle JM, Ragoussis J, Ratcliffe PJ (2009) Genome-wide association of hypoxia-inducible factor (HIF)-1alpha and HIF-2alpha DNA binding with expression profiling of hypoxia-inducible transcripts. J Biol Chem. 284: 16767-16775.

[43] Wiesener MS, Jurgensen JS, Rosenberger C, Scholze CK, Horstrup JH, Warnecke C, Mandriota S, Bechmann I, Frei UA, Pugh CW, Ratcliffe PJ, Bachmann S, Maxwell PH, Eckardt KU (2003) Widespread hypoxia-inducible expression of HIF-2alpha in distinct cell populations of different organs. FASEB J. 17: 271-273.

[44] Loboda A, Jozkowicz A, Dulak J (2010) HIF-1 and HIF-2 transcription factors--similar but not identical. Mol Cells. 29: 435-442.

[45] Hu CJ, Wang LY, Chodosh LA, Keith B, Simon MC (2003) Differential roles of hypoxia-inducible factor 1alpha (HIF-1alpha) and HIF-2alpha in hypoxic gene regulation. Mol Cell Biol. 23: 9361-9374.

[46] van Patot MC,Gassmann M (2011) Hypoxia: adapting to high altitude by mutating EPAS-1, the gene encoding HIF-2alpha. High Alt Med Biol. 12: 157-167.

[47] Bracken CP, Fedele AO, Linke S, Balrak W, Lisy K, Whitelaw ML, Peet DJ (2006) Cell-specific regulation of hypoxia-inducible factor (HIF)-1alpha and HIF-2alpha stabilization and transactivation in a graded oxygen environment. J Biol Chem. 281: 22575-22585.

[48] Imamura T, Kikuchi H, Herraiz MT, Park DY, Mizukami Y, Mino-Kenduson M, Lynch MP, Rueda BR, Benita Y, Xavier RJ, Chung DC (2009) HIF-1alpha and HIF-2alpha have divergent roles in colon cancer. Int J Cancer. 124: 763-771.

[49] Makino Y, Cao R, Svensson K, Bertilsson G, Asman M, Tanaka H, Cao Y, Berkenstam A, Poellinger L (2001) Inhibitory PAS domain protein is a negative regulator of hypoxia-inducible gene expression. Nature. 414: 550-554.

[50] Pugh CW, O'Rourke JF, Nagao M, Gleadle JM, Ratcliffe PJ (1997) Activation of hypoxia-inducible factor-1; definition of regulatory domains within the alpha subunit. J Biol Chem. 272: 11205-11214.

[51] Jiang BH, Zheng JZ, Leung SW, Roe R, Semenza GL (1997) Transactivation and inhibitory domains of hypoxia-inducible factor 1alpha. Modulation of transcriptional activity by oxygen tension. J Biol Chem. 272: 19253-19260.

[52] Kallio PJ, Okamoto K, O'Brien S, Carrero P, Makino Y, Tanaka H, Poellinger L (1998) Signal transduction in hypoxic cells: inducible nuclear translocation and recruitment of the CBP/p300 coactivator by the hypoxia-inducible factor-1alpha. EMBO J. 17: 6573-6586.

[53] Ema M, Hirota K, Mimura J, Abe H, Yodoi J, Sogawa K, Poellinger L, Fujii-Kuriyama Y (1999) Molecular mechanisms of transcription activation by HLF and HIF1alpha in response to hypoxia: their stabilization and redox signal-induced interaction with CBP/p300. EMBO J. 18: 1905-1914.

[54] Lando D, Peet DJ, Whelan DA, Gorman JJ, Whitelaw ML (2002) Asparagine hydroxylation of the HIF transactivation domain a hypoxic switch. Science. 295: 858-861.

[55] Pouyssegur J, Dayan F, Mazure NM (2006) Hypoxia signalling in cancer and approaches to enforce tumour regression. Nature. 441: 437-443.

[56] Bruick RK,McKnight SL (2001) A conserved family of prolyl-4-hydroxylases that modify HIF. Science. 294: 1337-1340.

[57] Maxwell PH, Wiesener MS, Chang GW, Clifford SC, Vaux EC, Cockman ME, Wykoff CC, Pugh CW, Maher ER, Ratcliffe PJ (1999) The tumour suppressor protein VHL targets hypoxia-inducible factors for oxygen-dependent proteolysis. Nature. 399: 271-275.

[58] Jaakkola P, Mole DR, Tian YM, Wilson MI, Gielbert J, Gaskell SJ, Kriegsheim A, Hebestreit HF, Mukherji M, Schofield CJ, Maxwell PH, Pugh CW, Ratcliffe PJ (2001) Targeting of HIF-alpha to the von Hippel-Lindau ubiquitylation complex by O2-regulated prolyl hydroxylation. Science. 292: 468-472.

[59] Huang J, Zhao Q, Mooney SM, Lee FS (2002) Sequence determinants in hypoxia-inducible factor-1alpha for hydroxylation by the prolyl hydroxylases PHD1, PHD2, and PHD3. J Biol Chem. 277: 39792-39800.

[60] Cockman ME, Masson N, Mole DR, Jaakkola P, Chang GW, Clifford SC, Maher ER, Pugh CW, Ratcliffe PJ, Maxwell PH (2000) Hypoxia inducible factor-alpha binding and ubiquitylation by the von Hippel-Lindau tumor suppressor protein. J Biol Chem. 275: 25733-25741.

[61] Lando D, Peet DJ, Gorman JJ, Whelan DA, Whitelaw ML, Bruick RK (2002) FIH-1 is an asparaginyl hydroxylase enzyme that regulates the transcriptional activity of hypoxia-inducible factor. Genes Dev. 16: 1466-1471.

[62] Chandel NS, McClintock DS, Feliciano CE, Wood TM, Melendez JA, Rodriguez AM, Schumacker PT (2000) Reactive oxygen species generated at mitochondrial complex III stabilize hypoxia-inducible factor-1alpha during hypoxia: a mechanism of O2 sensing. J. Biol. Chem. 275: 25130-25138.

[63] Li F, Sonveaux P, Rabbani ZN, Liu S, Yan B, Huang Q, Vujaskovic Z, Dewhirst MW, Li CY (2007) Regulation of HIF-1alpha stability through S-nitrosylation. Mol. Cell. 26: 63-74.

[64] Mansfield KD, Guzy RD, Pan Y, Young RM, Cash TP, Schumacker PT, Simon MC (2005) Mitochondrial dysfunction resulting from loss of cytochrome c impairs cellular oxygen sensing and hypoxic HIF-alpha activation. Cell. Metab. 1: 393-399.

[65] Pan Y, Mansfield KD, Bertozzi CC, Rudenko V, Chan DA, Giaccia AJ, Simon MC (2007) Multiple factors affecting cellular redox status and energy metabolism modulate hypoxia-inducible factor prolyl hydroxylase activity in vivo and in vitro. Mol Cell Biol. 27: 912-925.

[66] Hohler B, Lange B, Holzapfel B, Goldenberg A, Hanze J, Sell A, Testan H, Moller W, Kummer W (1999) Hypoxic upregulation of tyrosine hydroxylase gene expression is paralleled, but not induced, by increased generation of reactive oxygen species in PC12 cells. FEBS letters. 457: 53-56.

[67] Kolamunne RT, Clare M, Griffiths HR (2011) Mitochondrial superoxide anion radicals mediate induction of apoptosis in cardiac myoblasts exposed to chronic hypoxia. Archives of biochemistry and biophysics. 505: 256-265.

[68] Karlenius TC, Shah F, Di Trapani G, Clarke FM, Tonissen KF (2012) Cycling hypoxia up-regulates thioredoxin levels in human MDA-MB-231 breast cancer cells. Biochem Biophys Res Commun. 419: 350-355.

[69] Michelakis ED, Hampl V, Nsair A, Wu X, Harry G, Haromy A, Gurtu R, Archer SL (2002) Diversity in mitochondrial function explains differences in vascular oxygen sensing. Circ Res. 90: 1307-1315.

[70] Paky A, Michael JR, Burke-Wolin TM, Wolin MS, Gurtner GH (1993) Endogenous production of superoxide by rabbit lungs: effects of hypoxia or metabolic inhibitors. Journal of applied physiology. 74: 2868-2874.

[71] Welsh SJ, Bellamy WT, Briehl MM, Powis G (2002) The redox protein thioredoxin-1 (Trx-1) increases hypoxia-inducible factor 1alpha protein expression: Trx-1 overexpression results in increased vascular endothelial growth factor production and enhanced tumor angiogenesis. Cancer Res. 62: 5089-5095.

[72] Jones DT, Pugh CW, Wigfield S, Stevens MF, Harris AL (2006) Novel thioredoxin inhibitors paradoxically increase hypoxia-inducible factor-alpha expression but decrease functional transcriptional activity, DNA binding, and degradation. Clin Cancer Res. 12: 5384-5394.

[73] Csiki I, Yanagisawa K, Haruki N, Nadaf S, Morrow JD, Johnson DH, Carbone DP (2006) Thioredoxin-1 modulates transcription of cyclooxygenase-2 via hypoxia-inducible factor-1alpha in non-small cell lung cancer. Cancer Res. 66: 143-150.

[74] Welsh SJ, Williams RR, Birmingham A, Newman DJ, Kirkpatrick DL, Powis G (2003) The thioredoxin redox inhibitors 1-methylpropyl 2-imidazolyl disulfide and pleurotin inhibit hypoxia-induced factor 1alpha and vascular endothelial growth factor formation. Mol Cancer Ther. 2: 235-243.

[75] Naranjo-Suarez S, Carlson BA, Tsuji PA, Yoo MH, Gladyshev VN, Hatfield DL (2012) HIF-Independent Regulation of Thioredoxin Reductase 1 Contributes to the High Levels of Reactive Oxygen Species Induced by Hypoxia. PLoS One. 7: e30470.

[76] Beutler E, Blume KG, Kaplan JC, Lohr GW, Ramot B, Valentine WN (1977) International Committee for Standardization in Haematology: recommended methods for red-cell enzyme analysis. Br J Haematol. 35: 331-340.
[77] Li DL, Liu JJ, Liu BH, Hu H, Sun L, Miao Y, Xu HF, Yu XJ, Ma X, Ren J, Zang WJ (2011) Acetylcholine inhibits hypoxia-induced tumor necrosis factor-alpha production via regulation of MAPKs phosphorylation in cardiomyocytes. J Cell Physiol. 226: 1052-1059.
[78] Park KJ, Kim YJ, Choi EJ, Park NK, Kim GH, Kim SM, Lee SY, Bae JW, Hwang KK, Kim DW, Cho MC (2010) Expression pattern of the thioredoxin system in human endothelial progenitor cells and endothelial cells under hypoxic injury. Korean Circ. J. 40: 651-658.
[79] Semenza GL,Prabhakar NR (2007) HIF-1-dependent respiratory, cardiovascular, and redox responses to chronic intermittent hypoxia. Antioxid. Redox Signal. 9: 1391-1396.
[80] Yuan G, Nanduri J, Bhasker CR, Semenza GL, Prabhakar NR (2005) Ca2+/calmodulin kinase-dependent activation of hypoxia inducible factor 1 transcriptional activity in cells subjected to intermittent hypoxia. J. Biol. Chem. 280: 4321-4328.
[81] Yao K, Gietema JA, Shida S, Selvakumaran M, Fonrose X, Haas NB, Testa J, O'Dwyer PJ (2005) In vitro hypoxia-conditioned colon cancer cell lines derived from HCT116 and HT29 exhibit altered apoptosis susceptibility and a more angiogenic profile in vivo. Br J Cancer. 93: 1356-1363.
[82] Martinive P, Defresne F, Bouzin C, Saliez J, Lair F, Gregoire V, Michiels C, Dessy C, Feron O (2006) Preconditioning of the tumor vasculature and tumor cells by intermittent hypoxia: implications for anticancer therapies. Cancer Res. 66: 11736-11744.
[83] Cairns RA, Kalliomaki T, Hill RP (2001) Acute (cyclic) hypoxia enhances spontaneous metastasis of KHT murine tumors. Cancer Res. 61: 8903-8908.
[84] Liu Y, Song X, Wang X, Wei L, Liu X, Yuan S, Lv L (2010) Effect of chronic intermittent hypoxia on biological behavior and hypoxia-associated gene expression in lung cancer cells. J Cell Biochem. 111: 554-563.
[85] Nanduri J, Wang N, Yuan G, Khan SA, Souvannakitti D, Peng YJ, Kumar GK, Garcia JA, Prabhakar NR (2009) Intermittent hypoxia degrades HIF-2alpha via calpains resulting in oxidative stress: implications for recurrent apnea-induced morbidities. Proc Natl Acad Sci U S A. 106: 1199-1204.
[86] Peng YJ, Overholt JL, Kline D, Kumar GK, Prabhakar NR (2003) Induction of sensory long-term facilitation in the carotid body by intermittent hypoxia: implications for recurrent apneas. Proc Natl Acad Sci U S A. 100: 10073-10078.
[87] Hedley D, Pintilie M, Woo J, Nicklee T, Morrison A, Birle D, Fyles A, Milosevic M, Hill R (2004) Up-regulation of the redox mediators thioredoxin and apurinic/apyrimidinic excision (APE)/Ref-1 in hypoxic microregions of invasive cervical carcinomas, mapped using multispectral, wide-field fluorescence image analysis. Am. J. Pathol. 164: 557-565.
[88] Kim HJ, Chae HZ, Kim YJ, Kim YH, Hwangs TS, Park EM, Park YM (2003) Preferential elevation of Prx I and Trx expression in lung cancer cells following hypoxia and in human lung cancer tissues. Cell. Biol. Toxicol. 19: 285-298.
[89] Kim YJ, Ahn JY, Liang P, Ip C, Zhang Y, Park YM (2007) Human prx1 gene is a target of Nrf2 and is up-regulated by hypoxia/reoxygenation: implication to tumor biology. Cancer Res. 67: 546-554.

[90] Jewell UR, Kvietikova I, Scheid A, Bauer C, Wenger RH, Gassmann M (2001) Induction of HIF-1alpha in response to hypoxia is instantaneous. FASEB J. 15: 1312-1314.

[91] Kim SM, Kim JY, Lee S, Park JH (2010) Adrenomedullin protects against hypoxia/reoxygenation-induced cell death by suppression of reactive oxygen species via thiol redox systems. FEBS Lett. 584: 213-218.

[92] Malec V, Gottschald OR, Li S, Rose F, Seeger W, Hanze J (2010) HIF-1 alpha signaling is augmented during intermittent hypoxia by induction of the Nrf2 pathway in NOX1-expressing adenocarcinoma A549 cells. Free Radic Biol Med. 48: 1626-1635.

[93] Turoczi T, Chang VW, Engelman RM, Maulik N, Ho YS, Das DK (2003) Thioredoxin redox signaling in the ischemic heart: an insight with transgenic mice overexpressing Trx1. J. Mol. Cell. Cardiol. 35: 695-704.

[94] Krishnamachary B, Berg-Dixon S, Kelly B, Agani F, Feldser D, Ferreira G, Iyer N, LaRusch J, Pak B, Taghavi P, Semenza GL (2003) Regulation of colon carcinoma cell invasion by hypoxia-inducible factor 1. Cancer Res. 63: 1138-1143.

[95] Choi JY, Jang YS, Min SY, Song JY (2011) Overexpression of MMP-9 and HIF-1alpha in Breast Cancer Cells under Hypoxic Conditions. J Breast Cancer. 14: 88-95.

[96] Kim SJ, Miyoshi Y, Taguchi T, Tamaki Y, Nakamura H, Yodoi J, Kato K, Noguchi S (2005) High thioredoxin expression is associated with resistance to docetaxel in primary breast cancer. Clin. Cancer Res. 11: 8425-8430.

[97] Sasada T, Iwata S, Sato N, Kitaoka Y, Hirota K, Nakamura K, Nishiyama A, Taniguchi Y, Takabayashi A, Yodoi J (1996) Redox control of resistance to cis-diamminedichloroplatinum (II) (CDDP): protective effect of human thioredoxin against CDDP-induced cytotoxicity. J. Clin. Invest. 97: 2268-2276.

[98] Desoize B (2002) Cancer and metals and metal compounds: part I--carcinogenesis. Crit Rev Oncol Hematol. 42: 1-3.

[99] Schiff R, Reddy P, Ahotupa M, Coronado-Heinsohn E, Grim M, Hilsenbeck SG, Lawrence R, Deneke S, Herrera R, Chamness GC, Fuqua SA, Brown PH, Osborne CK (2000) Oxidative stress and AP-1 activity in tamoxifen-resistant breast tumors in vivo. J Natl Cancer Inst. 92: 1926-1934.

[100] Iwao-Koizumi K, Matoba R, Ueno N, Kim SJ, Ando A, Miyoshi Y, Maeda E, Noguchi S, Kato K (2005) Prediction of docetaxel response in human breast cancer by gene expression profiling. J. Clin. Oncol. 23: 422-431.

[101] Bussink J, Kaanders JH, Rijken PF, Raleigh JA, Van der Kogel AJ (2000) Changes in blood perfusion and hypoxia after irradiation of a human squamous cell carcinoma xenograft tumor line. Radiat Res. 153: 398-404.

[102] Moeller BJ, Cao Y, Li CY, Dewhirst MW (2004) Radiation activates HIF-1 to regulate vascular radiosensitivity in tumors: role of reoxygenation, free radicals, and stress granules. Cancer Cell. 5: 429-441.

[103] Moeller BJ, Batinic-Haberle I, Spasojevic I, Rabbani ZN, Anscher MS, Vujaskovic Z, Dewhirst MW (2005) A manganese porphyrin superoxide dismutase mimetic enhances tumor radioresponsiveness. Int J Radiat Oncol Biol Phys. 63: 545-552.

[104] Moeller BJ, Dreher MR, Rabbani ZN, Schroeder T, Cao Y, Li CY, Dewhirst MW (2005) Pleiotropic effects of HIF-1 blockade on tumor radiosensitivity. Cancer Cell. 8: 99-110.

[105] Williams KJ, Telfer BA, Xenaki D, Sheridan MR, Desbaillets I, Peters HJ, Honess D, Harris AL, Dachs GU, van der Kogel A, Stratford IJ (2005) Enhanced response to radiotherapy in tumours deficient in the function of hypoxia-inducible factor-1. Radiother Oncol. 75: 89-98.

[106] Kedersha NL, Gupta M, Li W, Miller I, Anderson P (1999) RNA-binding proteins TIA-1 and TIAR link the phosphorylation of eIF-2 alpha to the assembly of mammalian stress granules. J Cell Biol. 147: 1431-1442.

[107] Ozben T (2006) Mechanisms and strategies to overcome multiple drug resistance in cancer. FEBS Lett. 580: 2903-2909.

[108] Gottesman MM, Fojo T, Bates SE (2002) Multidrug resistance in cancer: role of ATP-dependent transporters. Nat Rev Cancer. 2: 48-58.

[109] Sarkadi B, Homolya L, Szakacs G, Varadi A (2006) Human multidrug resistance ABCB and ABCG transporters: participation in a chemoimmunity defense system. Physiol Rev. 86: 1179-1236.

[110] Tiwari AK, Sodani K, Dai CL, Ashby CR, Jr., Chen ZS (2011) Revisiting the ABCs of multidrug resistance in cancer chemotherapy. Curr Pharm Biotechnol. 12: 570-594.

[111] Comerford KM, Wallace TJ, Karhausen J, Louis NA, Montalto MC, Colgan SP (2002) Hypoxia-inducible factor-1-dependent regulation of the multidrug resistance (MDR1) gene. Cancer Res. 62: 3387-3394.

[112] Doublier S, Belisario DC, Polimeni M, Annaratone L, Riganti C, Allia E, Ghigo D, Bosia A, Sapino A (2012) HIF-1 activation induces doxorubicin resistance in MCF7 3-D spheroids via P-glycoprotein expression: a potential model of the chemo-resistance of invasive micropapillary carcinoma of the breast. BMC Cancer. 12: 4.

[113] Riganti C, Doublier S, Viarisio D, Miraglia E, Pescarmona G, Ghigo D, Bosia A (2009) Artemisinin induces doxorubicin resistance in human colon cancer cells via calcium-dependent activation of HIF-1alpha and P-glycoprotein overexpression. Br J Pharmacol. 156: 1054-1066.

Chapter 8

Expressional Alterations of Versican, Hyaluronan and Microfibril Associated Proteins in the Cancer Microenvironment

Hiroko Kuwabara, Masahiko Yoneda and Zenzo Isogai

Additional information is available at the end of the chapter

http://dx.doi.org/10.5772/55067

1. Introduction

The extracellular matrix (ECM) is composed of fibronectin, collagen, elastic fibers and microfibrils with many associated adaptor proteins and proteoglycans. The microenvironments of cancer tissues differ from those of normal tissues, and intimately communicate with the cancer cell surface. For example, in breast cancer stroma compared with a normal breast lobule, 2,338 genes are upregulated and 1,234 genes are downregulated in ductal carcinoma *in situ*, and a further 76 genes are upregulated and 229 genes are downregulated in invasive carcinoma [1]. Histologically, smooth muscle actin-positive fibroblasts appear in the cancer stroma. Cancer cells and their microenvironments seem to influence each other during early carcinogenesis, and the microenvironments appear to play important roles in cancer development. The tumor microenvironment is unique in containing higher amounts of versican and hyaluronan, and lower amounts of latent transforming growth factor β-binding proteins. These stromal changes in hyaluronan-binding proteins and microfibril-associated molecules may facilitate cancer spreading, and targeting of specific components of the cancer stroma could lead to effective anticancer therapies. In this chapter, we review the dynamics of ECM proteins such as versican, hyaluronan, fibrillin-1 and latent transforming growth factor β-binding proteins in cancer tissues. In addition, hyaluronan-binding proteins are discussed.

2. Versican

Versican is a type of ECM proteoglycan that was initially identified in cultured human fibroblasts, followed by isolation of its chicken homolog, PG-M, from chondrogenic condensation areas of developing limb buds [2]. Versican is a macromolecule composed of a specific core protein and covalently linked glycosaminoglycan chains named chondroitin sulfate (CS), which are linear, negatively charged polysaccharides comprising repeating disaccharides of acetylated hexosamines [2,3]. It is produced by cancer, lymphoma and leukemia cells, as well as activated peritumoral fibroblasts. Imunohistochemical staining with an anti-versican antibody (clone; 2B1 [4]) showed that versican is accumulated in the stroma of cancers such as melanoma, breast cancer and ovarian cancer (Figure 1). Versican regulates cell adhesion, proliferation, migration, survival, differentiation and angiogenesis, and its expression is increased with higher tumor grade and worse outcome [3].

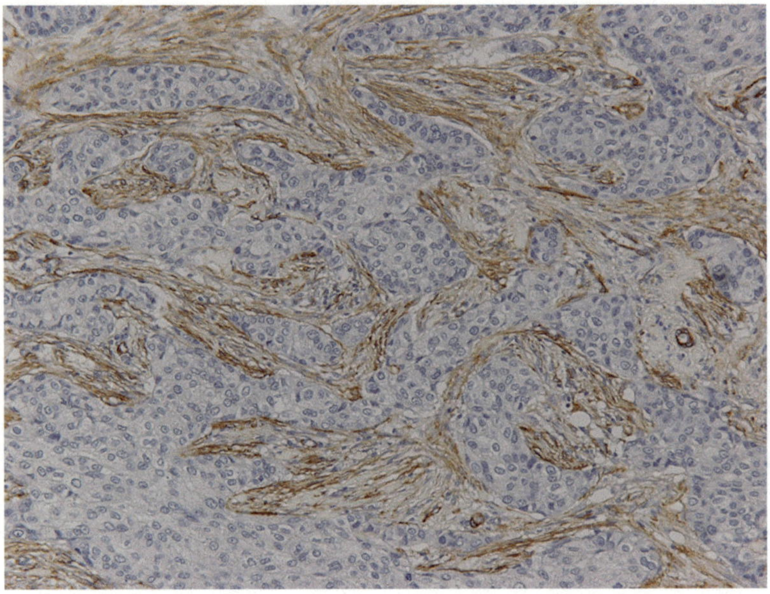

Figure 1. Anti-versican (2B1) immunohistochemistry of human invasive breast cancer. Versican is expressed in cancer stroma (x200).

Versican can be expressed as one of four splice variants (Figure 2) [5]. The amino- and carboxy-terminal globular domains (G1 and G3, respectively) are present in all isoforms, which differ in whether they contain two alternatively spliced CS-attachment regions (CS-α and CS-β). Specifically, versican V1 contains only the CS-β region, V2 contains only the CS-α region, V0 contains both CS regions and V3 contains neither of the CS regions. Each versican isoform has different functional roles. The V1 isoform enhances cell proliferation and protects NIH3T3 mouse fibroblasts against apoptosis [6]. We investigated the alterations in versican isoforms in breast cancer tissues in comparison with matched normal tissues using real-time reverse transcriptase-polymerase chain reaction (RT-PCR) [7]. Total RNA was isolated using an SV total RNA isolation system (Promega, Madison, WI). First-strand cDNA was synthesized from the total RNA using a SuperScript VILO cDNA Synthesis Kit (Invitrogen, Carlsbad, CA), and amplified using specific primers for versican V0, V1, V2 and V3. The housekeeping gene glyceraldhyde-3-phosphate dehydrogenase (GAPDH) was amplified as an internal control. The designed primers were as follows: V0, 5′-gcacaaaatttcaccctgacatt-3′ and 5′-cttctttagattctgaatctattggatgac-3′; V1, 5′-

cccagtgtggaggtggtctac-3′ and 5′-ctcaaatcactcattcgacgtt-3′; V2, 5′-tcagagaaaataagacaggacctgatc-3′, and 5′-catacgtaggaagtttcagtaggataaca-3′; and V3, 5′-ccctccccctgatagcagat-3′ and 5′-ggcacgggttcattttgc-3′. Real-time quantitative RT-PCR was performed using a Thermal Cycler Dice Real Time System (Takara Biochemicals, Shiga, Japan). Each PCR mixture contained 12.5 μl of Master Mix (SYBR Premix ExTaq™II; Takara Biochemicals), 0.01 mol/l forward and reverse primers, and 100 ng of first-strand cDNA in deionized water. After heating each sample to 95℃ for 10 s, 45 cycles of 95℃ for 5 s and 60 ℃ for 30 s were performed. The fluorescence was measured as a function of temperature. All samples were run in triplicate, and PCR amplifications of the GAPDH and target genes were run in parallel for each sample. The results were analyzed by the Thermal Cycler Dice Real Time System TP800 software, version 2.00. To obtain estimates of the mRNA expression levels of the target genes by real-time RT-PCR, the GAPDH mRNA expression level was given a value of 1.0 and used to normalize the other mRNA expression levels. The cancer and normal tissues expressed all four versican isoforms, with the V1 isoform showing the most abundant expression in both tissues (0.18±0.14 in cancer tissues and 0.032±0.028 in normal tissues) [7]. In the cancer tissues, the mRNA levels of V0 and V1 were increased by about 12-fold and 6-fold, respectively, compared with the normal tissues. The mRNA levels of V2 and V3 were very low in the normal tissues, and did not change in the cancer tissues. The versican V1-transfected Swarm rat chondrosarcoma cells show enhanced cell motility and migration, and produce tumors with more spindle-shaped cells and more myxomatous stroma in SD rats [8]. These findings suggest that versican V1 enhances the invasive capacity and leads to the formation of a cell-associated matrix in the cancer tissues. V2 has the opposite functions to V1, by inhibiting cell proliferation and lacking any association with apoptotic resistance, whereas V3 expression has a dual role in tumor growth and metastasis [9,10].

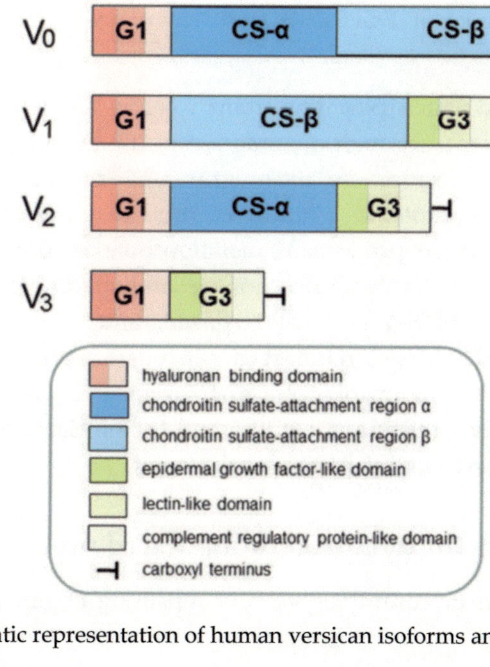

Figure 2. Schematic representation of human versican isoforms and domains.

Globular domains G1 and G3 include a hyaluronan binding portion and epidermis growth like repeats, respectively, and they play a crucial role in the function of versican [2,3]. For these reasons, G1 and G3 in breast cancer and non-cancerous lesions were compared by dot blot analyses [7]. Frozen samples (200 mg) were minced into small pieces using a Tissue Grinder System (Biomedical Polymers, Gardener, MA), homogenized in chilled lysis buffer comprising 4 M guanidine-HCl and 1 % protease inhibitor cocktail (Sigma, St. Louis, MO), and extracted at 4℃ for 48 h. After centrifugation, the supernatants were dialyzed against 50 mM Tris-HCl (pH 8.0) and 0.15 M NaCl at 4℃ overnight using Slide-A-Lyzer MINI Dialysis Units (Pierce, Rockford, IL). The protein contents in the lysates were measured using a Micro BCA Protein Assay Reagent Kit (Pierce), and aliquots containing 30 μg of protein were immobilized on nitrocellulose membranes (GE Healthcare, Buckinghamshire, UK) using a PR648 Slot Blot Manifold dot blot apparatus (GE Healthcare). The membranes were blocked with 10 % non-fat milk, and incubated with the 6084 antibody recognizing G1 [11] or the 2B1 antibody recognizing G3 [4]. In the breast cancer tissues, the staining intensities with the 6084 and 2B1 antibodies were increased by about two-fold and four-fold, respectively, compared with the non-cancerous tissues [7]. Immunohistochemical staining supported these findings.

The G1 and G3 domains are thought to be related to the proliferation and migration of cells. For example, the G1 domain stimulates cell migration and proliferation by destabilizing cell adhesion in NIH3T3 cells and astrocytoma cells [12,13]. The G3 domain promotes breast cancer cell proliferation, invasion and bone metastasis and enhances cancer apoptosis, by upregulating the epidermal growth factor receptor (EGFR)-mediating signaling pathway. Activation of phosphorylated extracellular regulated protein kinases (ERKs) is correlated with high levels of G3 expression [14]. The G3 domain contains two epidermal growth factor (EGF)–like motifs, and the activated EGF-EGFR-ERK pathway plays important roles in cell cycle progression and apoptosis.

Versican is cleaved by proteases, which play important roles in tissue remodeling and modulation of cell microenvironments through degradation of the ECM and processing of growth factors and adhesion molecules. A disintegrin and metalloproteinase with thrombospondin motifs (ADAMTS) proteins, a family of proteases, are composed of the following seven domains: signal peptide, prodomain, metalloproteinase domain, disintegrin domain, thrombospondin type 1 motif, cysteine-rich domain and spacer region. Versican is cleaved by ADAMTS-1 and ADAMTS-4 at Glu441-Ala442, and a 70-kDa neoepitope DPEAAE sequence is generated. ADAMTS-1 in breast cancer cells can promote their growth and metastasis through local accumulation of versican fragments and angiogenesis [15]. This indicates that the concentration of versican is influenced by the cleavage as well as the production, and ADAMTS plays a role in the cancer development.

3. Hyaluronan and receptors for hyaluronan-mediated motility

Hyaluronan (HA) is a nonsulfated glycosaminoglycan of repeating D-glucuronic acid and N-acetyl-D-glucosamine disaccharide units. It is a major constituent of the ECM, and plays an important role in tissue remodeling during development [16,17]. The high concentrations of HA in embryonic tissues are correlated with their rates of cell migration and proliferation, and HA accumulation induces epithelial-mesenchymal transition, at regions such as the future valve sites of the embryonic heart tube. In addition, HA can bind large amounts of water, and form viscous gels at relatively low concentrations. HA is synthesized by HA synthase (HAS) enzymes at the cytoplasmic face of the plasma membrane, and its secretion takes place by extrusion during polymer elongation [18]. HAS enzymes have three different isoforms, and HAS-2 and HAS-3 are common in cancer tissues [19]. HAS-2 in breast cancer stem-like cells (CSCs) promotes tumor progression in bone by stimulating the interactions of CSCs with macrophages and stromal cells [20]. HA plays a critical role in generating a favorable microenvironment by promoting the interactions of macrophages and CSCs, and HAS-2 may promote cancer cell proliferation.

HA synthesis is correlated with the level of HAS mRNA, suggesting that transcriptional regulation is important [21]. In addition to measuring the HAS mRNA levels, several different methods have been utilized for detecting HA. Histologically, the expression of HA was evaluated by staining with biotinylated HA-binding protein (5 μg/ml) prepared from bovine nasal cartilage. Another method used was HA-dependent pericellular coat assays. Cells were cultured in dishes, and the medium was then replaced with phosphate-buffered saline containing 1×10^{16} formalin-fixed horse erythrocytes. After 20 min, the dishes were observed and areas without erythrocytes were considered to be HA [22].

HA is rich in cancer stroma, including that of lung, bladder, prostate, colon and breast cancers (Figure 3), and stromal HA accumulation is typical for high-grade and poorly differentiated carcinoma [23]. An HA rich matrix supports tumor growth and spreading by regulating cell proliferation, and migration or by enhancing tumor angiogenesis in the cancer. In breast cancer in transgenic mice, HA overproduction accelerates tumor angiogenesis through stromal reactions, most notably in the presence of versican [24]. On the other hand, the HAS suppressor, 4-methylumbelliferone (MU), suppresses cell adhesion, locomotion, and matrix metalloproteinase (MMP)-9 and N-cadherin expression, and inhibits tumor metastasis [25-27]. HA is composed of high and low molecular weight forms that have been shown to have opposite functions. High- molecular-weight HA suppresses vascularization, and has anti-inflammatory and immunosuppressive functions. Low-molecular-weight HA, including HA oligosaccharides (less than 50 oligomers (mers)), has an angiogenic function, and induces cytokines and chemokines in inflammation and ECM degradation [28]. HA changes its biological activities depending on its molecular weight, and HA oligosaccharides (12 mers) suppress the growth of breast cancer [29]. MU and HA oligosaccharides may be candidates for anticancer therapies.

HA is present not only in the ECM, but also in the cellular cytoplasm and nucleus. Although the mechanism for HA internalization remains controversial, one possibility is that HA is transported in a retrograde manner through the Golgi, endoplasmic reticulum and cytoplasm. HA accumulation is seen in the cytoplasm of malignant cells, such as colon and gastric cancer cells and lymphoma cells. A high level of HA on tumor cells is a strong indicator of an unfavorable outcome [30]. The intracellular HA-binding proteins include

CDC37 (p50), receptors for HA-mediated motility (RHAMM), P-32 and intracellular HA-binding protein (IHABP)-4 [31]. RHAMM was isolated from culture supernatants of chick embryonic heart fibroblasts [32], and is present in the cell membrane, centrosomes and microtubules. RHAMM is overexpressed in the G2/M phase of cancer cells and in many kinds of cancers [33,34]. These observations suggest that HA and RHAMM play important intracellular roles in mitosis, maintaining the cell shape, and modulating centrosomes and microtubules, which enhance cell proliferation and migration.

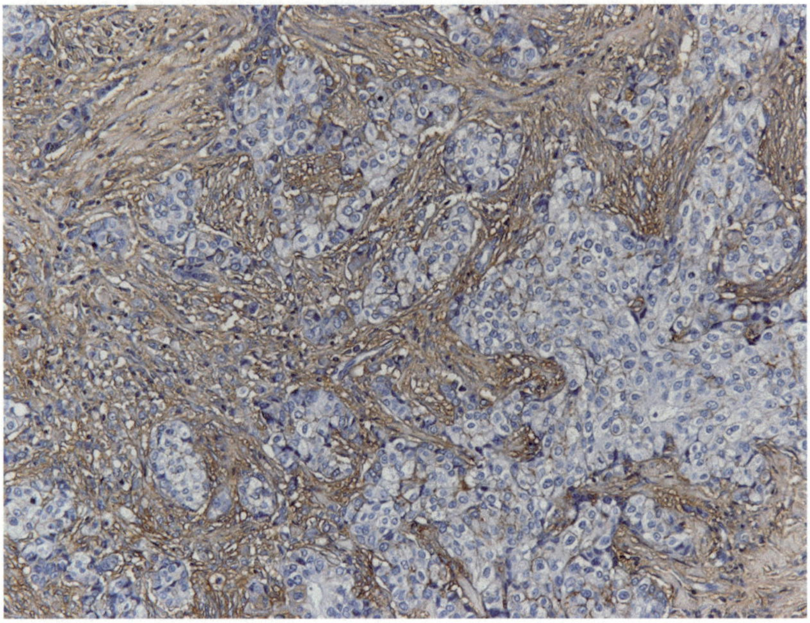

Figure 3. Histochemistry with biotinylated hyaluronan binding protein in human invasive breast cancer. Hyaluronan is expressed in cancer stroma (x200).

CDC37 and RHAMM form complexes with heat shock protein (Hsp) 90 and Hsp70, respectively [31,33]. The CDC37-Hsp90-HA complex stabilizes protein kinases such as Cdk4, p60Src kinase, casein kinase II, MPS1 kinase and Raf-1, and is important for trafficking of kinases from the cytoplasm to the nucleus. On the other hand, the complex of Hsp70 (GRP78 and GRP75) and RHAMM was confirmed by coimmunoprecipitation and glutathione-S-transferase (GST)-RHAMM fusion protein-binding assays [33]. For the GST-RHAMM fusion protein-binding assays, a membrane with transferred proteins from OHK cells (a malignant lymphoma cell line) after two-dimensional gel electrophoresis was used. The membrane was incubated with 0.05 μg/ml of GST-RHAMM fusion protein containing the central domain at room temperature for 1 h. After washing with PBS/Tween-20 at room temperature for 1 h, the localization of the RHAMM fusion protein binding was visualized using a peroxidase-conjugated anti-GST antibody (Amersham, Uppsala, Sweden) and an enhanced chemiluminescence system (Amersham). The membrane was then stripped by incubation in 0.05 M sodium phosphate (pH 6.5), 10 mM SDS and 0.1 M β-mercaptoethanol at 50℃ for 30 min, followed by a wash with PBS/Tween-20. The stripped membrane was then evaluated for another GST-RHAMM fusion protein (C-terminal domain) or GST. The transferred proteins from OHK cells were visualized with Coomassie brilliant blue R-250 and the spots corresponding to the proteins bound to RHAMM were excised from the membrane and submitted for sequencing. GRP78 and GRP75 were identified as RHAMM-binding proteins [33]. Double immunostaining revealed that GRP78 and GRP75 colocalized with RHAMM in the interphase of the cell cycle. The RHAMM-Hsp70 complex may stabilize microtubules in the interphase, and the separation of RHAMM and Hsp70 may play a role in cell division.

HA is cleaved into 10 to 15 disaccharide fragments by hyaluronidases (HYALs). In humans, four HYALs have been identified, namely HYAL1, HYAL2, HYAL3 and PH20 [35]. In lung cancer, wild-type HYAL1 was associated with a poorer prognosis, while the HYAL3-v1 variant was associated with a better prognosis [36]. Increased HYAL1 expression and hyaluronidase activity are associated with an unfavorable prognosis in bladder and prostatic cancers [37].

4. HA-versican-fibrillin-1 complex and HA-verscian complex

Versican interacts with HA and fibrillin-1 at its N-terminus and C terminus, respectively [2,38]. Fibrillin-1 is a major structural component of connective tissue microfibrils, and has significant roles in the maintenance of microfibrils and elastic fibers. The HA-versican-fibrillin-1 complex and its cleavage products exist in the ciliary nonpigmented epithelium and the vitreous body [39]. Regarding skin tissues, immunoblotting analyses of skin extracts with the 6084 antibody and biotin-conjugated HA revealed that versican was a major HA-binding component in the dermis [11]. MMP-12 (macrophage metalloelastase) degraded versican and abrogated its HA-binding ability. Immunohistochemical analyses revealed that the elastic materials in solar elastosis lesions were negative for 6084 antibody, but positive for 2B1 antibody, indicating loss of the HA-binding regions in the aggregated elastic fibers. In solar elastosis, which is seen in photoaged skin of elderly people, abrogation of the HA-binding ability of versican by MMP-12 is observed. On the other hand, assembly of HA-versican aggregates in the pericellular sheath of cancer cells promotes their motility [40]. Similar locations of HA, versican and fibrillin-1 were seen in the ECM of breast cancer tissues [7], but their exact functions in cancer were not elucidated.

5. Latent transforming growth factor β binding proteins

Latent transforming growth factor β binding protein (LTBPs) are large extracellular glycoproteins that are structurally related to fibrillins, and are major regulators of transforming growth factor-β (TGF-β) bioavailability and action [41]. TGF-β is a potent growth inhibitor in the early stage of carcinogenesis, controlling cellular growth and inducing apoptosis. In the advanced stage of carcinogenesis, TGF-β acts as an oncogenic factor and induces invasion-associated epithelial-mesenchymal transition. TGF-β is thought to enhance tumor growth and invasion through regulation of immune functions and angiogenesis, as well as the production of stromal components [42]. TGF-β is secreted as a latent complex containing one of the LTBPs. Latent TGF-β consists of the mature growth factor and the TGF-β propeptide, also known as the latency-associated peptide (LAP). The LTBPs and TGF-β propeptides have four and three isoforms, respectively. LTBP-1 and LTBP-3 bind all three TGF-β LAP isoforms with high affinity, while LTBP-4 shows a weak binding capacity only for the TGF-β1 LAP isoform. LTBP-1, LTBP-3 and LTBP-4 regulate TGF-β action at multiple levels [41]; (a) they ensure correct folding and efficient secretion; (b) they direct temporal and spatial deposition in the extracellular space; and (c) they regulate activation. These findings show that LTBPs have multiple roles with regard to TGF-β action, and the instability of the TGF-β associations with LTBPs yields inflammation and tumors. It has been reported that LTBP-1 and LTBP-3 expression is downregulated in hepatoma and mesothelioma, respectively, compared with normal tissues [43,44]. In breast cancer tissues, LTBP-4 was decreased (Figure 4) [7]. Downregulation of LTBP-3 expression in malignant mesothelioma contributes to increased TGF-β signaling activity [44], and upregulated TGF-β signaling following LTBP reduction seems to induce carcinoma. TGF-β signaling plays a key role in carcinogenesis, and the LTBP downregulation appears to be critical to cancer progression.

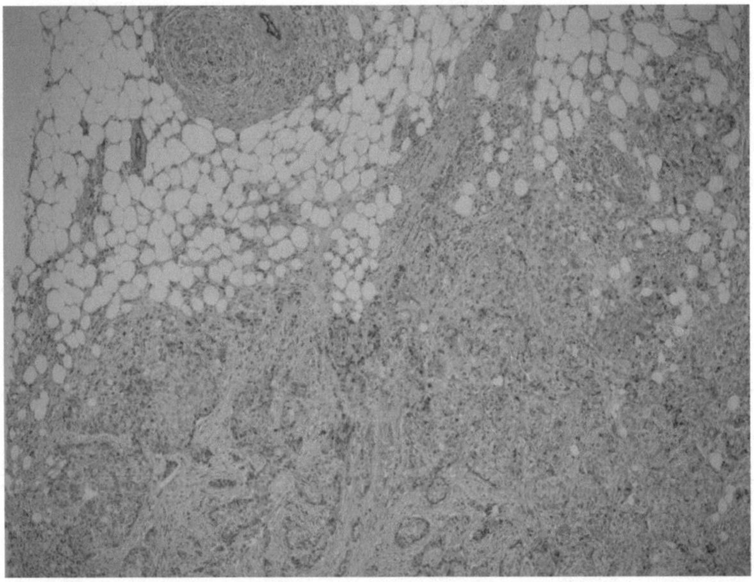

Figure 4. Anti LTBP-4 immunohistochemistry of human invasive breast cancer. LTBP-4 expression is absent (x100).

6. Conclusion

Versican, HA and LTBP distributions in the cancer ECM differ from those of normal tissues (Figure 5), and the ECM alteration facilitates cancer cell proliferation, migration and angiogenesis. In addition, these proteins can interact with each other, and exert a crucial role in the cancer progression. For these reasons, a novel cancer therapy that targets an individual ECM protein and the complex of these ECM proteins is proposed. One of our future research goals is to elucidate the function of HA-versican-microfibril complex in the cancer stroma.

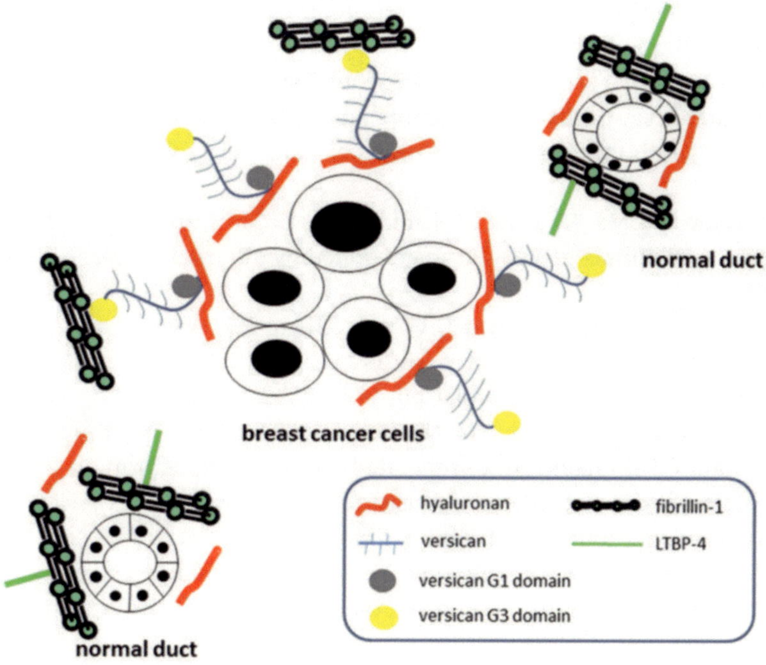

Figure 5. A diagram of the breast cancer tissue. Cancer stroma is rich in hyaluronan and versican, while normal tissues have LTBP-4.

Author details

Hiroko Kuwabara
Department of Pathology, Osaka Medical College, Japan

Masahiko Yoneda
Department of Nursing and Health, School of Nursing and Health, Aichi Prefectural University, Japan

Zenzo Isogai
Department of Advanced Medicine, National Center for Geriatrics and Gerontology, Japan

7. References

[1] Ma XJ, Dahiya S, Richardson E, Erlander M, Sgroi DC (2009) Gene expression profiling of the tumor microenvironment during breast cancer progression. Breast Cancer Res. 11: R7.

[2] Kimata K, Oike Y, Tani K, Shinomura T, Yamagata M, Uritani M, Suzuki S (1986) A large chondroitin sulfate proteoglycan (PG-M) synthesized before chondrogenesis in the limb bud of chick embryo. J. Biol. Chem. 261: 13517-13525.

[3] Wight TN (2002) Versican: a versatile extracellular matrix proteoglycan in cell biology. Curr. Opin. Cell Biol. 14: 617-623.

[4] Isogai Z, Shinomura T, Yamakawa N, Takeuchi J, Tsuji T, Heinegard D, Kimata K (1996) 2B1 antigen characteristically expressed on extracellular matrices of human malignant tumors is a large chondroitin sulfate proteoglycan, PG-M/versican. Cancer Res. 56: 3902-3908.

[5] Ito K, Shinomura T, Zako M, Ujita M, Kimata K (1995) Multiple forms of mouse PG-M, a large chondroitin sulfate proteoglycan generated by alternative splicing. J. Biol. Chem. 270: 958-965.

[6] Sheng W, Wang G, Wang Y, Liang J, Wen J, Zheng PS, Wu Y, Lee V, Slingerland J, Dumont D, Yang BB (2005) The roles of versican V1 and V2 isoforms in cell proliferation and apoptosis. Mol. Biol. Cell. 16: 1330-1340.

[7] Takahashi Y, Kuwabara H, Yoneda M, Isogai Z, Tanigawa N, Shibayama Y (2012) Versican G1 and G3 domains are upregulated and latent transforming growth factor-β binding protein-4 is downregulated in breast cancer stroma. Breast Cancer. 19: 46-53.

[8] Wasa J, Nishida Y, Shinomura T, Isogai Z, Futamura N, Urakawa H, Arai E, Kozawa E, Tsukushi S, Ishiguro N (2012) Versican V1 isoform regulates cell-associated matrix formation and cell behavior differentially from aggrecan in Swarm rat chondrosarcoma cells. Int. J. Cancer. 130: 2271-81.

[9] Serra M, Miquel L, Domenzain C, Docampo MJ, Fabra A, Wight TN, Bassols A (2005) V3 versican isoform expression alters the phenotype of melanoma cells and their tumorigenic potential. Int. J. Cancer. 114: 879-886.

[10] Miquel-Serra L, Serra M, Hernandez D, Domenzain C, Docampo MJ, Rabanal RM, de Torres I, Wight TN, Fabra A, Bassols A (2006) V3 versican isoform expression has a dual role in human melanoma tumor growth and metastasis. Lab. Invest. 86: 889-901.

[11] Hasegawa K, Yoneda M, Kuwabara H, Miyaishi O, Itano N, Ohno A, Zako M, Isogai Z (2007) Versican, a major hyaluronan-binding component in the dermis, loses its hyaluronan-binding ability in solar elastosis. J. Invest. Dermatol. 127: 1657-1663.

[12] Yang BL, Zhang Y, Cao L, Yang BB (1999) Cell adhesion and proliferation mediated through the G1 domain of versican. J. Cell Biochem. 72: 210-220.

[13] Ang LC, Zhang Y, Cao L, Yang BL, Young B, Kiani C, Lee V, Allan K, Yang BB (1999) Versican enhances locomotion of astrocytoma cells and reduces cell adhesion through its G1 domain. J. Neuropathol. Exp. Neurol. 58: 597-605.

[14] Du WW, Yang BB, Shatseva TA, Yang BL, Deng Z, Shan SW, Lee DY, Seth A, Yee AJ (2010) Versican G3 promotes mouse mammary tumor cell growth, migration, and metastasis by influencing EGF receptor signaling. Plos. One. 5: e13828.

[15] Ricciardelli C, Frewin KM, Tan IA, Williams ED, Opeskin K, Pritchard MA, Ingman WV, Russell DL (2011) The ADAMTS1 protease gene is required for mammary tumor growth and metastasis. Am. J. Pathol. 179: 3075-3085.

[16] Laurent TC, Fraser JR (1992) Hyaluronan. FASEB J 6: 2397-2404.

[17] Fraser JR, Laurent TC, Laurent UB (1997) Hyaluronan: its nature, distribution, functions and turnover. J. Intern. Med. 242: 27-33.

[18] Weigel PH, Hascall VC, Tammi M (1997) Hyaluronan synthases. J. Biol. Chem. 272: 13997-14000.

[19] Kuwabara H, Yoneda M, Nagai M, Nishio H, Tasaka T, Suzuki K, Mori H (2003) High levels of hyaluronan production by a malignant lymphoma cell line with primary effusion lymphoma immunophenotype OHK. Br. J. Haematol. 120: 1055-1057.

[20] Okuda H, Kobayashi A, Xia B, Watabe M, Pai SK, Hirota S, Xing F, Liu W, Pandey PR, Fukuda K, Modur V, Ghosh A, Wilber A, Watabe K (2012) Hyaluronan synthase HAS2 promotes tumor progression in bone by stimulating the interaction of breast cancer stem-like cells with macrophages and stromal cells. Cancer Res. 72: 537-547.

[21] Tammi RH, Passi AG, Rilla K, Karousou E, Vigetti D, Makkonen K, Tammi MI (2011) Transcriptional and post-transcriptional regulation of hyaluronan synthesis. FEBS. J. 278: 1419-1428.

[22] Kuwabara H, Yoneda M, Nagai M, Hayasaki H, Mori H (2004) A new polyclonal antibody that recognizes a human receptor for hyaluronan mediated motility. Cancer Lett. 210: 73-80.

[23] Tammi RH, Kultti A, Kosma VM, Pirinen R, Auvinen P, Tammi MI (2008) Hyaluronan in human tumors: Pathobiological and prognostic messages from cell-associated and stromal hyaluronan. Semin. Cancer Biol. 18: 288-295.

[24] Koyama H, Hibi T, Isogai Z, Yoneda M, Fujimori M, Amano J, Kawakubo M, Kannagi R, Kimata K, Taniguchi S, Itano N (2007) Hyperproduction of hyaluronan in neu-induced mammary tumor accelerates angiogenesis through stromal cell recruitment. Possible involvement of versican/PG-M. Am. J. Pathol. 170: 1086-1099.

[25] Yoshihara S, Kon A, Kudo D, Nakazawa H, Kakizaki I, Sasaki M, Endo M, Takagaki K (2005) A hyaluronan synthase suppressor, 4-methylumbelliferone, inhibits liver metastasis of melanoma cells. FEBS. Lett. 579: 2722-2726.

[26] Kuwabara H, Yoneda M, Hayasaki H, Nakamura T, Shibayama Y (2011) A hyaluronan synthase suppressor, 4-methylumbelliferone, inhibits the tumor invasion associated with N-cadherin decreasement. Pathol. Int. 61: 262-263.

[27] Nakamura R, Kuwabara H, Yoneda M, Yoshihara S, Ishikawa T, Miura T, Nozaka H, Nanashima N, Sato T, Nakamura T (2007) Suppression of matrix metalloproteinase-9 by 4-methylumbelliferone. Cell Biol Int 31: 1022-1026.

[28] Noble PW, McKee CM, Cowman M, Shin HS (1996) Hyaluronan fragments activate an NF-κB/I-κBα autoregulatory loop in murine macrophages. J. Exp. Med. 183: 2373-2378.

[29] Misra S, Ghatak S, Zoltan-Jones A, Toole BP (2003) Regulation of multidrug resistance in cancer cells by hyaluronan. J. Biol. Chem. 278: 25285-25288.

[30] Huang L, Grammatikakis N, Yoneda M, Banerjee SD, Toole BP (2000) Molecular characterization of a novel intracellular hyaluronan-binding protein. J. Biol. Chem. 275: 29829-29839.

[31] Yoneda M (2001) Key molecules to an understanding of intracellular hyaluronan function. Connect. Tissue. 33: 227-233.

[32] Turley EA (1982) Purification of a hyaluronan-binding protein fraction that modifies cell social behavior. Biochem. Biophys. Res. Commun. 108: 1016-1024.

[33] Kuwabara H, Yoneda M, Hayasaki H, Nakamura T, Mori H (2006) Glucose regulated proteins 78 and 75 bind to the receptor for hyaluronan mediated motility in interphase microtubules. Biochem. Biophys. Res. Commun. 339: 971-976.

[34] Ishigami S, Ueno S, Nishizono Y, Matsumoto M, Kurahara H, Arigami T, Uchikado Y, Setoyama T, Arima H, Kita Y, Kijima Y, Kitazono M, Natsugoe S (2011) Prognostic impact of CD168 expression in gastric cancer. BMC. Cancer. 11: 106.

[35] Stern R (2003) Devising a pathway for hyaluronan catabolism: are we there yet? Glycobiology 13: 105R-115R.

[36] de Sa VK, Olivieri E, Parra ER, Ab'Saber AM, Takagaki T, Soares FA, Carraro D, Carvalho L, Capelozzi VL (2012) Hyaluronidase splice variants are associated with histology and outcome in adenocarcinoma and squamous cell carcinoma of the lung. Hum. Pathol. 43: 675-683.

[37] Posey JT, Soloway MS, Ekici S, Sofer M, Civantos F, Duncan RC, Lokeshwar VB (2003) Evaluation of the prognostic potential of hyaluronic acid and hyaluronidase (HYAL1) for prostate cancer. Cancer Res. 63: 2638-2644.

[38] Isogai Z, Aspberg A, Keene DR, Ono RN, Reinhadt DP, Sakai LY (2002) Versican interacts with fibrillin-1 and links extracellular microfibrils to other connective tissur networks. J. Biol. Chem. 277: 4565-4572.

[39] Ohno-Jinno A, Isogai Z, Yoneda M, Kasai K, Miyaishi O, Inoue Y, Kataoka T, Zhao JS, Li H, Takeyama M, Keene DR, Sakai LY, Kimata K, Iwaki M, Zako M (2008) Versican and fibrillin-1 form a major hyaluronan-binding complex in the ciliary body. Invest. Ophthalmol. Vis. Sci. 49: 2870-2877.

[40] Ricciardelli C, Russell DL, Ween MP, Mayne K, Suwiwat S, Byers S, Marshall VR, Tilley WD, Horsfall DJ (2007) Formation of hyaluronan- and versican-rich pericellular matrix by prostate cancer cells promotes cell motility. J. Biol. Chem. 282: 10814-10825.

[41] Todorovic V, Rifkin DB (2012) LTBPs, more than just an escort service. J. Cell. Biochem. 113: 410-418.

[42] Imamura T, Hikita A, Inoue Y (2012) The roles of TGF-β signaling in carcinogenesis and breast cancer metastasis. Breast Cancer. 19: 118-124.

[43] Roth-Eichhorn S, Heitmann B, Flemming P, Kubicka S, Trautwein C (2001) Evidence for the decreased expression of the latent TGF-β binding protein and its splice form in human liver tumours. Scand. J. Gastroenterol. 11: 1204-1210.

[44] Vehvilainen P, Koli K, Myllarniemi M, Lindholm P, Soini Y, Salmenkivi K, Kinnula VL, Keski-Oja J (2011) Latent TGF-β binding proteins (LTBPs) 1 and 3 differentially regulate transforming growth factor-β activity in malignant mesothelioma. Hum. Pathol. 42: 269-278.

Chapter 9

Molecular Mechanisms of Metastasis: Epithelial-Mesenchymal Transition, Anoikis and Loss of Adhesion

M.E. Hernández-Caballero

Additional information is available at the end of the chapter

http://dx.doi.org/10.5772/55399

1. Introduction

During the process of tumorigenesis, some cells separate themselves from the tumor to invade distant tissues. Cellular migration in this process is similar to what occurs during embryonic development and wound healing. Unlike these two healthy processes, which involve the creation of a structure or the healing of tissue, metastasis results in the formation of a cellular mass that, if not eliminated, leads to the death of the organism. The process of metastasis includes the invasion of the basal membrane and nearby tissue by tumoral cells and the intravasation towards the blood vessels or infiltration of the lymphatic vessels. This is followed by the mechanisms of survival of tumor cells in these vessels and their extravasation to different tissues of the organism, where they may be able to proliferate. This pathogenic process requires a precise coordination of various signaling pathways that allows the tumor cells to move across the cell membrane, remodel the matrix, transport themselves by circulation [1] and create the appropriate conditions, at a distance, for establishing themselves in a different organ (Figure 1).

Although exploring this complex process of motility and invasion by tumoral cells is fundamental for deepening the understanding of metastasis [2], much remains a mystery despite the enormous amount of research contributions. Both *in vitro* and *in vivo*, the time required for analyzing the evolution of this pathogenesis is excessive. Today the best way to make functional evaluations of the genetic changes that take place in humans with metastasis is with animal models. Although time consuming, a complete follow up can be carried out of the entire process, from the moment of the appearance of a primary tumor, to the strategies used by cancerous cells to escape from the controls of adhesion, their interaction with endothelial cells during their migration, and the establishment of a secondary tumor through the preparation of a new microenvironment favorable to tumor growth in the affected organ.

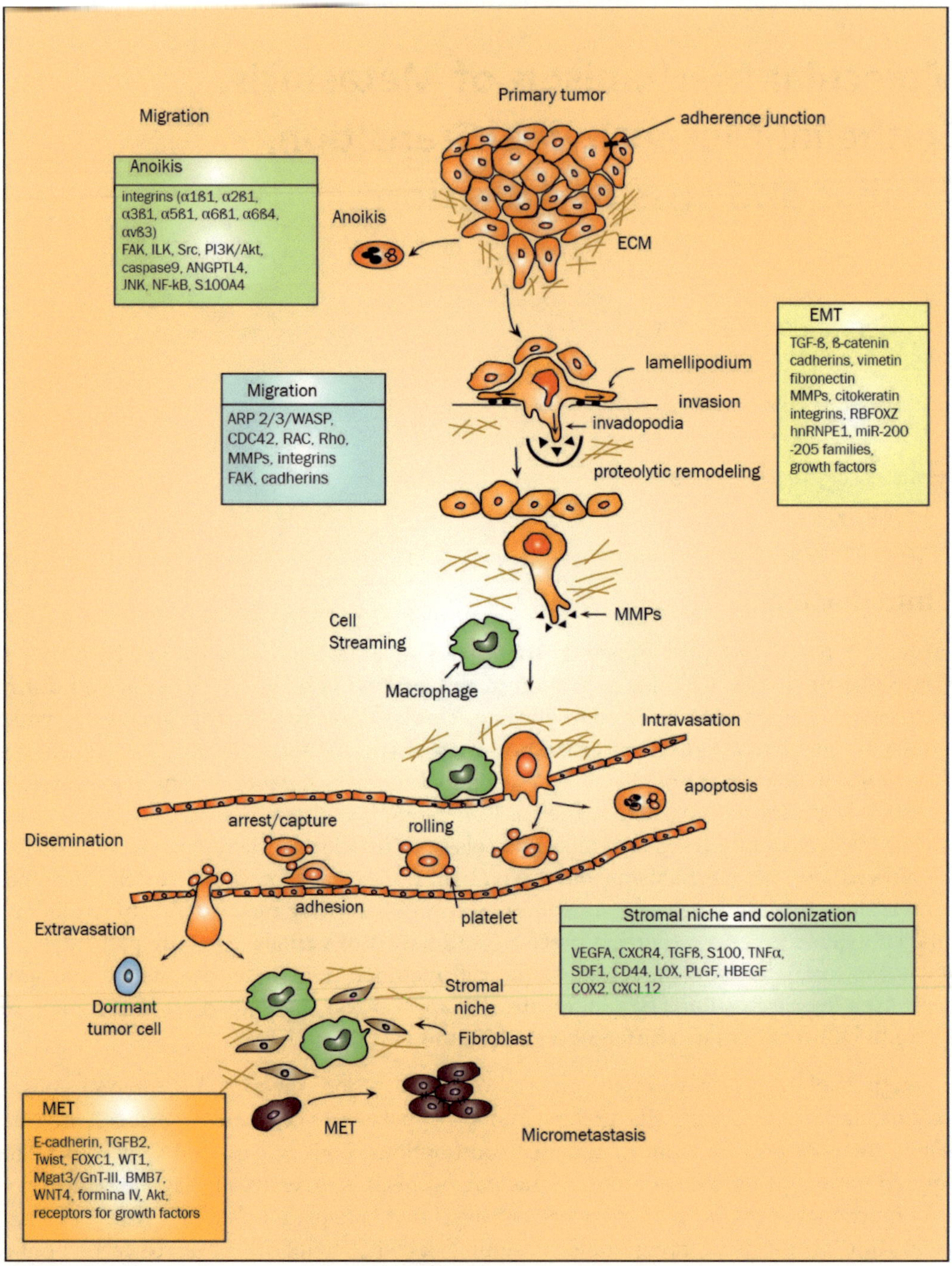

Figure 1. Separation of tumoral cells from a primary tumor and its migration to reach a blood or lymphatic vessel for dissemination to a secondary site is a very complex process that includes changes in the expression of multiple genes, which are genes involved in cell adhesion, survival, chemoattraction, growth factors, miRNAs. In the figure you can see some of the genes involved throughout this process.

2. Primary tumor migration

The majority of deaths from cancer are due to metastasis. Nevertheless, in any given moment only a small proportion of tumoral cells acquire the capacity of invasion and dissemination [3]. This capacity is favored by the activation of signaling pathways that trigger the metastatic cascade, which results from the continuous exposure to the development of the primary tumor, to growth factors, to angiogenesis and to accumulated genetic changes [4]. Since the probability that tumoral cells that travel to new sites give rise to a tumor is very small [5], the process of tumorigenesis is actually quite lengthy. Yachida et al [6], after analyzing autopsies of victims of metastatic pancreatic cancer, proposed a quantitative model of tumor development and metastasis. They consider that at least a decade must pass between the occurrence of the initial mutation and the birth of the parent cancerous cell that eventually results in a tumor. Another five years or more are required for the acquisition of a metastatic capacity. After this latter event, the process takes place very quickly, with the life expectancy of two years for the affected patient. Hence, the challenge is to detect a tumor after the onset of the parent cancerous cell but before metastasis.

Some years ago, Engel et al [7] found that the period from the onset of metastasis to the diagnosis of breast cancer was approximately 6 years. For the purpose of establishing such a diagnosis, two types of tumoral cells can be detected: those circulating in the blood and those disseminated in lymphatic nodes and bone marrow. Such tumor cells can persist for years, awaiting the adequate conditions in some organ to be able to establish themselves in a secondary tumor. In the event of the existence of both types of tumor cells in a patient, the likelihood of tumor development is quite high [8].

There are two proposed models for explaining metastasis. Firstly, there is the model of linear progression, which considers that tumoral cells pass through multiple successive rounds of mutations, resulting in the selection of the most apt for proliferation in a relatively autonomous manner, followed by the transport of these clones to a new site. Secondly, the model of parallel progression holds that tumor cells separate themselves from the primary tumor before the acquisition of the malignant phenotype, and that these cells then undergo a somatic progression and metastatic growth at a distant site [9, 10].

Detailed analysis of diverse data, including that from animal and computational models, suggests that dissemination is not a lengthy process, at least in breast cancer, prostate cancer or cancer of the esophagus [11,12]. Thus at least for these cancers, the model of parallel progression is best supported to explain metastasis from the primary tumor. Through the use of comparative genomic hybridization, Baudis [13] analyzed 5918 malignant epithelial neoplasias and observed typical imbalances: whereas there were recurrent findings of increases in 8q2, 20q, 1q, 3q, 5p, 7q and 17q, similar patterns of losses were seen in 3p, 4q, 13q, 17p and 18q, among others. These genetic similarities between primary and metastatic tumors tend to indicate a convergent evolution more than the result of selection starting from a clone [5]. Nowadays it is well known that tumoral cells abandon the primary tumor before cancer is diagnosed. The possibility that these cells develop a tumor in a distinct organ depends largely on the characteristics of the primary tumor.

2.1. Cell invasion

Tumor cells must acquire certain characteristics for cell migration to occur, such as polarity and disassociation from their point of origin. Afterwards, these cells must undergo cycles of extension and contraction, and at the same time they adhere to and are released from the substrate [14] to move from one site to another. During this process their form is radically modified.

The ability of cells to migrate, studied since 1863 after the discovery by Virchow, allowed them to carry out various processes including embryogenesis, angiogenesis and wound healing to immune response [15], Cell migration can be divided into stages according to the changes observed in the morphology of the cell: polarization, protrusion, adhesion, translocation of the cell body, and retraction of the rear portion. The physiology of cell migration is diverse, depending on the type of cell involved [16]. For instance, fibroblasts and melanocytes generally migrate mesenchymally, as individual cells that are highly adhesive and require proteolytic remodeling of the matrix [17,18.]. These cells form specialized protrusions of the membrane, among which are lamellipodia, which are actin projections of the cytoskeleton formed in the extreme front part of the mobile cell, and invadopodia (invasive pseudopods), which are proteolytically active protrusions of the plasmatic membrane that are responsible for the focal degradation of the components of the extracellular matrix (ECM). The latter type, characteristic of highly invasive tumor cells, contains sites of matrix metalloproteinases (MMPs) [19]. Wolf et al [20] observed that tumor cells do not always require MMPs, since they can escape through openings in the ECM by means of a great contractile force. Also among specialized protrusions of the membrane of metastatic fibroblasts and melanocytes are philopodia and podosomes. The former protrusions are in the shape of thin bundles of actin, and are in charge of probing the environment in search of signals [21]. The latter are functionally the same as invadopodia, forming in macrophages and osteoclasts associated with a tumor, and aiding in the process of invasion. The capacity of malignant cells to migrate in a directional manner is due to the presence of receptors on their surface that allows them to follow the gradient of chemokines [22]. Among the most common type of chemokines are CXCR4 and CCR7, which have been found in diverse types of cancer and are attracted by CXCL12 and CCL21, respectively [23].

2.2. Mechanisms of invasion

Yilmaz et al [24] suggest classifying the invasion by cancerous cells as individual or collective. The use of one or another type of mobility depends on the type of malignant tumor and the surrounding tissue, defined by distinct patterns in the activity of extracellular proteases, matrix-cell adhesion mediated by integrins, cell-cell adhesion mediated by cadherins, cellular polarity and cytoskeletal arrangements [25]. Epithelial cells, which are the most common source of diverse cancers, can exhibit multiple phenotypes of migration. They commonly have a stationary behavior and form layers of cells interconnected with strong bonds. They are capable of moving individually, as a layer, or as a tubular structure. The latter type of structure is found during embryonic development [26]. Among epithelial tumoral cells, all these three types can be found for any particular tissue, suggesting that these pathogenic cells have the capacity to change from individual to collective migration, according to the environment that they face.

2.3. Individual cell migration

The movement of cells inside of living organisms is highly complex and strictly coordinated. For instance, hematopoietic cells exhibit a highly individualized ameboid movement, with little adhesion and without causing remodeling of the matrix. Tumor cells are capable of taking advantage of the strategies of healthy cells, moving in the same individual manner for example as a leukocyte or fibroblast. Individual migration of cells can have some variants: ameboid or mesenchymal [27, 28], solitary or in single file. When cells are transported to a new location, their form is modified. They often, but not always, adopt a bottle form. The constriction of their apexes can have two functions: (i) the cells can transport much of their intracellular content and begin the movement out of the epithelium, and (ii) they can reduce the amount of non-adhesive apex membrane, since by passing through the epithelial layer to arrive to the new location the apical point breaks. Additionally, this form allows for passage through the epithelium layer with a reduced space left behind. The apical constriction is driven by contractions based on actinomiosine, while the apical membrane is reduced by endocytosis. The cells must carry out a process of de-epithelialization, which means that they lose an essential property of epithelial cells—contact with neighboring cells.

Apart from the eventual loss of the adherence of the apical point, the adjoining surfaces forming the bottle neck are also broken up [29]. Due to employment of intravital multiphoton imaging, it has been possible to observe tumor cells in movement, and therefore to see breast cancer cells utilizing ameboid movement to transport themselves rapidly (~4μm/min) [30]. During transport these cells acquire a polarized phenotype, bearing Ca^{2+} in front of and behind the cell, which allows for the retraction of the rear portion [31]. This process of retraction is supported by the contraction of miosine II and by the disassembly of focal adhesion at the rear of the cell, due to the breakage mediated by calpain of the proteins of focal bonds, including integrins, talin, vinculin and focal adhesion kinase (FAK) [32]. Focal adhesion is composed of a structural point and adhesion signaling between the ECM and the cytoskeleton. The velocity of the formation and disassembly of the focal adhesions is what determines the efficiency of cellular migration [33]. In tumor cells the loss of E-cadherin facilitates the formation of focal adhesion and better communication with the ECM. The small STPases (Rho, Rac, CDC42) are among the key molecules for initiating remodeling of the cytoskeleton. The remodeling of actin is mediated by actin-related proteins (such as ARP2/3) [34]. The other type of individual migration, mesenchymal migration, can be used by cells that undergo a transition from the epithelial to mesenchymal cell type, the latter of which is present in 10-40% of carcinomas [35]. This type of migration requires proteolysis of ECM proteins so that the cells can move through the matrix-filled spaces of the tumor [19].

2.4. Collective cell invasion

Targeted multicellular migration can be of two types: (i) collective cellular migration, in which the cells undergoing transport maintain close contact with one another, and (ii) streaming, in which these cells are not always in direct contact [22, 23]. This latter type is carried out by cells during the stage of gastrulation in embryonic development and in wound healing. Collective cell migration, where the cells are bonded together in layers, is more common than individual migration under normal physiological conditions [36]. The best understood collective cell migration is that of wound healing. Neurons and smooth muscle cells also move collectively, as a cohesive group and in a coordinated and integrated manner. The cells involved in this movement retain much of their epithelial characteristics, such as the cell to cell adhesion, averting the need for an epithelial-mesenchymal transition that leads to a modification of cellular shape [37]. In all types of collective migration, the foremost cells of the migratory group actively participate in chemotaxis and degradation of the matrix in order to make way for passage. These leading cells are linked to the cells behind them, dragging them through the remodeled matrix [36].

In tumor cell collective migration, the leading cell can be a tumor cell with proteolytic activity or a stromal cell of the tumoral microenvironment [38]. Among the most relevant proteins for collective cell migration are the β1 and β3 integrins grouped in the ruffling edges of the cell group in movement. These proteins are responsible for providing the adhesion and dynamic strength necessary for transporting the cell group. The leading cells have the greatest proteolytic capacity in relation to the ECM, and it is their production of the metalloproteinases MT1-MMP and MMP-2 that enable proteolysis, as these proteins cut collagen fibers and form a pathway for collective migration and expansion of the migratory group [39, 40]. In squamous carcinomas of the larynx, lungs, esophagus, cervix and skin, among other tissues, collective invasion has been associated with the presence of podoplanin and CDC42 proteins [41-43].

3. The epithelial to mesenchymal transition (EMT)

Regarding the acquisition of mobility, a fundamental process in the transformation to a malignant cell, the best understood phenomenon is the epithelial-mesenchymal transition. The epithelial layer is formed by cells with apical-basal polarity that maintain the laminar structure intact through various types of adhesion, thus forming the barrier necessary for the good functioning of the epithelial layers. This barrier, known as the apical joint complex, is formed and maintained by cell to cell contact at the cell surfaces that surround the apical-lateral dominion. This complex includes the adhesive joints (AJ), which promote the integrity of the tissue by maintaining a strong bond between the cells [44] and have cadherins as their principal component [45]. The resulting tight joints (TJ) form a physical barrier to the movement of ions, macromolecules, immune cells and pathogens between the epithelial cells [46] and desmosomes. The AJ as well as the TJ are closely related with the actin cytoskeleton and are functionally regulated by filaments of the circumference of actomyosin [47]. Their dynamic interaction is important during the morphogenesis of epithelial tissues in embryonic development, in tissue repair [48], and in the maintenance of an effective epithelial barrier in an adult [49].

During early embryonic development, there is a process of essential differentiation resulting in the establishment of the germinal layers in the epithelial-mesenchymal transition (EMT) [29]. The EMT, discovered by Frank Lillie in 1908, is an important mechanism for the reorganization of the germinal layers [50]. This process, whose essential characteristics are the interruption of intercellular contacts and the acquisition of a fibroblast-type conjugated morphology, converts well-organized epithelial cells into isolated cells with a mesenchymal morphology that are capable of transporting themselves [51] to become established in new tissues, thus allowing for inductive interactions during embryogenesis. Currently, it is thought that three subtypes of EMT exist: EMT type 1 is related to embryonic development, EMT type 2 to wound healing, and EMT type 3 to tumor cells [52]. As Thiery [53] points out, it took a long time for EMT to be recognized as a mechanism of tumor progression due to the difficulty of detecting the process in patients. Today, it is known that tumor cells utilize the EMT as a key element in the invasive process, a phenomenon very similar to embryonic EMT. There are diverse pathways in common between embryonic and tumoral EMT, including the stimulation by TGF-β that induces phosphorylation of β-catenin, which in turn activates transcription factors such as Snail [54], as well as diverse growth factors and proteins. This is accompanied by a loss of diverse epithelial proteins such as E-Cadherin, α and β-catenins, Claudin, ocludin and citokeratins, and at the same time an overexpression of mesenchymal proteins such as vimentin, fibronectin, metalloproteinases, actin and integrins αv and β1 [55, 56]. E-cadherin is a key protein because it facilitates the adhesion of epithelial cells and desmosomes [57], which in turn prevents cellular mobility and metastatic dissemination.

The cadherin switch is essential to increase mobility, but is not always necessary for the morphological changes that accompany the EMT [58]. The expression of cadherins can be inactivated by somatic mutations, hypermethylation and desacetylation of histones or transcriptional repression. Some researchers have considered that the expression of N-cadherin is more important for metastasis than that of E-cadherin [59], based on the fact that the former is a mesenchymal protein marker found overexpressed in cells with the EMT. Camand et al [60] found that a decrease in the N-cadherin levels, through regulation of focal adhesion formation, promotes a more rapid migration in healthy and tumoral glia cells. In the latter cells, this contributes to the invasive capacity of astrocyte tumors.

Integrins, a determining factor in the process of cellular adhesion, can also induce EMT. Recently, Gupta et al [61] proposed that integrin α9β1 is implicated in EMT by accelerating lung tumor cell migration, mediated by scr, in a TGFβ-independent manner. To date, a wide variety of proteins and factors have been discovered that regulate EMT. Indeed, it is thought that hundreds of genes significantly modify their expression during EMT [52]. One example is Twist, a potent inducer of EMT that was originally identified as an inducer of the mesoderm in Drosophila [62]. Its expression in epithelial cells causes the loss of cell to cell adhesion mediated by E-cadherin, which leads to cell decomposition. It also activates BMI1 polycomb proteins, which induce stem-like properties and thus annul the p53- and Rb-dependent pathways that would otherwise allow the cells to enter in premature senescence induced by oncogenes. Twist also suppresses the production of let-7i, which in turn allows cells to acquire mobility in the last stage of EMT [63, 64]. The overexpression and activation of the signaling pathways of HER-2/Neu and TGFβ activate EMT in tumoral cells of breast cancer.

EMT is also regulated by alternative splicing, such as that of ENAH, a regulating protein of the cytoskeleton of actin. The transcript present in epithelial cells contains a small exon 11a, which is absent in mesenchymal cell lines and during the EMT [65]. RBFOX2 is a splicing factor which together with ESRP1 and ESRP2, proteins for binding with RNA that are specific to the epithelium, promote splicing of transcripts that are important in EMT [66]. The loss of ESRPs in epithelial cells induces morphological changes similar to EMT [67]. On the other hand, Shapiro et al [68] found a partial induction of the splicing program in mesenchymal cells by means of the ectopic expression of ESRP1 or by elimination of RBFOX2 in immortalized epithelial mammary cells. Mesenchymal isoform IIIc of FGFR2, isoform 3 of catenin p120, and isoform CD44s of CD44 are all expressed in mesenchymal cells and in tumoral cells with the EMT, as reviewed in [69].

Just as the process of EMT resembles that observed during embryonic development, it seems that both pathways are regulated by an intricate interaction of transcriptional and post-transcriptional programs, as was discovered by observing that the ribonucleoprotein, heterogeneous nuclear E1 (hnRNP E1) is a selective transductional regulator of transcripts of EMT induced by TGFβ. Due to its capacity to bind to RNA, hnRNP E1 adheres to 3'-UTR BAT structural elements present in the transcripts of mRNA necessary for EMT, and upon doing so silences these elements. This silencing, mediated by hnRNP E1, occurs during the stage of elongation when hnRNP E1 impedes the release of the elongation factor eukaryote 1 A1 (eEF1A1) of the ribosomal site A. The phosphorylation of hnRNP by Akt2, mediated by TGFβ, restores the transduction of white transcripts of EMT. The attenuation of the expression of hnRNP E1 in non-invasive breast cancer cell lines induces not only EMT but also metastasis [70,71]. Furthermore, the steroid hormones such as androgens have also been observed to be implicated in the maintenance of cellular characteristics, evidenced by the fact that Sun et al [72] found that the absence of androgens in prostate tumors is associated with a worse prognosis and acquisition of cell characteristics typical of mesenchymal or stem cells.

With triple negative breast cancer (ER^-, PR^- $HET2^-$), there is an overexpression of N-cadherin and EMT, leading to a worse prognosis. Regulation by miRNAs is not an exception in EMT, particularly the miRNAs of the miR-200 (miR-200a, miR-200b, miR-200c, miR-141 and miR-429) and miR-205 family. These miRNAs participate in the regulation of EMT induced by TGFβ by mediating the production of ZEB1 and ZEB2 [73,74]. Recently miR-29b was added to the list of miRNAs that regulate EMT, due to the fact that an increase in miR-29b in PC3 prostate cancer cells inhibits the capacity of these tumoral cells to invade and colonize [75]. In addition to TGFβ, other growth factors such as EGF, HGF, PDGF, FGF2, TNFα and IGF can induce EMT by activating the expression of transcriptional repressors of E-cadherin or by activating the transduction signaling pathways, such as MAPK, PI3K, Wnt/β-catenin, NF-κB and Notch [69 and references there].

3.1. EMT reversion

After tumoral cells are disseminated, they must reactivate their epithelial properties by means of the reversion of the process of EMT, known as the mesenchymal-epithelial transition (MET). In the metastatic process, just as EMT is essential for the initial transformation of cells from being part of the epithelial tissue to being released from intercellular connectedness and ready for transport, MET is critical for the later stages of metastasis. Possibly this latter change is triggered by the local environment after extravasation towards the parenchyma of the invaded organs [76]. Although EMT has been extensively studied, there is much yet to be discovered about the molecular mechanisms that regulate MET. One of the keys to the process of MET is the re-expression of E-cadherin, which enables tumor cells to interact with the tissue of the recently colonized organ [77]. Leontovich et al [78] demonstrated that the constitutive activation of Raf-1 induces the overexpression of HER-2/Neu, leading in turn to the development of metastasis in xenografts of MCF7 ERα+ cells. This metastasis was linked to the activation of the MET pathway, and curiously it was characterized by a reduction in the expression of genes implicated in EMT, such as TGFB2, TWIST and FOXC1. On the other hand, Phino et al [79] found that the levels of glycosylation of E-cadherin regulated by Mgat3/GnT-III were diminished in EMT, and that they were recovered when the cells once again acquired an epithelial phenotype. Other genes identified in MET are WT1, BMB7, WNT4 and the protein formina IV of the cytoskeleton [53 and references there]. Diverse miRNAs have been found to be deregulated in tumors, particularly metastamir, which is implicated in metastasis [80]. Wang & Wang [81] summarized the types of metastamir that are deregulated in breast cancer cells: miR-9, -10b, -21, -29a, -31, -103/107, -126, -335, -210, and -373. All of these are involved in migration, aggressiveness and the worst prognoses. An increase in the levels of miR-200 induces MET by reducing motility and aggressiveness [82]. Likewise, the expression of miR124 modifies the morphology and capacity of metastasis of MDA-MB-231 cells, as well as by decreasing the levels of vimentina, a mesenchymal marker [83]. The regulation of diverse transcription factors, receptors for growth factors (including FGFR2b, FGFR2c, EGFR and HER2), and the activation of Akt are other elements in the reversion of MET.

3.2. Collective to ameboid transition and the mesenchymal to ameboid transition

Through the process of metastasis, cells can undergo changes in the way in which they transport themselves. In explants of melanoma, it has been observed that the inhibition of the integrin β1 provokes the separation of groups of cells, which thus become individual ameboid cells. These cells acquire the capacity to migrate, independently of proteases and/or integrins, similar to that observed in ameboid movement. Hence, the transition from collective invasion to ameboid movement of individual cells is an interchangeable and bidirectional process that depends on environmental factors, making evident the great plasticity that tumoral cells can have [84]. The mesenchymal-ameboid transition can serve as a compensatory mechanism of migration after the inhibition of pericellular proteolysis. This transition provokes a change from a cellular form similar to a fibroblast to a round or elliptical shape, and at the same time spurs a change in the cytoskeletal organization as well as the distribution of integrins [85].

4. The tumor microenvironment

During the process of migration, cancerous cells pass through different microenvironments, including the stroma, the endothelium of blood vessels, the lymphatic vessels and the tissue of the organ where the secondary tumor forms [86]. In each of these sites, the microenvironment exerts a strict control over the behavior of tumor cells [87].

Cells can cross the basal membrane (BM) during embryonic development and immune vigilance, either as part of the embryonic process or more routine morphological processes such as leukocyte activity [88]. The BM is a dense layer of the extracellular matrix that is highly reticular and rich in laminina, collagen type IV, perlecan, nidogen-1 and nidogen-2. Its structural function is to delimit epithelial and endothelial tissue, and to give polarity to cells [89, 90]. After the loss of intercellular adhesion, cells acquire a mobile phenotype and produce metalloproteinases that allow them to digest the BM. Hence, the BM is the first barrier that tumor cells must cross [2]. As a tumor invades an organ, there is a dynamic interaction between invasive cells, the invaded tissue and the BM that separate the two. Although it has not been easy to study this process *in vitro*, the transmigration of leukocytes has proved to be a very useful model, allowing for the identification of regions of the perivascular BM that have less resistance to invasion. These regions contain reduced levels of laminin and collagen IV [91]. It is not yet clear how carcinoma cells initiate the invasive process after abandoning the primary tumor, but there is evidence that points to the participation of invadopodium in the proteolysis of vascular BM.

4.1. Interactions with the extracellular matrix

A critical component of the cellular microenvironment is the extracellular matrix (ECM), a biopolymer complex that provides healthy and tumor cells with biophysical and biochemical signals that influence their function and survival [92]. Cells are capable of sensing and responding to changes in the conformation of the ECM through a process of mutual feedback that involves cellular contractile mechanisms. Each cell type responds to the rigidity that is characteristic of its host [93]. Integrins are crucial participants in the communication of cells with the ECM, because they act as a conduit between extracellular ligands and the cytoskeleton. Therefore they have the capacity of responding to the rigidity of the external substrate through a counter-response exerted by the actomiosin network. They act as mechanosensors that undergo conformational changes in response to mechanical forces, resulting in increased adhesion between the cells and the ECM, the formation of focal adhesions, and the dispersion of the cells [94]. The extracellular signals mediated by integrins are transduced internally through focal adhesion components [95].

Tumor cells have the capability of ignoring the conformational changes that take place in the ECM, and this capability is associated with the activation of integrin β1 and the phosphorylation of FAK in a manner dependent on fibronectin and the overexpression of αvβ3 [96]. Lysyl oxidase (LOX), a copper-dependent amine oxidase that catalyzes the crosslinking of collagen, elastin and fibrin in the ECM, can modulate metastasis by facilitating extravasation or by conditioning the metastatic niche, the latter done by increasing the rigidity of the ECM and fibrillar collagen [97]. As can be seen, although the ECM is considered a barrier for the dissemination of tumor cells, its remodeling by tumor cells actually converts it into a promoter of the same process. The release of proteins from the ECM by tumor MMPs can create a promigratory stimulus, in part by increasing the rigidity of the tissue, which in turn augments the motility of tumor cells [98].

4.2. The cancer-associated fibroblast and the tumor associated macrophages and immune cells

Diverse signals emanating from tumor cells allow them to recruit and activate host cells, particularly monocytes, fibroblasts and mesenchymal stem cells, all of which are abundant in the microenvironment of a tumor. Among these cell types, fibroblasts are the most abundant and important in the interaction with the tumor. The carcinoma associated fibroblasts (CAFs) are miofibroblasts with contractile properties and a staining capacity for alpha-smooth muscle actin (α-SMA). Several studies have reported that they can potentiate tumorigenesis by expressing proteins that favor migration or by altering the stromal environment in a way that facilitates colonization. Brentnall et al [99] point out that the overexpression of paladin by the activation of k-ras can transform normal fibroblasts into miofibroblasts in 5 days. As a result, the expression of paladin alters the morphology and behavior of cells, leading to an increased cellular migration, the degradation of the ECM by the formation of invadopodia, and the creation of tunnels through which cancerous cells can transport themselves. Malanchi et al [100] found that to facilitate the process of colonization, infiltrating tumor cells need to induce the expression of stromal periostina (POSTN) in the target organ for a secondary tumor. POSTN is a component of the ECM that is expressed by fibroblasts, both in healthy tissue as well as in the stroma of a primary tumor. Møller et al [101] reported that fibulin 5, whose expression is downregulated by factors released by fibroblasts in tumors, is capable of suppressing metastatic colonization of the lungs and liver by inhibiting the production of metalloproteinase 9 and by reducing the invasive behavior of fibroblasts. Hence, tumor cells avoid the expression of this protein.

Epithelial cells produce multiple factors that recruit various cells able to facilitate the infiltration of tumors, including tumor-associated macrophages (TAMs), tumor-associated neutrophils (TANs), lymphocytes, mesenchymal stem cells, endothelial cells and the aforementioned CAFs. In the case of macrophages, experimental evidence exists supporting the idea that they can differentiate into pro-inflammatory macrophages (M1) or anti-inflammatory macrophages (M2), depending on the stimulus [102,103]. TAMs are similar to M2 macrophages, promoting tumor progression by their incapacity to induce T cells, their increased expression of manose and scavenger receptors, as well as their release of pro-tumorigenic factors (e.g., TGF-β1, IL-10 and MMPs) and pro-angiogenic factors [104]. As they generally accumulate in hypoxic zones, the pro-angiogenic program of TAMs is triggered, resulting in the secretion of VEGF, IL-1b, TNF-a, angiogenin and semaphorin 4D. By secreting urokinasetype plasminogen activator (uPA) and its receptor, uPAR, TAMs can participate in the degradation of the ECM [105].

The non-neoplasic cells present in the stroma of the tumor produce a series of chemokines and growth factors that form a complex network of communication within the tumoral microenvironment. One factor produced by the CAFs is CXCL12, which promotes the migration of tumor cells towards blood vessels [106]. TAMs co-migrate with tumor cells in a paracrine-dependent manner. They produce EGF, which increases the migration of breast cancer cells that express EGFRs. In response, these tumor cells secrete CSF1, thereby attracting the TAMs that express CSF1Rs [107]. Campbell et al [108] found that the TAMS positive to CD68 and PCNA are associated with a worse prognosis for breast cancer patients.

Macrophages are capable of regulating other stromal cells and of exerting influence through them. For instance, the loss of signaling by TGF-β in mammary fibroblasts produces an increase in the secretion of CCL2, which in turn results in a progression of 4T1 tumors, either through direct action on cancerous cells or through the recruitment of macrophages [109]. The infiltration of lymphocytes is associated with metastasis and an increased expression of the activator of the NF-κB (RANK) receptor and of its ligand (RANKL). In particular, T regulatory cells (Treg) infiltrated in a breast cancer tumor stimulate metastasis in breast cancer through the signaling by RANKL-RANK to IKK-α, causing the suppression of the inhibitor of the antimetastatic serine proteinase and maspin, and favoring the survival of circulating tumor cells [110]. It is possible that CAFs express CCL5, thus attracting Treg cells that express CCR1 and produce RANKL. Treg cells secrete IL-4 and IL-13, which in this case would result in the activation of TAMs and consequently the promotion metastasis in RANK-positive tumors [111]. Neutrophils, on the other hand, participate in the preparation of the tumoral microenvironment. They produce enzymes that remodel the ECM, and also produce ROS, which in turn activates NF-κB and in this way allows tumor cells to attenuate their apoptotic response and increase their mutation rate [112].

5. Survival of tumoral cells and modulation of cell survival

The metastatic process has various rate-limiting steps, and consequently only a minority of tumor cells is able to reach distant sites [86]. It has been suggested that approximately 0.01% of circulating tumor cells can manage to produce a metastasis [113]. Talin 1 is one of the proteins whose altered expression allows for the survival of tumor cells. It can recruit focal adhesion proteins ILK, FAK and Src through its interaction with integrin β, resulting in the promotion of the survival, invasion and angiogenesis of tumor cells. Its overexpression allows prostate cancer tumor cells to activate survival signals and resist death by anoikis [114]. In this sense, the PI3K/Akt and Wnt/β-catenin signaling pathways, along with mutations in p53 and other genes, play an important role in the avoidance of death by metastatic cells.

The adhesion of tumor cells to the ECM is not sufficient for inducing a survival signal. The changes in the cytoskeleton associated with adhesion signaling are critical for tumor cell survival. Halder & Johnson [115] indicate that the newly established Hippo suppressor pathway (which regulates the size of organs by maintaining a balance between proliferation and apoptosis in physiological conditions) might be involved in tumor proliferation. The Hippo pathway phosphorylates and inhibits the transcriptional coactivator Yes-associated protein (YAP), a key oncogene for the regulation of the size of organs. This inactivation is triggered by the reorganization of the cytoskeleton. Once the cell has separated, the Hippo kinases Lats 1/2 are activated, causing the inhibition of YAP, and therefore resulting in anoikis. It has been found that with metastatic prostate cancer, the levels of expression of Lats 1/2 are significantly downregulated [116], whereas, Lamar et al [117] demonstrated that increased YAP activity promotes metastasis and tumor growth at both the primary site and the metastatic site.

5.1. Integrins in cell survival and apoptosis (anoikis)

A loss of balance between cell division and cell death is common in cancer, due to a decrease in apoptotic cell death that leads to the progression of a tumor. There are various ways by which a malignant tumor cell averts or resists apoptosis.

The distinctive morphological characteristic of apoptosis is the condensation of chromatin and the posterior fragmentation of the nucleus, accompanied by a reduction of cell volume, a retraction of pseudopods, and the formation of vacuoles, all leading to a loss of integrity of the cell membrane [110]. The biochemical changes that occur during apoptosis are: (i) the activation of caspases, (ii) the rupture of DNA and proteins, and (iii) changes in the membrane related to its recognition by phagocytes [111].

Tumor cells can avert apoptosis by altering the balance of pro-and anti-apoptotic proteins, decreasing the function of caspases, and altering the signaling of receptors related to cell death [112]. A cancerous cell in an ectopic site, whether near a primary tumor or in route to a secondary organ, can employ various mechanisms to avert the process of apoptosis known as anoikis [113]. Through anoikis, a healthy cell in an inappropriate location activates its programmed death by separating itself from its neighbors and its microenvironment, and thus is eliminated. Anoikis is therefore a barrier against the formation and survival of potentially oncogenic clones. Only non-adherent cells, such as leukocytes and mature hematopoietic cells, are protected from anoikis [114].

The principal effector mechanisms of anoikis are autophagy and apoptosis [115]. A critical step in the series of changes through which a tumor cell passes to avoid apoptosis is a change in the expression of integrins, which are a family of receptors that receive signals from the ECM. This change is based on genetic and epigenetic alterations that can only occur in the microenvironment of a tumor [116], allowing tumor cells to ignore signals by the ECM and act as if they were in the appropriate microenvironment. Besides this extrinsic pathway, tumor cells can also avoid apoptosis by damaging the mitochondria, an intrinsic pathway allowing these cells to hyperactivate mechanisms of survival and proliferation

[117]. Another important factor in anoikis is the integrity of the cytoskeleton [118], since many pro-apoptotic proteins, including BIM and BMF, co-locate with the cytoskeleton.

In vertebrates, integrins are a family of receptors composed of 18 subunits α and 8 subunits β, whose combination gives rise to 24 types of these receptors [119]. Changes in the integrins that act as receptors for the ECM are essential for the avoidance of anoikis. The normal functioning of these receptors not only provides a physical bond with the ECM, but also establishes a platform that depends on signals from adhesion molecules, including adaptor proteins and kinases [120, 121]. For instance, the integrins $\alpha1\beta1$, $\alpha2\beta1$, $\alpha3\beta1$, $\alpha5\beta1$, $\alpha6\beta1$, $\alpha6\beta4$ and $\alpha v\beta3$ have a profound impact on cell survival [122].

A particularly important structure in this sense is hemidesmosome, in which there are complexes of integrin-talin-paxilin-actin that receive signals from the ECM and transduce these signals through various proteins such as focal adhesion kinase (FAK) in order to avoid anoikis. FAK, the kinase linked to the integrin ILK, tyrosine kinase Src, PI3K, the extracellular signal-related kinase (ERK) and the adaptor protein Shc are key to the transduction of signals mediated by integrins for protection against anoikis [123]. The FAK binds to the cytoplasmic tails of the integrins and is autophosphorylated at the Y397 residue in order to transmit a survival signal [124]. After the adhesion of integrins with the appropriate proteins of the ECM, FAK and ILK recruit and activate PI3K/Akt, ERK and the Jun kinase (JNK) pathway [125].

The separation of these cells, which move towards the vascular lymphatic space, as well as their implantation in a site with an unknown ECM can cause the separation of the α and β subunits of the heterodimeric receptors of integrin, which in turn leads to the deactivation of FAK, of the family of tyrosine kinases Src, and of ILK. Whereas this attenuates pro-survival pathways, including the mitogen-activated protein kinase/ERK, Akt/phosphatase, tensin homologue (PTEN), and the nuclear factor κB (NF-κB) [126], it at the same time stimulates other mechanisms of survival. The latter mechanisms include the activation of PKB/Akt, which can inhibit anoikis at multiple levels. This inhibition takes place by the inactivation of caspase 9, by a scavenging process that is dependent on the phosphorylation of the pro-apoptotic Bad protein by the 14-3-3 protein, by the activation of NF-κB, and by the inhibition of transcription factors Fork-head [127-130].

It has been seen that the response to anoikis can be recovered by silencing FAK with siRNAs in pancreatic cancer cells [131]. Recently it was found that the inhibition of the proteins of the subfamily of Rho and the expression of Akt in the B16F10 cell line inactivates the FAK pathway and induces anoikis in resistant cells [132]. Whereas healthy epithelial cells express the receptor for collagen $\alpha2\beta1$ and receptors for laminin $\alpha3\beta1$ and $\alpha6\beta1$, hyperproliferative cells overexpress integrins $\alpha v\beta5$ and $\alpha v\beta6$ and squamous carcinoma cells overexpress $\alpha v\beta6$. The latter integrin is required for the adhesion of melanoma cells to dermic collagen and for survival in the environment of the new tissue [133-137]. Goldstein et al [138] found that the substitution of valine by glutamic acid at aminoacid 600 of B-RAF (B-RAFV600E), which is found in 66% of melanomas, is an event that leads to resistance to anoikis by continuous activation of MEK/ERK and the inhibition of BIM, a pro-apoptotic protein. Whereas in a healthy cell BIM levels are increased upon its separation from its tissue as a mechanism to activate its programmed death, this does not occur in tumor cells. Although the overexpression of integrin $\alpha v\beta 3$ is associated with an increase in invasiveness, it has also been implicated in the induction of anoikis, which suggests that it has a dual role in tumorigenesis [139, 140].

ANGPTL4, a regulator of the metabolism of lipids, leads to the activation of Rac1 and FAK by binding to integrins β1 and β5. This phenomenon protects against anoikis through the activation of Src, Akt/PKB and ERK. Hence, the binding of ANGPTL4 with integrins is capable of deceiving the mechanism of programmed death by generating a false impression of anchorage [141]. The phosphorylation of ERK2 by FAK, though, leads to the phosphorylation of BIM, marking the latter for ubiquitination and degradation. Another critical protein for resisting anoikis is the α5 integrin, which as shown by Shen et al [142], has its expression in gastric cancer regulated by the S100A4 protein. S100A4 permits the survival of tumor cells and favors the overexpression of the α5 integrin.

By interacting with integrins, the microenvironment modulates their function in an important way. Marchan et al [143] found that β3 expressed in pancreatic cancer cells has important effects, including the promotion of migration in single-layer cell cultures, the induction of anoikis *in vitro*, and the suppression of tumor growth *in vivo*. At the same time that tumor cells avoid programmed death by anoikis, they acquire a mesenchymal phenotype that allows them to begin migration.

6. Transendothelial or lymphatic migration and extravasation

Tumor cells must go in and out of blood vessels by crossing endothelial layers as part of the metastatic process, and in order to do this they undergo dramatic changes in their shape, driven by a reorganization of their cytoskeleton. The most difficult part of these changes in malignant cells, which adopt elastic and viscous properties for this purpose, is the deformation of the nucleus in interphase, because it is 10 times more rigid than the cytoplasm [144].

Intravasation is the principal route for the dissemination of tumor cells coming from carcinomas. Once inside of a blood vessel, the survival of tumor cells is affected by various factors, including hemodynamic forces, immunological stress, and collisions with blood cells. Consequently, only a very small number of tumor cells manage to leave blood vessels [145]. The majority of tumor cells that enter the bloodstream are detained in the microvasculature of the first organ they pass through [146].

It has been demonstrated that in breast cancer tumors, intravasation depends on the paracrine loop between tumor cells and TAMs [100]. In one clinical study of patients with breast cancer, the half-life of tumor cells in the bloodstream was from 1 to 2.4 h [147]. Png et al [148] pointed out that endothelial cells play an important initial role in metastasis by providing signals that promote this process. These researchers identified molecules such as secretory IGFBP2, the transference protein PITPNC1, and the kinase MERK as necessary for mediating the recruitment of metastatic endothelial cells.

Brown & Ruoslahti [149] suggested that there are molecules that favor the capture of tumor cells in blood vessels. In the case of breast cancer cells, the expression of metadherin favors homing in the pulmonary vasculature. In the majority of tumors of epithelial origin, the first sign of metastasis is found in regional lymphatic nodes. Once inside the lymphatic vessels, tumor cells can produce local or regional metastasis, or can enter in a quiescent state, whose duration depends in great part on the immune system. Immune vigilance can induce quiescence in individual cells by detaining the cell cycle through signals mediated by cytokines [150, 151]. It is estimated that 80% of metastasis of solid tumors, such as in breast cancer and melanoma, are disseminated through the lymphatic system [151].

In the bloodstream a tumor cell can be detained or can succeed in passing through the wall of a blood vessel. If the tumor cell has a diameter greater than that of a given blood vessel, mechanical or occlusive detainment will occur. This mechanism of detention has been observed in mouse models of brain cancer metastasis [152]. On the other hand, if the tumor cell has a diameter less than that of the blood vessel, it must bond to the wall of this channel in order to be able to leave the bloodstream. There is evidence that tumor cells are associated with platelets, which can mask and protect these cells from being located by natural killer cells [153]. Platelets can also facilitate the accumulation of VEGF at the bond between a tumor cell and the endothelium tissue, favoring vascular hyperpermeability and consequently extravasation [154].

7. Colonization

During the progression of cancer, the colonization of distant organs by circulating tumor cells marks the difference between a possibly curable tumor and a systemic and generally incurable disease [155]. After an analysis of breast cancer tumors, Paget [156] concluded that the local microenvironment of some organs must be favorable for the dissemination of tumor cells or their progenitors. On the one hand, the microenvironment of the target organ is a determinant for the survival of tumor cells, and on the other hand the accumulation of these malignant cells in a given organ can create an adequate stromal microenvironment to allow metastasis [157].

In the preparation of an adequate niche, the primary tumor secretes VEGFA to mobilize progenitor hematopoietic cells from bone marrow (HPCs) toward the bloodstream, and from there to the site of metastasis. The same process occurs with fibronectin, metalloproteinases and growth factors, all of which can be synthesized by the primary tumor and released to the bloodstream, later to accumulate in the target organ. In this way, these molecules prepare a premetastatic microenvironment, to which the HPCs arrive and continue this process of adaptation for the purpose of their own survival.

Tumor cells and macrophages are recruited towards the premetastatic niche due to the chemokines synthesized by cells associated with cancer [158]. It has been shown that chemokines are chemotactic molecules important for colonization of a given organ [159, 160]. Wendel et al [161], by utilizing intravital observation techniques, were able to demonstrate that the receptor of chemokine CXCR4 plays an important role in the extravasation of breast cancer tumor cells towards their target organs.

The anatomy of some organs provides a barrier to metastasis. In the case of the lungs, endothelial capillaries are surrounded by a basal membrane [162]. In the blood-brain barrier, capillaries have tight junctions and astrocyte foot processes [163]. Capillaries in bone marrow and the liver, on the other hand, are fenestrated, making them susceptible to invasion [162].

Another important factor in the ability of a tumor to invade a distant organ is the type of primary tumor. Breast cancer tumors positive for estrogen receptors, as well as ocular prostate cancer tumors and melanoma tumors, can give metastatic signals decades after elimination of the primary tumor [7, 164-166]. This is due to the fact that tumor cells are disseminated from the primary tumor various years before detection of the primary tumor. Adenocarcinoma of pancreatic and lung cancer have malignant cells that rapidly acquire the capacity to infiltrate and colonize without requiring a process of quiescence to generate a macrometastasis [167, 168]. Furthermore, tumor cells in general can adopt two distinct states of quiescence while awaiting a favorable microenvironment. They can exist as individual cells (cellular quiescence) or as small indolent groups (tumor mass quiescence), in either case maintaining a balance between proliferation and death during the period of latency [169].

7.1. Most frequent organs for metastasis

Although no organ is totally protected from the development of metastasis, this process tends to take place more frequently in certain regions of the body, including the lymphatic nodes (lymphatic metastasis), lungs, liver, bone marrow, brain (haematogenic metastasis), peritoneum and pleura [145]. Each type of cancer is more prone to certain organs. When it occurs, metastasis exists in at least 2 organs, with an average of 5.6 metastases per patient.

With breast cancer, metastasis generally is a slow process that occurs in the lymph nodes, lungs, bone marrow, liver or brain. Only in 6-18% of breast cancer patients does metastasis takes place in the gastrointestinal tract, with the stomach and small intestine being the most frequent hosts. On the other hand, colorectal cancer rarely metastasizes to bone marrow [170]. Adrenal glands are the preferred site for metastasis of lung cancer tumors with small cells [171]. In North and South America, lung and breast cancer are the first and second source of metastasis to the brain. Generally the earliest metastasis takes place with lung cancer [172], with 80% of such events occurring in the cerebellar hemispheres [173]. However, the most frequent metastasis to the cerebellar hemispheres occurs in breast cancer patients [174]. This frequency can be explained in part by the production of osteoclast-activating factors, such as the parathyroid hormone related protein (PTHrP), IL-1, IL-6, IL-11 and GM-CSF by breast cancer tumor cells [175]. These osteoclasts release growth factors derived from bones, such as TGF-β and IGF-1 [176]. Contrarily, the metastasis of tumor cells from prostate cancer to bone marrow generally stimulates the formation of bone, regulated by the production of osteoblast-activating factors such as endothelin-1, BMPs and PDGF. In this way, the activated osteoblasts can maintain the proliferation and survival of the tumor cells [177].

Cyclooxygenase COX 2, EGFR, the ligand HBEGF and α2,6-sialyltransferase ST6GALNAC5 are mediators of the passage of cancerous cells through the blood-brain barrier. Nevertheless, only ST6GALNAC5 mediates metastasis of breast cancer tumor cells to the brain, facilitating the both the passage through the blood-brain barrier and the adhesion of these cells to brain endothelial cells [178]. A recent study [179] reported that the greatest number of metastasis to the brain occur in breast cancer patients of African origin. The least frequent teratogenic metastases are found in the kidneys, gonads, spleen, subcutaneous fat and especially in the walls of the gastrointestinal tract, uterus, heart and skeletal muscle [180].

The gradients of chemokines can explain the tropism of some types of cancer. It has been suggested that in organs with high levels of chemokine expression, these latter molecules can attract metastatic tumor cells that express the corresponding receptor. This model has been demonstrated in the metastasis of breast and prostate cancer tumors to bone marrow due to the presence of CXCR4-CXCL12. With solid and hematopoietic tumors, chemokines CCL21 and CCL19 are present in metastasis to lymphatic nodules with the corresponding receptor CCR7 [18].

8. Conclusion

The capacity of tumor cells to be transported to organs distant from the primary tumor is driven by two types of factors: the complex interactions between tumor cells and their surroundings, and the changes in such cells that allow them to adapt to their environment. Among the latter factors is the hallmark of tumor cells: their capacity to avoid apoptosis. At the onset of the metastatic process, the epithelial-mesenchymal transition is critical for a tumor cell to escape the controls of adhesion and be released for transport from the primary tumor. It must then be able to move across the cell membrane, remodel the extracellular matrix, transport itself by circulation, and establish itself in a distant organ. The mesenchymal-epithelial transition is critical for this last stage in which the tumor cell survives in a new organ. Although very few tumor cells are able to achieve this task, metastasis unfortunately is a common occurrence with cancer patients due to the continuous exposure to the development of the primary tumor, to growth factors, to angiogenesis and to accumulated genetic changes. The great complexity of the regulatory network that is implicated in the susceptibility of an organ to metastasis, as well as the capacity of tumor cells to dodge the immune response and influence the microenvironment of a given organ to make it favorable to metastasis, makes the study of metastasis for the purpose of drug design for cancer treatment a titanic task. The advantage is that there are now thousands of researchers and hundreds of thousands of reports in the field of metastasis. Furthermore, metastasis is a lengthy process, often taking a decade. Hence, the challenge is to detect a tumor after the onset of the parent cancerous cell but before metastasis.

Author details

ME Hernández-Caballero
Sección de Estudios de Posgrado, Escuela Superior de Medicina, Instituto Politécnico Nacional, Mexico City, Mexico

9. References

[1] Friedl P, Wolf K (2003) Tumour-cell invasion and migration: diversity and escape mechanisms. Nat Rev Cancer. 3: 362-374.
[2] Bravo-Cordero JJ, Hodgson L, Condeelis J (2011) Directed cell invasion and migration during metastasis. Curr Opin Cell Biol. 2011 Dec 30.
[3] Wang W, Goswami S, Lapidus K, Wells AL, Wyckoff JB, Sahai E, et al. (2004) Identification and testing of a gene expression signature of invasive carcinoma cells within primary mammary tumors. Cancer Res. 64: 8585-94.
[4] Wirtz D, Konstantopoulos K Searson PC (2011) The physics of cancer: the role of physical interactions and mechanical forces in metástasis. Nat Rev Cancer. 11: 512-522.
[5] Klein CA (2009) Parallel progression of primary tumours and metastases. Nat Rev Cancer. 9: 302-312
[6] Yachida S, Jones S, Bozic I, Antal T, Leary R, Fu B, et al. (2010) Distant metastasis occurs late during the genetic evolution of pancreatic cancer. Nature. 467:1114-7.
[7] Engel J, Eckel R, Kerr J, Schmidt M, Fürstenberger G, Richter R, et al. (2003) The process of metastasisation for breast cancer. Eur. J. Cancer. 39: 1794–1806.
[8] Hynes RO (2011) Metastatic Cells Will Take Any Help They Can Get. Cell. 20: 689-690.
[9] Klein G (1998) Foulds' dangerous idea revisited: the multistep development of tumors 40 years later. Adv. Cancer Res. 72: 1–23.
[10] Friberg S, Mattson S (1997) On the growth rates of human malignant tumors: implications for medical decision making. J. Surg Oncol. 65: 284–297.
[11] Haustein V, Schumacher U (2012) A dynamic model for tumour growth and metastasis formation. J Clin Bioinforma. 2: 11-23.
[12] Ghotra VP, He S, de Bont H, van der Ent W, Spaink HP, van de Water B, Snaar-Jagalska BE, Danen EH (2012) Automated whole animal bio-imaging assay for human cancer dissemination. PLoS One. 7: e31281.
[13] Baudis M (2007) Genomic imbalances in 5918 malignant epithelial tumors: an explorative meta-analysis of chromosomal CGH data. BMC Cancer 7, 226-241.
[14] Rørth P (2011) Whence directionality: guidance mechanisms in solitary and collective cell migration. Dev Cell. 20: 9-18.
[15] Ridley AJ, Schwartz MA, Burridge K, Firtel RA, Ginsberg MH, Borisy G, et al. (2003) Cell migration: integrating signals from front to back. Science. 302: 1704–1709.
[16] Yoshida K, Soldati T (2006) Dissection of amoeboid movement into two mechanically distinct modes. J Cell Sci. 119: 3833-44.

[17] Abraham VC, Krishnamurthi V, Taylor DL, Lanni F (1999) The actin-based nanomachine at the leading edge of migrating cells. Biophys J. 77: 1721-32.

[18] Dunn GA, Zicha D (1995) Dynamics of fibroblast spreading.. J Cell Sci. 108: 1239-49.

[19] Nabeshima K, Inoue T, Shimao Y, Sameshima T (2002). Matrix metalloproteinases in tumor invasion: role for cell migration. Pathol. Int. 52: 255–264.

[20] Wolf K, Mazo I, Leung H, Engelke K, von Andrian UH, Deryugina EI, et al. (2003) Compensation mechanism in tumor cell migration: mesenchymal–amoeboid transition after blocking of pericellular proteolysis. J Cell Biol. 160: 267–277.

[21] Arjonen A, Kaukonen R, Ivaska J (2011) Filopodia and adhesion in cancer cell motility. Cell Adh Migr. 5: 421-30.

[22] Müller A, Homey B, Soto H, Ge N, Catron D, Buchanan ME, et al. (2001) Involvement of chemokine receptors in breast cancer metastasis. Nature. 410: 50–56.

[23] Lazennec G, Richmond A (2010) Chemokines and chemokine receptors: new insights into cancer-related inflammation. Trends Mol. Med. 16: 133–144.

[24] Yilmaz M, Christofori G, Lehembre F (2007) Distinct mechanisms of tumor invasion and metastasis. Trends Mol Med 13: 535–541.

[25] Yilmaz M, Christofori G (2010) Mechanisms of motility in metastazising cells. Mol Cancer Res. 8: 629-642.

[26] Friedl P (2004) Prespecification and plasticity: shifting mechanisms of cell migration. Curr Opin Cell Biol. 16: 14-23.

[27] Friedl P, Wolf K (2010) Plasticity of cell migration: a multiscale tuning model. J Cell Biol. 188:11-9.

[28] Sahai E (2005) Mechanisms of cancer cell invasion. Curr Opin Genet Dev. 15: 87–96.

[29] Shook D, Keller R (2003) Mechanisms, mechanics and function of epithelial-mesenchymal transitions in early development. Mech Dev 120: 1351–1383.

[30] Condeelis J, Segall JE (2003) Intravital imaging of cell movement in tumours. Nat Rev Cancer. 3: 921-930.

[31] Brundage RA, Fogarty KE, Tuft RA, Fay FS (1991) Calcium gradients underlying polarization and chemotaxis of eosinophils. Science. 254: 703–706.

[32] Ridley, A. JSchwartz MA, Burridge K, Firtel RA, Ginsberg MH, Borisy G, et al. (2003) Cell migration: integrating signals from front to back. Science. 302: 1704–1709.

[33] Prevarskaya N, Skryma R, Shuba Y (2011) Calcium in tumour metastasis: new roles for known actors. Nat Rev Cancer. 11: 609-18.

[34] Wolf K, Wu YI, Liu Y, Geiger J, Tam E, Overall C, et al. (2007) Multi-step pericellular proteolysis controls the transition from individual to collective cancer cell invasion. Nat Cell Biol. 9: 893–904.

[35] Thiery JP, Acloque H, Huang RY, Nieto MA (2009) Epithelial–mesenchymal transitions in development and disease. Cell. 139: 871–890.

[36] Rørth P (2007) Collective guidance of collective cell migration. Trends Cell Biol. 17: 575–579.

[37] Olson MF (2010) Follow the leader: LIM kinases pave the way for collective tumor cell invasion. Cell Cycle. 9: 4417-8.

[38] Ilina O, Friedl P (2009) Mechanisms of collective cell migration at a glance. J Cell Sci. 122: 3203–3208.

[39] Nabeshima K, Inoue T, Shimao Y, Okada Y, Itoh Y, Seiki M, Koono M (2000) Front-cell-specific expression of membrane-type 1 matrix metalloproteinase and gelatinase A during cohort migration of colon carcinoma cells induced by hepatocyte growth factor/scatter factor. Cancer Res. 60: 3364-9.

[40] Friedl P, Wolf K (2008) Tube travel: the role of proteases in individual and collective cancer cell invasion. Cancer Res. 68: 7247–9.

[41] González-Alva P, Tanaka A, Oku Y, Miyazaki Y, Okamoto E, Fujinami M, et al. (2010) Enhanced expression of podoplanin in ameloblastomas. J Oral Pathol Med. 39: 103-9.

[42] Gaggioli C, Hooper S, Hidalgo-Carcedo C, Grosse R, Marshall JF, Harrington K, et al. (2007) Fibroblastled collective invasion of carcinoma cells with differing roles for RhoGTPases in leading and following cells. Nat Cell Biol. 9: 1392–1400.

[43] Wicki A, Lehembre F, Wick N, Hantusch B, Kerjaschki D, Christofori G (2006) Tumor invasion in the absence of epithelial-mesenchymal transition: podoplanin mediated remodeling of the actin cytoskeleton. Cancer Cell. 9: 261–272.

[44] Harris TJC, Tepass U (2010) Adherens junctions: from molecules to morphogenesis. Nat Rev Mol Cell Biol. 11: 502–514.

[45] Takeichi M (1991) Cadherin cell adhesion receptors as a morphogenetic regulator. Science. 251: 1451–1455.

[46] Shen L, Weber CR, Raleigh DR, Yu D, Turner JR (2011). Tight junction pore and leak pathways: a dynamic duo. Annu Rev Physiol. 73: 283–309.

[47] Hartsock A, Nelson WJ (2008) Adherens and tight junctions: structure, function and connections to the actin cytoskeleton. Biochim Biophys Acta. 1778: 660–669.

[48] Baum B, Georgiou M (2011) Dynamics of adherens junctions in epithelial establishment, maintenance, and remodeling. J Cell Biol. 192: 907–917.

[49] Turner JR (2009) Intestinal mucosal barrier function in health and disease. Nat Rev Immunol. 9: 799–809.

[50] Lillie, FR (1908) The Development of the Chick. Henry Holt and Co, New York.

[51] Vincent-Salomon A, Thiery JP (2003) Host microenvironment in breast cancer development: epithelial-mesenchymal transition in breast cancer development. Breast Cancer Res. 5: 101–106.

[52] Kalluri R, Weinberg RA (2009) The basics of epithelial-mesenchymal transition. J Clin Invest. 119: 1420-8.

[53] Thiery JP (2002) Epithelial-mesenchymal transitions in tumour progression. Nat Rev Cancer. 2: 442–54.

[54] Batlle E, Sancho E, Franci C, Dominguez D, Monfar M, Baulida J et al. (2000) The transcription factor snail is a repressor of E-cadherin gene expression in epithelial tumour cells. Nat Cell Biol. 2: 84-89.

[55] Yang J, Weinberg RA (2008) Epithelial-mesenchymal transition: at the crossroads of development and tumor metastasis. Dev Cell. 14: 818-29.

[56] Kang Y, Massague J (2004) Epithelial-mesenchymal transitions: twist in development and metastasis. Cell.118: 277-9.

[57] Adams CL & Nelson WJ (1998) Cytomechanics of cadherinmediated cell-cell adhesion. Curr Opin Cell Biol. 10: 572–577.

[58] Maeda M, Johnson KR, Wheelock MJ (2005) Cadherin switching: essential for behavioral but not morphological changes during an epithelium-tomesenchyme transition. J Cell Sci. 118: 873–887.

[59] Nakajima S, Doi R, Toyoda E, Tsuji S, Wada M, Koizumi M, et al. (2004) N-cadherin expression and epithelial-mesenchymal transition in pancreatic carcinoma. Clin Cancer Res 10: 4125–4133.

[60] Camand E, Peglion F, Osmani N, Sanson M, Etienne-Manneville S (2012) N-cadherin expression level modulates integrin-mediated polarity and strongly impacts on the speed and directionality of glial cell migration. J Cell Sci. Jan 24.

[61] Gupta SK, Oommen S, Aubry MC, Williams BP, Vlahakis NE (2012) Integrin $\alpha9\beta1$ promotes malignant tumor growth and metastasis by potentiating epithelial-mesenchymal transition. Oncogene. Feb 27. doi: 10.1038/onc.2012.41.

[62] Thisse B, el Messal M, Perrin-Schmitt F (1987) The twist gene: isolation of a Drosophila zygotic gene necessary for the establishment of dorsoventral pattern. Nucleic Acids Res. 15: 3439–3453.

[63] Yang J, Mani SA, Donaher JL, Ramaswamy S, Itzykson RA, Come C, et al. (2004) Twist, a master regulator of morphogenesis, plays an essential role in tumor metastasis. Cell. 117: 927–939.

[64] Yang WH, Lan HY, Huang CH, Tai SK, Tzeng CH, Kao SY, et al. (2012) RAC1 activation mediates Twist1-induced cancer cell migration. Nat Cell Biol. Mar 11. doi: 10.1038/ncb2455.

[65] Pino MS, Balsamo M, Di Modugno F, Mottolese M, Alessio M, Melucci E, et al. (2008) Human Mena+11a isoform serves as a marker of epithelial phenotype and sensitivity to epidermal growth factor receptor inhibition in human pancreatic cancer cell lines. Clin Cancer Res. 14: 4943–4950.

[66] Yeo GW, Coufal NG, Liang TY, Peng GE, Fu XD, Gage FH (2009) An RNA code for the FOX2 splicing regulator revealed by mapping RNA-protein interactions in stem cells. Nat Struct Mol Biol. 16: 130–137.

[67] Warzecha CC, Jiang P, Amirikian K, Dittmar KA, Lu H, Shen S, et al. (2010) An ESRPregulated splicing programme is abrogated during the epithelial-mesenchymal transition. Embo J. 29: 3286–3300.

[68] Shapiro IM, Cheng AW, Flytzanis NC, Balsamo M, Condeelis JS, Oktay MH, et al. (2011) An EMT-driven alternative splicing program occurs in human breast cancer and modulates cellular phenotype. PLoS Genet. 7: e1002218.

[69] Tiwari N, Gheldof A, Tatari M, Christofori G (2012) EMT as the ultimate survival mechanism of cancer cells. Semin Cancer Biol. Mar 8.

[70] Chaudhury A, Hussey GS, Howe PH (2011) 3'-UTR-mediated post-transcriptional regulation of cancer metastasis: beginning at the end. RNA Biol. 8: 595-9.

[71] Hussey GS, Chaudhury A, Dawson AE, Lindner DJ, Knudsen CR, Wilce MC, et al. (2011) Identification of an mRNP complex regulating tumorigenesis at the translational elongation step. Mol Cell. 41: 419-31.

[72] Sun Y, Wang BE, Leong KG, Yue P, Li L, Jhunjhunwala S, et al. (2011) Androgen Deprivation Causes Epithelial-Mesenchymal Transition in the Prostate: Implications for Androgen-deprivation Therapy. Cancer Res. 2011 Nov 22.

[73] Park SM, Gaur AB, Lengyel E, Peter ME (2008) The miR-200 family determines the epithelial phenotype of cancer cells by targeting the E-cadherin repressors ZEB1 and ZEB2. Genes Dev. 22: 894–907.

[74] Gregory PA, Bert AG, Paterson EL, Barry SC, Tsykin A, Farshid G, et al. (2008) The miR- 200 family and miR-205 regulate epithelial to mesenchymal transition by targeting ZEB1 and SIP1. Nat Cell Biol. 10: 593–601.

[75] Ru P, Steele R, Newhall P, Phillips NJ, Toth, K, Ray RB (2012) MicroRNA-29b Suppresses Prostate Cancer Metastasis by Regulating Epithelial–Mesenchymal Transition Signaling. Mol Cancer Ther. Mar 8.

[76] Foroni C, Broggini M, Generali D, Damia G (2011) Epithelial-mesenchymal transition and breast cancer: Role, molecular mechanismsand clinical impact. Cancer Treat Rev. Nov 25.

[77] Wells A, Yates C, Shepard CR (2008) E-cadherin as an indicator of mesenchymal to epithelial reverting transitions during the metastatic seeding of disseminated carcinomas. Clin Exp Metastasis. 25: 621–8.

[78] Leontovich AA, Zhang S, Quatraro C, Iankov I, Veroux PF, Gambino MW, Det al. (2012) Raf-1 oncogenic signaling is linked to activation of mesenchymal to epithelial transition pathway in metastatic breast cancer cells. Int J Oncol. Mar 19.

[79] Pinho SS, Oliveira P, Cabral J, Carvalho S, Huntsman D, Gärtner F et al. (2011) Loss and Recovery of Mgat3 and GnT-III Mediated E-cadherin N-glycosylation Is a Mechanism Involved in Epithelial-Mesenchymal-Epithelial Transitions. PLoS One. 7: e33191.

[80] Hurst DR, Edmonds MD, Welch DR (2009b) Metastamir: the field of metastasis regulatory microRNA is spreading. Cancer Res. 69: 7495–7498.

[81] Wang L, Wang J (2011) MicroRNA-mediated breast cancer metastasis: from primary site to distant organs. Oncogene. Oct 3. doi: 10.1038/onc.2011.444.

[82] Korpal M, Lee ES, Hu G, Kang Y (2008) The miR-200 family inhibits epithelial-mesenchymal transition and cancer cell migration by direct targeting of E-cadherin transcriptional repressors ZEB1 and ZEB2. J Biol Chem. 283: 14910–14914.

[83] Lv XB, Jiao Y, Qing Y, Hu H, Cui X, Lin T, et al. (2011) miR-124 suppresses multiple steps of breast cancer metastasis by targeting a cohort of pro-metastatic genes *in vitro*. Chin J Cancer. 30: 821-30.

[84] Hegerfeldt Y, Tusch M, Bröcker EB, Friedl P (2002) Collective cell movement in primary melanoma explants: plasticity of cell-cell interaction, beta1-integrin function, and migration strategies. Cancer Res. 62: 2125-30.

[85] Wolf K, Mazo I, Leung H, Engelke K, von Andrian UH, Deryugina EI, et al. (2003) Compensation mechanism in tumor cell migration: mesenchymal–amoeboid transition after blocking of pericellular proteolysis. J. Cell Biol. 160: 267–277.

[86] Chambers AF, Groom AC, MacDonald IC (2002) Dissemination and growth of cancer cells in metastatic sites. Nature Rev. Cancer. 2: 563–572.

[87] Dvorak HF, Weaver VM, Tlsty TD, Bergers G (2011) Tumor microenvironment and progression. J Surg Oncol.103: 468e74.

[88] Rowe RG, Weiss SJ (2008) Breaching the basement membrane: who, when and how? Trends Cell Biol. 18: 560-574.

[89] Hotary K, Li XY, Allen E, Stevens SL, Weiss SJ (2006) A cancer cell metalloprotease triad regulates the basement membrane transmigration program. Genes Dev. 20: 2673–2686.

[90] Timpl R, Brown JC (1996) Supramolecular assembly of basement membranes. Bioessays. 18:123–132.

[91] Wang S, Voisin MB, Larbi KY, Dangerfield J, Scheiermann C, Tran M, et al. (2006) Venular basement membranes contain specific matrix protein low expression regions that act as exit points for emigrating neutrophils. J Exp Med. 203:1519-1532.

[92] Pedersen JA, Swartz MA (2005) Mechanobiology in the third dimension. Ann Biomed Eng. 33: 1469e90.

[93] Engler AJ, Carag-Krieger C, Johnson CP, Raab M, Tang HY, Speicher DW, et al. (2008) Embryonic cardiomyocytes beat best on a matrix with heart-like elasticity: scar-like rigidity inhibits beating. J Cell Sci. 121: 3794–3802.

[94] Friedland JC, Lee MH, Boettiger D (2009) Mechanically activated integrin switch controls alpha5beta1 function. Science. 323: 642–644.

[95] Schwartz MA (2001) Integrin signaling revisited. Trends Cell Biol. 11: 466– 470.

[96] Indra I, Beningo KA (2011) An *in vitro* correlation of metastatic capacity, substrate rigidity, and ECM composition. J Cell Biochem. 112: 3151-8.

[97] Levental KR, Yu H, Kass L, Lakins JN, Egeblad M, Erler JT, Fong SF, Csiszar K, Giaccia A, Weninger W, et al: Matrix crosslinking forces tumor progression by enhancing integrin signaling. Cell 2009, 139: 891-906.

[98] S. Kumar, Weaver V (2009) Mechanics, malignancy, and metastasis: the force journey of a tumor cell, Cancer Metastasis Rev. 28: 113-27.

[99] Brentnall TA, Lai LA, Coleman J, Bronner MP, Pan S, Chen R (2012) Arousal of cancer-associated stroma: overexpression of palladin activates fibroblasts to promote tumor invasion. PLoS One. 7: e30219.

[100] Malanchi I, Santamaria-Martínez A, Susanto E, Peng H, Lehr HA, Delaloye JF, Huelsken J (2011) Interactions between cancer stem cells and their niche govern metastatic colonization. Nature. 481: 85-9.

[101] Møller HD, Ralfkjær U, Cremers N, Frankel M, Pedersen RT, Klingelhöfer J, et al. (2011) Role of fibulin-5 in metastatic organ colonization. Mol Cancer Res. 9: 553-63.

[102] Caras I, Tucureanu C, Lerescu L, Pitica R, Melinceanu L, Neagu S, et al, (2011) Influence of tumor cell culture supernatants on macrophage functional polarization: in vitro models of macrophage-tumor environment interaction. Tumori. 97: 647-54.

[103] Sica A, Porta C, Riboldi E, Locati M (2010) Convergent pathways of macrophage polarization: The role of B cells. Eur J Immunol. 40: 2131-3.

[104] Sica A, Larghi P, Mancino A, Rubino L, Porta C, Totaro MG, et al, (2008) Macrophage polarization in tumour progression. Sem Cancer Biol. 18: 349-355.

[105] Romer J, Nielsen BS, Ploug M (2004) The urokinase receptor as a potential target in cancer therapy. Curr Pharm Des. 10: 2359-2376.

[106] Lazennec G, Richmond A (2010) Chemokines and chemokine receptors: new insights into cancer-related inflammation. Trends Mol Med. 16: 133-44.

[107] Wyckoff J, Wang W, Lin EY, Wang Y, Pixley F, Stanley ER, et al. (2004) A paracrine loop between tumor cells and macrophages is required for tumor cell migration in mammary tumors. Cancer Res. 64: 7022–7029.

[108] Campbell MJ, Tonlaar NY, Garwood ER, Huo D, Moore DH, Khramtsov AI, et al. (2010) Proliferating macrophages associated with high grade, hormone receptor negative breast cancer and poor clinical outcome. Breast Cancer Res Treat. 128: 703-11.

[109] Hembruff SL, Jokar I, Yang L, Cheng N (2010) Loss of transforming growth factor-beta signaling in mammary fibroblasts enhances CCL2 secretion to promote mammary tumor progression through macrophage-dependent and -independent mechanisms. Neoplasia. 12: 425-33.

[110] Tan W, Zhang W, Strasner A, Grivennikov S, Cheng JQ, Hoffman RM, et al. (2011) Tumour-infiltrating regulatory T cells stimulate mammary cancer metastasis through RANKL-RANK signalling. Nature. 470: 548-53.

[111] DeNardo DG, Barreto JB, Andreu P, Vasquez L, Tawfik D, Kolhatkar N, et al. (2009) CD4(+) T cells regulate pulmonary metastasis of mammary carcinomas by enhancing protumor properties of macrophages. Cancer Cell. 16: 91-102.

[112] Li N, Karin M (1999) Is NF-kapaB the sensor of oxidative stress? FASEB J. 13: 1137-1143.

[113] Panteleakou Z, Lembessis P, Sourla A, Pissimissis N, Polyzos A, Deliveliotis C, et al. (2009). Detection of circulating tumor cells in prostate cancer patients: methodological pitfalls and clinical relevance. Mol Med. 15: 101-114.

[114] Sakamoto S, McCann RO, Dhir R, Kyprianou N (2010) Talin1 promotes tumor invasion and metastasis via focal adhesion signaling and anoikis resistance. Cancer Res. 70: 1885-95.

[115] Halder G, Johnson RL (2011) Hippo signaling. Growth control and beyond. Development. 138: 9–22.

[116] Zhao B, Li L, Wang L, Wang CY, Yu J, Guan KL (2012) Cell detachment activates the Hippo pathway via cytoskeleton reorganization to induce anoikis. Genes Dev. 26: 54-68.

[117] Lamar JM, Stern P, Liu H, Schindler JW, Jiang ZG, Hynes RO (2012) The Hippo pathway target, YAP, promotes metastasis through its TEAD-interaction domain. Proc Natl Acad Sci U S A. 109: E2441–E2450.

[118] Kroemer G, El-Deiry WS, Golstein P, Peter ME, Vaux D, Vandenabeele P, et al. (2005) Classification of cell death: recommendations of the Nomenclature Committee on Cell Death. Cell Death Differ. 12: 1463-1467.

[119] Galluzi L, Maiuri MC, Vitale I, Zischka H, Castedo M, Zitvogel L, et al. (2007) Cell death modalities: classification and pathophysiological implications. Cell Death Differ. 14: 1237-1266.

[120] Wong R (2011) Apoptosis in cancer: from pathogenesis to treatment. J Exp Clin Cancer Res. 30: 87-100.

[121] Kumar R, Vadlamudi RK, Adam L (2000) Apoptosis in mammary gland and cancer. Endocr Relat Cancer. 7: 257-269.

[122] Giannoni E, Buricchi F, Grimaldi G, Parri M, Cialdai F, Taddei ML et al. (2008) Redox regulation of anoikis: reactive oxygen species as essential mediators of cell survival. Cell Death Differ. 15: 867–878.

[123] Eisenberg-Lerner A, Bialik S, Simon HU, Kimchi A (2009) Life and death partners: apoptosis, autophagy and the cross-talk between them. Cell Death Differ. 16: 966–975.

[124] Simpson CD, Anyiwe K, Schimmer D (2008) Anoikis resistance and tumor metastasis. Cancer Lett. 272: 177–185.

[125] Guadamillas MC, Cerezo A, Del Pozo MA (2011) Overcoming anoikis--pathways to anchorage-independent growth in cancer. J Cell Sci. 124: 3189-97.

[126] Puthalakath H, Huang DC, O'Reilly LA, King SM, Strasser A (1999) The proapoptotic activity of the bcl-2 family member bim is regulated by interaction with the dynein motor complex. Mol Cell. 3: 287–96.

[127] Loftus JC, Liddington RC (1997) Cell adhesion in vascular biology. New insights into integrin–ligand interaction. J Clin Invest. 99: 2302–6.

[128] Gilmore AP (2005) Anoikis. Cell Death Differ. 12(Suppl. 2): 1473–1477.

[129] Hynes RO (2002) ntegrins: bidirectional, allosteric signaling machines. Cell. 110: 673-87.

[130] Alahari SK, Reddig PJ, Juliano RL (2002) Biological aspects of signal transduction by cell adhesion receptors. Int Rev Cytol. 220: 145–184.

[131] Hanks SK, Ryzhova L, Shin NY, Brábek J (2003) Focal adhesion kinase signaling activities and their implications in the control of cell survival and motility. Front Biosci. 8: d982–996.

[132] Calalb MB, Polte TR, Hanks SK (1995) Tyrosine phosphorylation of focal adhesion kinase at sites in the catalytic domain regulates kinase activity: a role for Src family kinases. Mol Cell Biol. 15: 954–63.

[133] Ilic D, Almeida EA, Schlaepfer DD, Dazin P, Aizawa S, Damsky CH (1998) Extracellular matrix survival signals transduced by focal adhesion kinase suppress p53-mediated apoptosis. J Cell Biol. 143: 547–560.

[134] Horbinski C, Mojesky C, Kyprianou N (2010) Live free or die: tales of homeless (cells) in cancer. Am J Pathol. 177: 1044-52.

[135] Cardone MH, Roy N, Stennicke HR, Salvesen GS, Franke TF, Stambridge E, et al. (1998) Regulation of cell death protease caspase-9 by phosphorylation. Science. 282: 1318–1321.

[136] Datta SR, Katsov A, Hu L, Fesik SW, Yaffe MB, Greenberg ME (2000) 14–3–3 proteins and survival kinases cooperate to inactivate BAD by BH3 domain phosphorylation. Mol Cell. 6: 41–51.

[137] Romashkova JA, Makarov SS (1999) NF-κB is a target of AKT in antiapoptotic PDGF signalling. Nature. 401: 86–90

[138] Kops GJ, Burgering BM (1999) Forkhead transcription factors: new insights into protein kinase B (c-akt) signaling. J Mol Med. 77: 656–665.

[139] Duxbury MS, Ito H, Zinner MJ, Ashley SW, Whang EE (2004) Focal adhesion kinase gene silencing promotes anoikis and suppresses metastasis of human pancreatic adenocarcinoma cells. Surgery. 135: 555–62.

[140] Goundiam O, Nagel MD, Vayssade M (2012) Akt and RhoA inhibition promotes anoikis of aggregated B16F10 melanoma cells. Cell Biol Int. 36: 311-9.

[141] Carter WG, Wayner EA, Bouchard TS, Kaur P (1990) The role of integrins α2β1 and α3β1 in cell–cell and cell–substrate adhesion of human epidermal cells. J Cell Biol. 110: 1387–1404.

[142] Breuss JM, Gallo J, DeLisser HM, Klimanskaya IV. Folkesson HG, Pittet JF, et al (1995) Expression of the β6 integrin subunit in development, neoplasia and tissue repair suggests a role in epithelial remodeling. J Cell Sci. 108: 2241–2251.

[143] Haapasalmi K, Zhang K, Tonnesen M, Olerud J, Sheppard D, Salo T, et al (1996) Keratinocytes in human wounds express αvβ6 integrin. J Invest Dermatol. 106: 42–48.

[144] Regezi JA, Ramos DM, Pytela R, Dekker NP, Jordan NC (2002) Tenascin and β6 integrin are overexpressed in floor of mouth in situ carcinomas and invasive squamous cell carcinomas. Oral Oncol. 38: 332–336.

[145] Montgomery AM, Reisfeld RA, Cheresh DA (1994) Integrin αvβ3 rescues melanoma cells from apoptosis in three-dimensional dermal collagen. Proc Natl Acad Sci USA. 91: 8856–8860.

[146] Goldstein NB, Johannes WU, Gadeliya AV, Green MR, Fujita M, Norris DA, et al. (2009) Active N-Ras and B-Raf inhibit anoikis by down-regulating Bim expression in melanocytic cells. J Invest Dermatol. 129: 432–7.

[147] Albelda SM, MetteSA, Elder DE, Stewart R, Damjanovich L, Herlyn M, et al (1990) Integrin distribution in malignant melanoma: association of the beta 3 subunit with tumor progression. Cancer Res. 50: 6757–6764.

[148] Kozlova NI, Morozevich GE, Chubukina AN, Berman AE (2001) Integrin alphavbeta3 promotes anchorage-dependent apoptosis in human intestinal carcinoma cells. Oncogene. 20: 4710–4717.

[149] Zhu P, Tan MJ, Huang RL, Tan CK, Chong HC, Pal M, et al. (2011) Angiopoietin-like 4 protein elevates the prosurvival intracellular O2(-):H2O2 ratio and confers anoikis resistance to tumors. Cancer Cell. 19: 401–415.

[150] Shen W, Chen D, Fu H, Liu S, Sun K, Sun X (2011) S100A4 protects gastric cancer cells from anoikis through regulation of αv and α5 integrin. Cancer Sci. 102: 1014-8.

[151] Marchán S, Pérez-Torras S, Vidal A, Adan J, Mitjans F, Carbó N, et al. (2011) Dual effects of β3 integrin subunit expression on human pancreatic cancer models. Cell Oncol (Dordr). 34: 393-405.

[152] Tseng Y, Lee JS, Kole TP, Jiang I, Wirtz D (2004) Micro-organization and visco-elasticity of the interphase nucleus revealed by particle nanotracking. J Cell Sci. 117: 2159-67.

[153] Fidler IJ, Yano S, Zhang RD, Fujimaki T, Bucana CD (2002) The seed and soil hypothesis: vascularisation and brain metastases. Lancet Oncol. 3: 53-7.

[154] Weiss L, Orr FW, Honn KV (1988) Interactions of cancer cells with the microvasculature during metastasis. FASEB J. 2: 12–21.

[155] Meng S, Tripathy D, Frenkel EP, Shete S, Naftalis EZ, Huth JF, et al. (2004) Circulating tumor cells in patients with breast cancer dormancy. Clin Cancer Res. 10: 8152–62.

[156] Png KJ, Halberg N, Yoshida M, Tavazoie SF (2011) A microRNA regulon that mediates endothelial recruitment and metastasis by cancer cells. Nature. 481: 190-4.

[157] Brown DM, Ruoslahti E (2004) Metadherin, a cell surface protein in breast tumors that mediates lungmetastasis. Cancer Cell. 5: 365-74.

[158] Eyles J, Puaux AL, Wang X, Toh B, Prakash C, Hong M, et al. (2010) Tumor cells disseminate early, but immunosurveillance limits metastatic outgrowth, in a mouse model of melanoma. J Clin Invest. 120: 2030–2039.

[159] Leong SP, Nakakura EK, Pollock R, Choti MA, Morton DL, Henner WD et al. (2011) Unique patterns of metastases in common and rare types of malignancy. J Surg Oncol. 103: 607-614.

[160] Kienast Y, von Baumgarten L, Fuhrmann M, Klinkert WE, Goldbrunner R, Herms J, et al. (2010) Real-time imaging reveals the single steps of brain metastasis formation. Nature Med. 16: 116–122.

[161] Palumbo JS, Talmage KE, Massari JV, La Jeunesse CM, Flick MJ, Kombrinck KW, et al.(2005) Platelets and fibrin(ogen) increase metastatic potential by impeding natural killer cellmediated elimination of tumor cells. Blood. 105: 178–185.

[162] Nash G, Turner L, Scully M, Kakkar A (2002) Platelets and cancer. Lancet Oncol. 3, 425–430.

[163] Nicolson GL (1988) Cancer metastasis: TC and host organ properties important in metastasis to specific secondary sites. Biochem Biophys Acta. 948: 175–224.

[164] Paget S (1889) The distribution of secondary growths in cancer of the breast. Lancet. 1: 571–573.

[165] Psaila B, Kaplan RN, Port ER, Lyden D (2006-2007) Priming the 'soil' for breast cancer metastasis: the pre-metastatic niche. Breast Dis. 26: 65-74.

[166] Perelmuter VM, Manskikh VN (2012) Preniche as Missing Link of the Metastatic Niche Concept Explaining Organ_Preferential Metastasis of Malignant Tumors and the Type of Metastatic Disease. Biochemistry. 77: 11-118.

[167] Ali S, Lazennec G (2007) Chemokines novel targets for breast cancer metastasis. Cancer Metastasis Rev. 26: 401–420.

[168] Baruch-Ben A (2008) Organ selectivity in metastasis: regulation by chemokines and their receptors. Clin Exp Metastasis. 25: 345–356.
[169] Wendel C, Hemping-Bovenkerk A, Krasnyanska J, Mees ST, Kochetkova M, Stoeppeler S, et al. (2012) CXCR4/CXCL12 participate in extravasation of metastasizing breast cancer cells within the liver in a rat model. PLoS One. 7: e30046.
[170] Inoue S, Osmond DG (2001) Basement membrane of mouse bone marrow sinusoids shows distinctive structure and proteoglycan composition: a high resolution ultrastructural study. Anat Rec. 264: 294–304.
[171] Weil RJ, Palmieri DC, Bronder JL, Stark AM, Steeg PS (2005) Breast cancer metastasis to the central nervous system. Am J Pathol. 167: 913–920.
[172] Lee YT. (1985) Patterns of metastasis and natural courses of breast carcinoma. Cancer Metastasis Rev. 4: 153–172.
[173] Johansson JE, Andrén O, Andersson SO, Dickman PW, Holmberg L, Magnuson A, et al. (2004) Natural history of early, localized prostate cancer. JAMA. 291: 2713–2719.
[174] Triozzi PL, Eng C, Singh,AD (2008) Targeted therapy for uveal melanoma. Cancer Treat. Rev. 34: 247–258.
[175] Nieto J, Grossbard ML, Kozuch P (2008) Metastatic pancreatic cancer 2008: is the glass less empty? Oncologist. 13: 562–576.
[176] Feld R, Rubinstein LV, Weisenberger TH (1984) Sites of recurrence in resected stage I non-small-cell lung cancer: a guide for future studies. J. Clin. Oncol. 2: 1352–1358.
[177] Aguirre-Ghiso JA (2007) Models, mechanisms and clinical evidence for cancer dormancy. Nat Rev Cancer. 7: 834–846.
[178] Weiss L (1992) Comments on hematogenous metastatic patterns in humans as revealed by autopsy. Clin Exp Metastasis 10: 191–199.
[179] Gassmann P, Haier J (2008) The tumor cell-host organ interface in the early onset of metastatic organ colonization. Clin. Exp. Metastasis. 25: 171–181.
[180] Barnholtz-Sloan JS, Sloan AE, Davis FG, Vigneau FD, Lai P, Sawaya RE (2004) Incidence proportions of brain metastases in patients diagnosed in the Metropolitan Detroit Cancer Surveillance System. J Clin Oncol. 22: 2865–2872.
[181] Delattre JY, Krol G, Thaler HT (1988) Distribution of brain metastases. Arch Neurol. 45: 741–744.
[182] Eichler AF, Kuter I, Ryan P, Schapira L, Younger J, Henson JW et al. (2008) Survival in patients with brain metastases from breast cancer: the importance of HER-2 status. Cancer. 112: 2359–2367.
[183] Kang Y, Siegel PM, Shu W, Drobnjak M, Kakonen SM, Cordon-Cardo C, et al. A multigenic program mediating breast cancer metastasis to bone. Cancer Cell. 3: 537–49.
[184] Roodman GD (2004) Mechanisms of bone metastasis. N Engl J Med. 350: 1655–64.
[185] Ibrahim T, Flamini E, Mercatali L, Sacanna E, Serra P, Amadori D (2010) Pathogenesis of osteoblastic bone metastases from prostate cancer. Cancer. 116: 1406–18.
[186] Bos PD, Zhang XH, Nadal C, Shu W, Gomis RR, Nguyen DX, et al. (2009) Genes that mediate breast cancer metastasis to the brain. Nature. 459: 1005-9.

[187] Hengel R, Sidhu G, Choi J, Weedon J, Nwokedi E, Axiotis CA, et al. (2012) Attributes of brain metastases from breast and lung cancer. Int J Clin Oncol. Mar 2.

[188] Lalor PF, Edwards S, McNab G, Salmi M, Jalkanen S, Adams DH (2002) Vascular adhesion protein-1 mediates adhesion and transmigration of lymphocytes on human hepatic endothelial cells. J Immunol. 169: 983-92.

Section 3

Animal Model Systems to Study Carcinogenesis

Chapter 10

Lobe-Specific Carcinogenesis in the Transgenic Adenocarcinoma of Mouse Prostate (TRAMP) Mouse Model

Jinhui Zhang, Lei Wang, Yong Zhang and Junxuan Lü

Additional information is available at the end of the chapter

http://dx.doi.org/10.5772/54904

1. Introduction

Prostate cancer (PCA) is the most commonly diagnosed cancer affecting men in many countries and it has been estimated that there would be 33, 000 deaths due to PCA in the United States in 2011 alone [1]. The standard chemotherapy for metastatic castration-resistant prostate cancer (CRPC) is the taxane anticancer drug docetaxel in combination with the steroid prednisone. In the past two years, autologous immunotherapy sipuleucel-T (Provenge), the new taxane drug cabazitaxel (Jevtana) and a P450 C17 inhibitor drug abiraterone acetate (Zytiga) were also approved by the US FDA (Food and Drug Administration) [2]. Unfortunately, those drugs can only offer limited survival benefit but have significant side effects that negatively affect the quality of life of the patients.

In contrast to chemotherapy, cancer chemoprevention uses naturally occurring or synthetic chemicals to block, delay or reverse carcinogenesis, progression and metastasis and is increasingly being recognized as essential for winning the war on PCA. Animal models are essential for development of effective chemoprevention. Currently, the mouse models used for PCA research include human xenograft models in immunocompromised mice, mouse prostate reconstitution models, transgenic models and single stem cell-based prostate regeneration (see a comprehensive review by Jeet *et al.* [3]). Considering the facts that PCA is a complex disease of uncertain etiology and multifocal phenotypic heterogeneity, a desirable model should recapitulate some critical features of human PCA: initiation of PCA with PIN (prostatic intraepithelial neoplasia), followed by progression to invasive adenocarcinoma, and subsequent metastasis with defined kinetics. Although no single model is perfect, transgenic models are widely used to delineate the mechanisms of prostate carcinogenesis and evaluate the chemopreventive efficacy of candidate agents because the lesions/cancers develop "naturally" *in situ* in the genetically engineered hosts and can be followed over a long time course [4].

2. TRAMP model represents at least two lineages of prostate carcinogenesis

The transgenic adenocarcinoma of mouse prostate (TRAMP) model was originally developed by Dr. Greenberg in 1995 [5]. It belongs to the first generation of models based on SV40 viral oncogenes [3]. In this TRAMP model, the rat probasin promoter (-426 to 28 bp) drives the expression of SV40 large T-antigen (T-Ag) and small t-antigen in the prostate. T-Ag abrogates P53 and Rb tumor suppressor proteins by direct binding. Simultaneously, small t-antigen interacts with protein phosphatase 2A [6] to regulate activity of the mitogen activated protein kinase activation pathway and the AP-1 transcription factor activity [7]. T-Ag and small t-antigen act spontaneously to propel the genesis of prostate epithelial lesions and malignant carcinomas and metastases. The TRAMP model is by far the most widely used PCA transgenic model for chemoprevention studies because of its simplicity in breeding compared to next generations of transgenic models based on deletions, insertions or mutations of mouse genes to mimic their changes in human PCA.

For more than one decade since its inception, the TRAMP model has been believed to represent a single lineage of epithelial lesion progression with well-defined kinetics and molecular marker alterations. The progression was thought to start from low and high grade PIN, to well-differentiated (WD) and moderately-differentiated (MD) adenocarcinoma in the dorsolateral prostate lobes (DLP) and finally by stoichastic phenotypic conversion, to poorly differentiated adenocarcinomas (PD-Ca) with lymph node and other distant metastases [8]. Many subsequent publications interpreted the histology results and molecular characterizations using such a paradigm.

However, several recent studies have suggested that the poorly-differentiated neuro-endocrine (NE)-like carcinomas (NECa) [9, 10] belonged to a distinct lineage from the epithelial lesions, which included low and high grade PIN, WD to MD "adenocarcinomas" of the original classification by Dr. Greenburg [8]. Those epithelial lesions were recently termed "atypical hyperplasias of T-Ag" (AHT) to distinguish from the human prostate cancer pathogenesis because they did not invade adjacent tissues [9]. In addition, the incidence of the NECa was found to be profoundly affected by the genetic background of the host mice [9]. In the C57BL/6 background, the lifetime incidence of NECa was estimated to be about 20% whereas in the FVB background, 87% NECa incidence was recorded by as early as 16 weeks of age and reached 100% by 20 weeks of age [9]. Furthermore, these NECa mostly arose in the ventral prostate (VP) lobes instead of the DLP in both strains [9, 10]. Tissue reconstitution experiments carried out by Chiaverotti *et al* indicated that NECa did not arise from the trans-differentiation of pre-existing AHT [9]. Tang *et al* reported that stress induced by anti-cancer treatments (castration and/or docetaxol) increased the incidence of NECa in TRAMP mice ((C57BL/6

x FVB) F1) [11]. However, the conclusion might be questionable since no mouse in the control group had NECa by the time of death, although they all developed adenocarcinoma in their prostates.

These findings significantly challenged the classical notion of single-lineage disease progression in the TRAMP DLP [8, 12]. Since the TRAMP model has been increasingly used for prostate cancer chemoprevention studies, it is very critical to further characterize the lobe-specificity of lesion lineages and NECa incidence in the prostate to consolidate the advantages of this model and minimize its limitations for both etiological and chemoprevention studies. To experimentally approach this, our group estimated the incidence of NECa based on 90 TRAMP mice in the C57BL/6 background spanning the age range of 16-50 weeks from several study cohorts [13-15]. We also characterized the histological features of different lineages of carcinogenesis in this model using archived tissue blocks from those studies [13-15]. In addition, by using state-of-the-art proteomics, we sought insights on mechanisms underlying carcinogenesis of different lineages and possible targets of chemopreventive reagents [15-17]. Here, we review our results as well as from other researchers' work to provide an objective analysis of the utility of this preclinical model for cancer chemoprevention studies.

3. Histological characteristics of prostate carcinogenesis in TRAMP model

In our studies, the female heterozygous C57BL/TGN TRAMP mice (line PB Tag 8247NG) were purchased from The Jackson Laboratory (Bar Harbor, ME), and were cross-bred with non-transgenic C57BL/6 males [13-15]. H&E and immuno-histological (IHC) staining were routinely performed in our lab and the results are summarized in Table 1 [15]. Figure 1a shows the H&E staining of representative morphological features of DLP and VP with micro NECa in TRAMP mice [15]. As can be seen in Figure 1b-1e, the AR-expressing glandular prostate epithelial lesions, which are now termed atypical hyperplasias of T-Ag (AHT), express nuclear T-Ag, epithelial membrane-staining of E-cadherin and are negative for synaptophysin (SYP), which is a neuroendocrine cell marker [15]. Staining of Ki67 (Figure1f), a proliferative index protein, showed a descending order of NE-Ca >> DLP AHT > VP epithelium. In the prostate from wild-type mice, single layer luminal epithelial cells were stained positive for nuclear AR, membrane E-cadherin with rare Ki-67 positive proliferating cells, while negative for T-Ag and SYP (Figure 2) [13-15]. In contrast, poorly-differentiated prostate carcinomas (PD) as classified by Greenberg [5] had distinct morphological features compared to AHT described above, regardless of the microscopic size found within the VP lobe (Figure 1, right panels) or those weighing over many grams [15]. Those lesions/tumors expressed strong T-Ag and SYP (except negative in trapped glandular epithelial islands), and were negative for AR and E-cadherin (except positive in the trapped glandular epithelial islands) [15].

We analyzed all tumors and prostates in our cohorts with the above panel of biomarkers. The incidence of macroscopic tumors (>1 gram) in TRAMP mice of 16-18, 22-24 and 26 weeks of age (WOA) were 10%, 20% and 30%, respectively. They were all poorly differentiated NECa expressing SYP [13, 15]. In another study, 31 C57BL/6 TRAMP mice in the control group (no chemo-preventive agents administrated) were followed up to 50 WOA. Ten large tumors traceable to the prostate were found (32.3%) and they were all SYP positive poorly differentiated NECa [13]. Overall, we observed that there was a trend for increasing detection of visible macroscopic NECa in TRAMP mice and the life-time NECa incidence rate was 1 out of 3 TRAMP mice from our experiments. This value was slightly higher than that reported by Chiaverotti (20%) [9]. The possible reason might be a smaller number of and younger C57BL/6 TRAMP mice used in their study [9].

We attempted to identify the anatomical origin of the NECa. Out of 18 NECa's in a cohort of 90 C57BL/6 TRAMP mice of 22 to 24 WOA, 12 were traceable to the VP (66.7%), two tiny tumors were traced to DLP (11.1%), whereas 1 large tumor was found in the anterior prostate (AP) (5.6%). The other three tumors were not traceable to any lobe location due to their overwhelming large sizes. These data were consistent with two recent studies showing a preponderance of SYP positive NECa arising from VP in the TRAMP mice of both C57BL/6 and FVB backgrounds [9, 10]. In contrast, the weight of macroscopic tumor-free VP lobes was only slightly increased in TRAMP mice compared to their wild type littermates at 24 WOA (Table 2 [15]), whereas the DLP lobes underwent significant expansion (more than doubled) in the TRAMP mice in one study where these lobes were compared side by side [14, 15].

The Greenberg group had reported the prevalence of seminal vesicles (SV) problems such as papillary fibroadenoma in the TRAMP mice with C57BL/6 background shortly after the strain was established [12, 18]. Later on, several publications also described the histogenesis and pathology of SV neoplasms in the TRAMP mice [19, 20]. In one long-term survival experiment carried out by our group [13], 54.8% (17 out of 31) TRAMP mice in the control group developed tumors in their SV and SV tumor loads became significantly increased beyond 30 WOA [13, 15]. Tani *et al* reported that most of the tumors contained phyllode lesions, which were typically composed of single layer epithelial linings that were negative for T-Ag, but positive for E-cadherin and AR staining and stromal cells that were neoplastic. These stromal cells frequently exhibited mitotic figures (BrdU incorporation) and SV40-TAg protein expression in the nuclei and were positive for desmin immuno-histological staining [19]. Since they did not observe conclusive evidence of malignancy such as invasion or metastasis, they recommended diagnosis of the SV tumors as epithelial–stromal tumors. The descriptions matched phyllodes-tumors in the C57B/6 TRAMP mice reported by Hsu *et al* [18]. However, in our long term studies, tumors/lesions were found in pelvic lymph nodes, liver, lung or kidney of mice without significantly increased prostate size but much enlarged SV in very rare cases (<5%), suggesting metastatic lesions from the SV tumors [13, 15]. Tables 1&2 summarize the expression of biomarkers (by immunohisto staining) and tumor incidence in different lineages of carcinogenesis in TRAMP mice [15].

Protein Biomarker	Wild type Prostrate	TRAMP AHT*	TRAMP NECa/Metastasis	TRAMP Seminal vesicle Epithelial-stromal tumors/Metastasis
T-Antigen	-	+++	+++	+
Androgen Receptor	++	+++	-	+
Synaptophysin	-	-	+++	-
E-cadherin	+++	+++	-	-/+
Ki-67 (MIB-1)	<1%	++	+++	++

*AHT-atypical hyperplasia of T-antigen of glandular epithelia

Table 1. Summary of Immunohistochemical Marker Expression in Prostate lesions and metastases in C57BL/6 TRAMP mice [15]

	Prostate lobes			
Prostate lobes	**Dorsolateral**	**Lobe uncertain***	**Ventral**	**Anterior**
Synaptophysin(+) NE carcinoma	2/18	3/18	12/18	1/18
# (%)	11.10%	16.70%	66.70%	5.60%
Average tumor weight	0.09	4.98	1.65	1.1
(Weight range), g	(0.07, 0.11)	(3.44, 4.38, 7.11)	(0.02- 4.84)	
TRAMP lobe weight at 24 weeks, mg	79.2±3.7 (n =17)**		15.3±1.1 (n=17)**	
Wild type lobe weight at 24 weeks, mg	31.7±2.9 (n=8)**		12.5±1.7 (n=8)**	
t-test	*p*<0.001		*p*>0.05	

*These 3 big tumors are hard to distinguish the exact originating sites.
**Presented as mean±SEM. t-test analysis between the TRAMP and wild type mice.

Table 2. Lobe specificity of NECa distribution in 90 TRAMP mice at ≤24 weeks of age (from different experiments) [15]

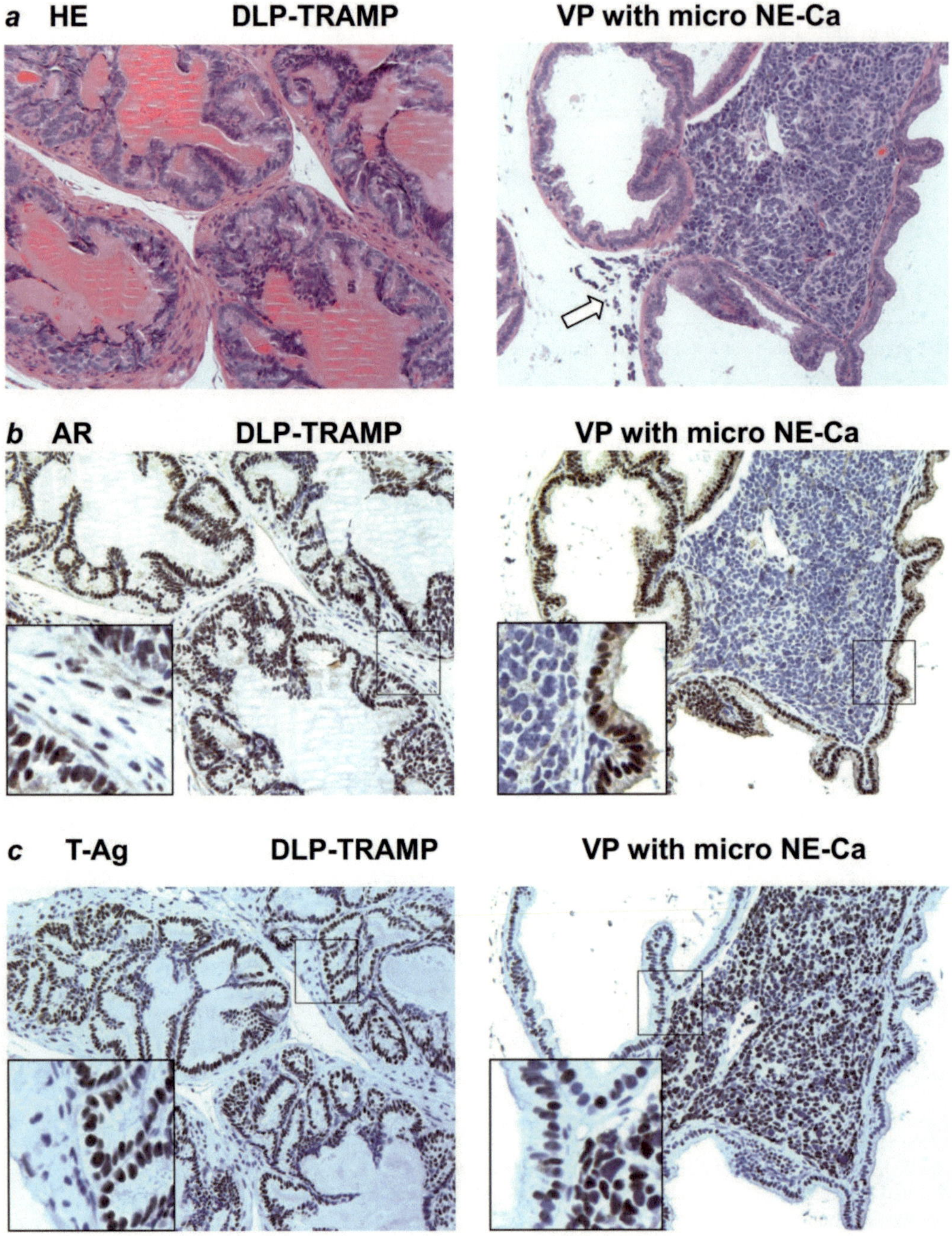
a HE
DLP-TRAMP
VP with micro NE-Ca
b AR
DLP-TRAMP
VP with micro NE-Ca
c T-Ag
DLP-TRAMP
VP with micro NE-Ca

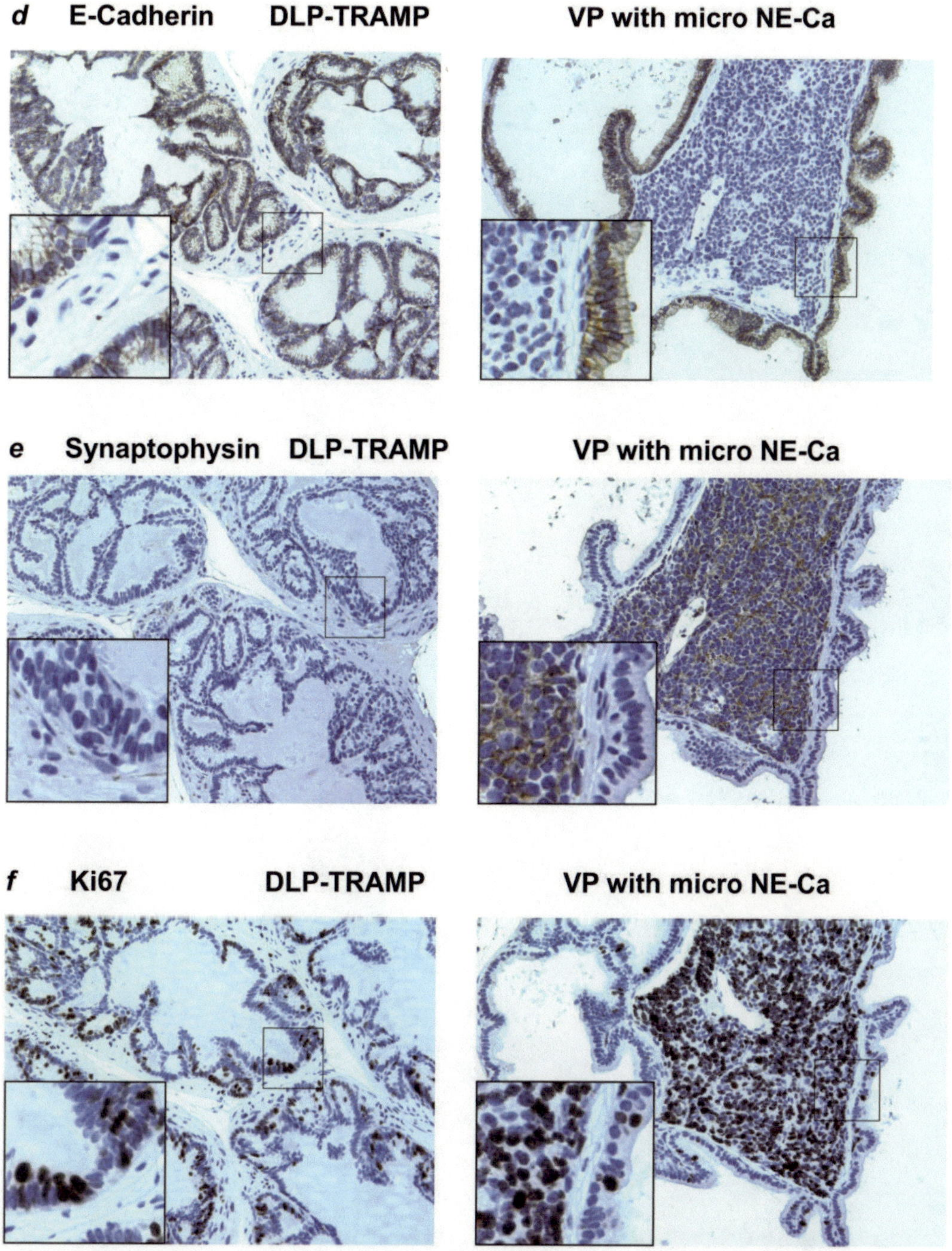

Figure 1. Immunohistochemical profiling of key protein markers in dorsal lateral (DLP) and ventral prostate (VP) with a microscopic neuroendocrine carcinoma (NECa) from a TRAMP B6 mouse. Serial sections were stained for hematoxylin and eosin (HE, a), androgen receptor (AR, b), SV40-T antigen (T-Ag, c), E-cadherin (d), synaptophysin (e) or Ki67 (Mib1) proliferation-associated protein (f). Magnification, 100x. Insets in panels show a higher magnification of staining patterns (400x) [15].

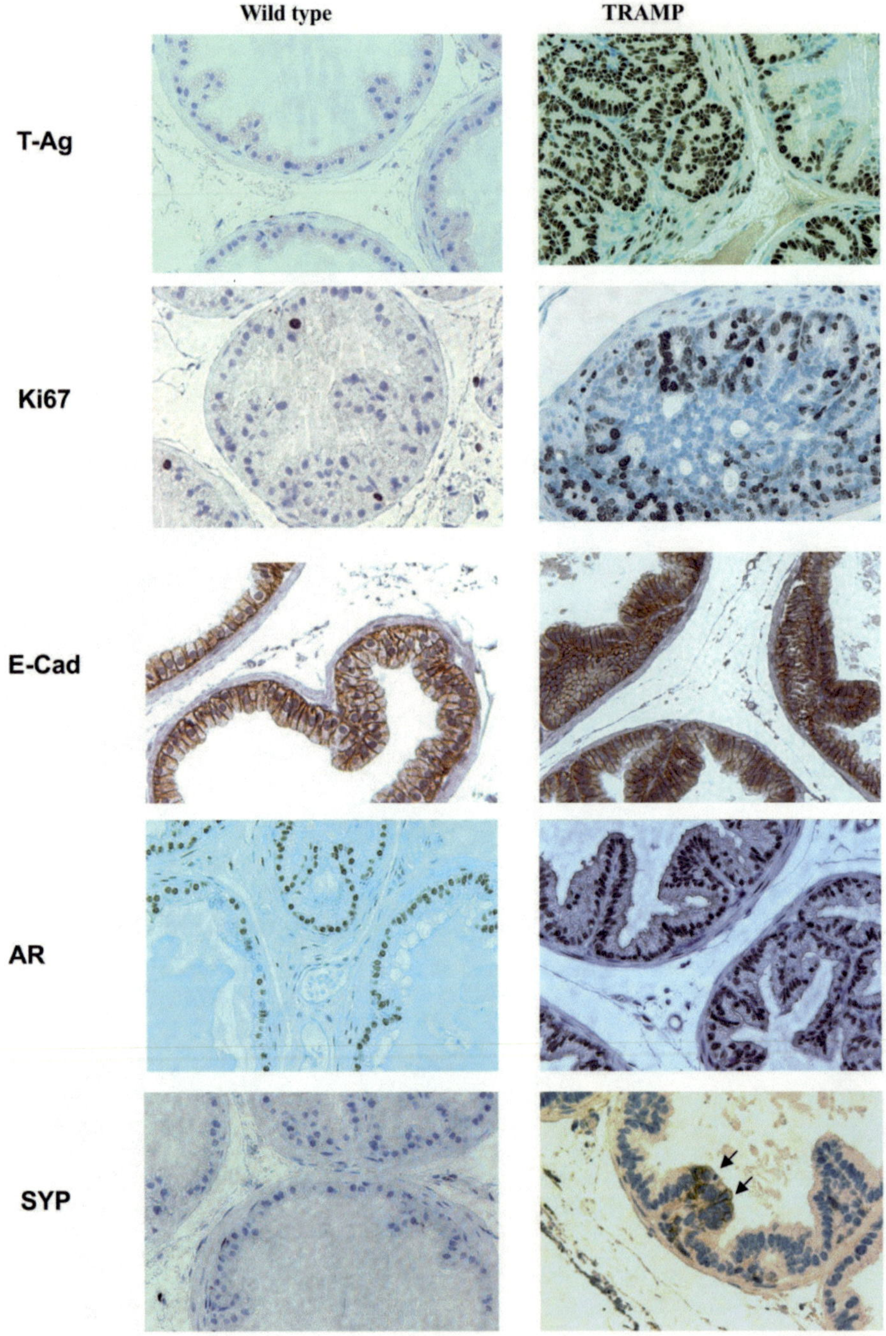

Figure 2. IHC staining patterns of wild type and TRAMP prostate for T-antigen (T-ag, nuclear), Ki67 proliferative antigen (nuclear), E-cadherin (E-Cad, cell membrane), and androgen receptor (AR, nuclear) and Synaptophysin (Syp, arrows point to representative positive NE-cells, cytosolic and cell membrane) [15].

4. Molecular changes in prostate carcinogenesis in TRAMP model

Classical methods detecting the steady levels of mRNAs and proteins, as well as "omics" approaches such as microarray, antibody array and two-dimension electrophoresis based proteomics have been used to study the molecular changes associated with TRAMP carcinogenesis using prostate or serum as starting materials. The Greenberg group reported increased expression of basic fibroblast growth factor (FGF2) in the prostates (whole prostate) of TRAMP mice ([C57BL/6 X FVB] F1) [21]. They found that the expression of the 25-kDa isoform of FGF2 was 2-fold higher in PIN and WD and MD tumors than in normal DLP and VP; the expression of the 22-kDa isoform of FGF2 was not elevated in PIN lesions, but was observed to be increased in WD, MD, PD and androgen-independent tumors. Interestingly, the 18-kDa isoform of FGF2 was only expressed in the samples representing PD and androgen-independent disease. These observations implicated specific changes in the FGF axis with the initiation and progression of PCA. The important role of FGF2 in PCA progression was further investigated in an *in vivo* study [22]. In that study, TRAMP mice (C57BL/6 background) were crossed with FGF2 knockout (*FGF2*$^{-/-}$, SV129 background) mice, and tumor progression in TRAMP mice that were either hemi- or homozygous for inactivation of the *FGF2* allele was compared with wild-type TRAMP mice. They found that even inactivation of one *FGF2* allele resulted in increased survival, less PD phenotype in primary tumors and a decrease in metastasis [22]. Later on, Agarwal's group reported that the chemopreventive effect of dietary silibinin against TRAMP carcinogenesis (C57BL/6 background) was accompanied with a decreased plasma FGF2 level [23]. The observation further suggested FGF2 as a target for chemoprevention of PCA. Similarly, the roles of ERKs, EGFR, NF-κB, clusterin, cyclins, insulin-like growth factor-I (IGF-I), DNMTs and other molecular pathways in the TRAMP carcinogenesis have also been reported by different groups [24-30].

Considering extracellular proteolysis as an important biochemical event in the invasion and metastasis of PCA, Bok *et al* studied the expression of matrix metalloproteases (MMP) and other related proteins in TRAMP mice (C57BL6/FVB mix) using gelatin zymography [31]. In their study, distinct lobes of the prostate (ventral, lateral, dorsal and anterior), seminal vesicles, as well as lymph nodes (LN) with metastases were isolated by micro-dissection if possible. They found increased expression of mainly pro-MMP 9 and pro-MMP2 in early TRAMP tumors, but substantial elevation of activated MMP9 and MMP2 only in late TRAMP tumors. In addition, they found a progressive increase in the activities of cysteine, serine and certain membrane-bound proteases (cathepsin B, MT-SP1, MT1-MMP) from normal to advanced prostate tumors. Interestingly, a gradual decrease in urokinase plasminogen activator (uPA) expression with tumor progression was also observed. Overall, the study suggested proteases as potential targets for the therapy and secondary prevention of PCA. Ruddat *et al* profiled the proteome of TRAMP ([C57BL/6TRAMPx-FVB] F1) prostate by 2-D electrophoresis followed by peptide identification by MALDI-TOF [32]. In their study, the WD dorsal prostate (from mice approximately 14 WOA) was compared with normal dorsal prostate tissue. The prostates from mice approximately 25 WOA with PD CA were not further dissected since it is not practical to differentiate the lobes in an advanced stage. The data revealed that there were few significant changes in the protein abundances in the WD dorsal prostates compared to wild-type dorsal prostates, with the exception of increases in proliferating cell nuclear antigen (PCNA) and beta tubulin, two proteins implicated in cell proliferation, and a more than 2-fold increase in an anti-apoptotic protein Hsp60. In contrast, there were substantial changes in protein abundance in the PD tumors compared to wild-type dorsal prostates. While some of those changes could be related to the disappearance of stromal tissue such as decreased expression of myosin light chain alkali, desmin and tropomyosin beta 2, the most notable was the overall decrease in calcium homeostasis proteins such as calreticulin and Hsp70 (10-fold decrease) and creatine kinase bb (40-fold decrease) in the cancerous tissue. The expression patterns of desmin, Hsp70 and calreticulin were further confirmed by Western blot. Although some of their results have been cross-validated by us (e.g. down-regulation of calreticulin and tropomyosin beta 2, to be discussed later) [16, 17], many of these changes could be due to the differences between the cells in the two different carcinogenesis lineages rather than the purported changes due to progression of diseases of the Greenberg paradigm.

Using Affymetrix GeneChip Mouse Genome 430 2.0 micorarrays, Haram *et al* profiled the mRNAs from eight TRAMP (C57BL/6 background, 30±4 WOA)) tumors and DLP or VP of nine wild-type mice [33]. Statistical analysis indicated that 3,870 transcripts such as cyclin A2, cyclin B1, cyclin B2, cyclin E1, cyclin E2, cyclin F, Forkhead box M1, Aurora Kinase A and B were up-regulated in TRAMP tumors and 2,945 transcripts such as cyclin D2 and probasin were down-regulated in TRAMP tumors. Real-time RT-PCR confirmed the expression of the 11 genes mentioned above. In each real-time PCR experiment, three to four normal samples (typically one dorsolateral and three ventral) and four tumors (the same four tumor samples in every experiment) were used. Moreover, cross-referencing differentially expressed TRAMP genes to public human prostate array datasets revealed 66 genes with concordant expression in mouse and human PCA. Among the 66 genes, Sox4 and Tubb2a, which were reported to be up-regulated in primary PCA compared to normal prostates, were further validated by real-time RT-PCR. In addition to providing information regarding the mechanisms of TRAMP carcinogenesis, the concordance analysis between TRAMP and human PCA associated genes also supported the utility of the model. In another study, Morgenbesser *et al* studied the dynamic changes of mRNA profiles in TRAMP ([C57BL/6 TRAMP x FVB] F1) mice, especially the genes involved in the acquisition of androgen-independent and metastatic tumor growth, using both microarray and SAGE approaches [34]. The following cohorts were used in their study: C18 (prostates from wild-type mice at 18 WOA); C24 (prostates from wild-type mice at 24 WOA); T12 and T18 were prostates from TRAMP mice at 12 and 18 WOA representing PIN and MD stages of disease, respectively; T24 were PD, androgen-dependent (AD) primary tumors from TRAMP mice at 24 WOA whereas T(12)24 were PD, androgen-independent (AI) primary tumors from 24-week-old TRAMP mice that were castrated at 12 WOA. In their paper, differentially expressed genes between AD tumors and normal prostates, AI tumors and normal prostates, as well as AD and AI tumors were presented. The dynamic changes of ten transcripts (e.g. tissue inhibitor of metalloproteinase 4, GATA-binding protein 2, ER-resident protein ERdj5, paralemmin, MYC-associated zinc finger protein) over the progress of

TRAMP carcinogenesis were further validated by real-time RT-PCR. Their analyses uncovered many transcripts that had not previously been implicated in PCA progression, especially in the transition from androgen-dependent to androgen-independent status. Again, these studies were conducted under the Greenberg paradigm of single lineage disease progression. Many of these changes could be due to the differences between the cells in the two different carcinogenesis lineages rather than the purported changes due to progression of the disease.

Therefore, it will be prudent to carefully read the descriptions of the tissue samples used in the published papers. For example, many older publications prepared lysate from the whole prostate whereas very few focused on particular lobes [24, 31, 32]. Recently, researchers started to carefully look into the molecular pathways involved in two lineages of carcinogenesis (different prostate lobes, mainly DLP and VP) in TRAMP mice after the lineage differences of the prostate carcinogenesis had been recognized [9, 13]. For instance, Slack-Davis *et al* studied the requirement for focal adhesion kinase (FAK) signaling in cancer progression in TRAMP mice with C57BL/6 background [35]. They found that loss of FAK or its inhibition with PF-562271 (small molecular inhibitor for FAK) did not alter the progression to AHT. However, continued FAK expression (and activity) is essential for the androgen-independent formation of NECa.

Our group [15] dissected prostate lobes and visible tumors separately in most of our experiments in order to assess the lobe-specific biochemical changes. Using these dissected lobes/tumors as starting materials, we studied the expression of classical biomarkers by immuno-blot. The expression patterns of proliferative cell nuclear antigen (PCNA) (Figure 3a) confirmed the Ki67 staining patterns by IHC staining described above [15]. Consistent with the lack of proliferation of normal prostate epithelium, PCNA was non-detectable in the DLP and VP in the wild type mice at 16-18 WOA, whereas significantly higher levels of PCNA were detected in the DLP and VP and NECa of TRAMP mice. Since the Ki67 proliferation index in the VP epithelium appeared to be lower than in TRAMP DLP as evidenced by IHC (Figure 1f), the higher level of PCNA in TRAMP VP (Figure 3b) than in DLP might be due to the presence of micro NECa foci in the TRAMP VP lobes (NECa has much higher Ki67 index, Figure 1f) [15]. We also confirmed the contrasting patterns of AR, SYP and E-cadherin expression patterns in the DLP AHT vs. NECa. Although the expression of AR and E-cadherin were increased in both DLP and VP in TRAMP mice at 16-18 WOA, there were more AR and E-cadherin in VP than in DLP of littermate wild type mice (Figure 3b) [15]. These patterns are in agreement with that published by the Greenberg group [8, 12] and others [9]. In addition, we found that the level of cleaved PARP (endogenous substrate for caspase 3) was higher in the NECa than in the DLPs of TRAMP and wild type mice (Figure 3a). The STAT3 level in TRAMP DLP was higher than in the wild type DLP and the NECa. However, there might be an isoform of STAT3 with higher molecular weight in the NECa, indicated by a mobility-retarded band (Figure 3a, arrow) [15]. Our observation was consistent with phosphorylative modification and activation of STAT3 in NECa, as reported by Aziz *et al* [36]. The changes of these biomarkers further support molecular differences between NECa and DLP AHT.

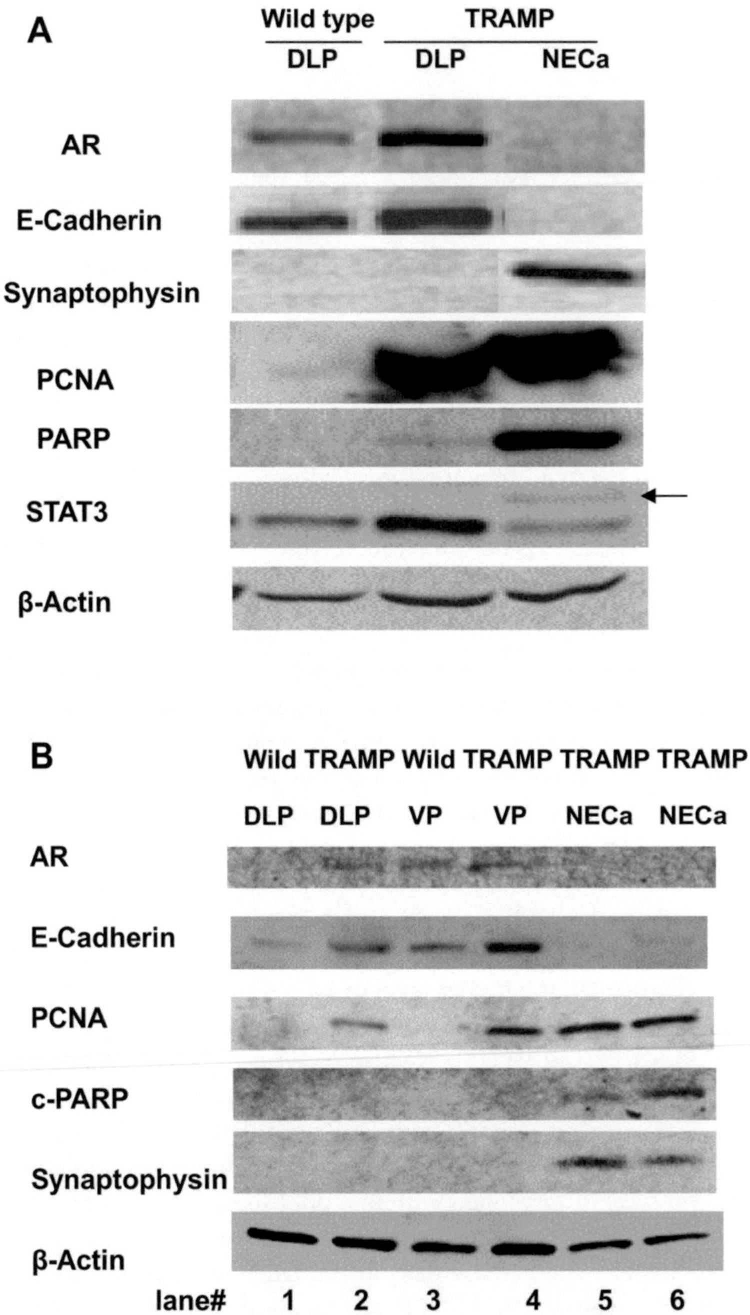

Figure 3. Western blot analyses of protein biomarkers in (A) wild type mouse prostate and in TRAMP DLP (DLP) and in NE-Carcinomas (NECa); in (B) DLP and VP of wild type and TRAMP mice at 16-18 WOA. AR, androgen receptor; PCNA, proliferating cell nuclear antigen; PARP, polyADPribose polymerase; STAT3, signal transduction and activator of transcription-3. Arrow marks mobility retarded STAT3 that is likely phosphorylated [15].

To provide more information on potential molecular correlates of the differences in DLP and VP for epithelial lesions and NE-carcinogenesis, we compared the expression level of proteins in respective lobes of wild type vs. TRAMP mice of 18 WOA by the iTRAQ proteomic approach, as we recently reported [16, 17]. We employed two-dimensional liquid chromatography coupled with tandem mass spectrometry (2D-LC-MS/MS) with iTRAQ labeling, which enables the concurrent identification and quantification of proteins through peptides generated upon tryptic digestion. The principle and advantages of the platform have been described in our previous publications [16, 17, 37]. In total, we identified 1068 proteins expressed in the DLP and VP of TRAMP mice and wild type mice. Among them, 483 and 748 proteins were identified at FDRs of 1% and 5% respectively. We found that the expression levels of 84 proteins were different between DLP and VP in wild-type mice [17]. For example, heat shock protein 5/glucose-regulated protein78 (GRP78), transglutaminase 4 (TGM4), experimental autoimmune prostatitis antigen 2 (EAPA2), probasin, beta-tropomyosin, calponin-1, as well as high mobility group box 1 & 2 were preferentially expressed in DLP, whereas there were higher levels of prostatic spermine-binding protein (SBP), serine peptidase inhibitor Kazal type 3 (SPINK3), polymeric immunoglobulin receptor (PIGR), solute carrier family 12 member 2, epidermal growth factor (EGF) and clusterin in the VP lobe. The expression pattern of GRP78 and clusterin were validated by immuno-blots [17]. The mRNA abundances of prostatic proteins in each lobe of mice or rats have been investigated by Fujimoto *et al* and Berquin *et al* using PCR and microarray, respectively [38-40]. Our results not only agreed with theirs but also extended to more lobe specific proteins. Importantly, we found that different sets of proteins were involved in lobe specific carcinogenesis in TRAMP mice. The expression levels of 118 proteins were significantly altered in DLP and/or VP during TRAMP carcinogenesis. 55 and 36 proteins were uniquely changed in DLP or VP respectively and only 27 proteins were found to be significantly modulated in both lobes during TRAMP carcinogenesis [17]. The majority (24 out of 27 proteins) shared the same trend, albeit the extent of change was not exactly the same. Shared changes in DLP and VP might indicate possible common molecular events associated with carcinogenesis such as elevated proliferation (e.g. up regulation of HMGB1&2 and nuclear proteins such as histone(s)), oxidative stress (e.g. decreased antioxidant enzyme PRDX6) and disruption of stroma (e.g. down-regulation of SMMHC (myosin-11) and calponin-1) [17]. The three proteins, namely clusterin, polymeric immunoglobulin receptor and aldose reductase, which were differentially expressed in DLP versus VP, were more likely related to lobe-specific mechanisms of carcinogenesis. Interestingly, although some of prostatic proteins had been reported to be regulated by androgen signaling [38], EAPA2 and calreticulin were down-regulated in DLP whereas zinc-alpha-2-glycoprotein was only down-regulated in VP during carcinogenesis. These observations suggested that AR signaling could play different roles in carcinogenesis of different lobes of TRAMP mice.

To shed light on the key expression signatures or "master switches" that may not be virtually identified due to technical limitation, we analyzed the lists of differentially expressed proteins in each lobe by IPA software for pathway connections based on gene ontogeny and functionality [17]. Proteins with altered expression in DLP during carcinogenesis were preferentially clustered into Immunological Disease/Cancer/Antigen Presentation and Post-Translational Modification/Protein Folding/Cancer networks. 14-3-3 zeta/delta (YWHAZ, up-regulated only in DLP), NF-κB, epidermal growth factor (EGF, up-regulated only in DLP), ERK1/2, PKCs were identified as distinct inferred network nodes for those networks. On the other hand, proteins with altered expression in VP were mapped to Connective Tissue Disorders/Developmental Disorder/Genetic Disorder and Cancer/Cell Cycle/Cellular Development pathways with ERK1/2 and FGF2 identified as distinct network nodes in the two networks. We further used immunoblot to study the expression pattern of FGF2 proteins, which were not identified by LC-MS/MS but unraveled by IPA analysis as important proteins in the TRAMP carcinogenesis of the VP lobe. The data indicated that different isoforms of FGF2 were expressed in each lobe and FGF2 was only up-regulated in the VP lobe of TRAMP mice [17]. To our knowledge, we are the first to systematically compare the different protein profile changes between DLP and VP lobes during TRAMP carcinogenesis. Our results further support the concept that the C57BL/6 TRAMP mouse represents two lineages of prostate carcinogenesis in DLP and VP lobes. Further efforts to narrow down possible target proteins and investigation on the functional significance of those proteins will not only help understand the mechanisms of TRAMP carcinogenesis, but also facilitate the understanding and use of TRAMP model in the field of prostate cancer chemoprevention.

5. Effects of chemopreventive agents on prostate carcinogenesis in TRAMP model and possible mechanisms

Because the breeding strategy of TRAMP mice is straightforward, TRAMP mice have been widely used in evaluating potential preventive modalities by many groups in the past decade. Besides the effect of androgen deprivation therapy (ADT) on the progression of PCA by surgical castration of TRAMP mice [41, 42], the effects of many agents with chemo-preventive potential including green tea [26, 43], NSAIDs [44, 45], flutamide [46], retinoic acid [47], vitamin E analog [48], genistein [24, 49], epigallocatechin-3-gallate (EGCG) [50], silibinin [23, 51], dietary restriction [52] and immunotherapy [53, 54], have been studied using this model. While most of the publications reported anti-cancer effects of their test compounds, El Touny *et al* showed that feeding TRAMP mice (TRAMP-FVB) with a diet containing 0.25% genistein from 12 to 20 WOA induced an aggressive progression of PCA, as evidenced by a 16% increase in the number of WD and PD prostates, coinciding with a 70% incidence of pelvic lymph node metastases as opposed to 0% in the control group [49].

The recognition of different lineages of carcinogenesis in the TRAMP prostate has important implications on the interpretation of chemoprevention data. Due to the distinct characteristics of AHT in DLP and NECa in VP, their sensitivity to different chemo-preventive agents might not be the same. Knowledge of lineage-specific effects of each agent will be essential for selecting additional models to confirm the efficacy and to ultimately benefit clinical translation studies. In addition, it can provide valuable insights into mechanism studies for molecular pathway(s) and targets specific to the particular lineage of carcinogenesis. Using this paradigm, our group evaluated the chemopreventive efficacy of next-generation selenium compounds methylseleninic acid (MSeA) and methylselenocysteine (MSeC) in TRAMP mice with C57BL/6 background [13]. In a short-term experiment, TRAMP mice of 8 WOA were given an oral dose of MSeA or MSeC at 3 mg Se/kg daily and were euthanized at either 18 or 26 WOA. By 18 WOA, the genitourinary tract and DLP weights for both treatment groups were lower than for the control ($p< 0.01$). At 26 weeks, 4 of 10 control mice had genitourinary weight >2 g whereas only 1 of 10 in each of the treatmente groups did. The efficacy was accompanied by delayed lesion progression, increased apoptosis, and decreased proliferation without appreciable changes of T-antigen expression in the DLP. In another experiment, giving MSeA to TRAMP mice from 10 or 16 WOA increased their survival to 50 weeks of age and delayed the death due to SYP-positive NECa, SYP-negative prostate lesions and seminal vesicle hypertrophy [13]. Interestingly, although MSeA and MSeC were considered as precursors of methylselenol, the proteins they modulated in the DLP of TRAMP mice were quite different as indicated by proteomic profiling. The data suggest that MSeA and MSeC should be developed as separate agents rather than as equal precursors of methylselenol [16]. Very recently, our group also demonstrated that oral administration of the alcoholic extract of *Angelica gigas* (AGN), a traditional Korean herb, had strong inhibitory effect on two lineages of carcinogenesis in TRAMP mice, especially the NECa [55, 56]. In contrast to the examples of MSeA, MSeC and AGN described above, we also published a lack of efficacy of a novel sulindac derivative sulindac sulfide amide (SSA) against NECa, whereas it exerted a significant protection against the DLP epithelial lesions [14]. Consistent with the fact that NECa originated from VP independently of AR, suppressing AR signaling in DLP was one of the important mechanisms underlying the chemopreventive effect of SSA, both *in vivo* and *in vitro* [14]. Similar to our strategy, Harper *et al* gave TRAMP mice (C57BL/6) water containing 0.06% EGCG starting at 5 WOA and dissected DLP and VP carefully when mice were euthanized at 12 WOA [50]. They found that EGCG significantly reduced the incidence of HG-PIN (Grade 3) from 100% to 17% in the VP of TRAMP mice but did not have a protective effect in DLP. At 28 WOA, it was difficult to dissect DLP and VP separately and EGCG did not have any inhibitory effect against TRAMP carcinogenesis in general.

As mentioned above, the life-time NECa incidence has been estimated to be approximately 30% in TRAMP mice with C57BL/6 background. Rest of the mice will be free of NECa and may therefore model the epithelial lineage lesions that are more relevant to the human prostate epithelial adeno-carcinogenesis, since the majority of human PCA are adenocarcinomas.

On the other hand, NECa occurs in nearly 100% of the TRAMP mice in the FVB background and the DLP undergoes more epithelial lesion growth than does the VP [9, 12]. This might have contributed to the assumption that a single lineage of carcinogenesis progressed from DLP epithelial lesions to poorly differentiated Ca (i.e., NECa) by the Greenberg group. Based on the current information, the C57BL/6 background will be a preferred choice over the FVB background for chemoprevention studies since the former allows a clear separation of estimation of the impact of the test agents on both lineages of lesions in the prostate, provided that the studies are terminated before SV tumors in the C57BL/6 TRAMP mice become a serious complication to survival.

Since many studies had followed the Greenberg paradigm for interpretation of their results, it will be prudent to carefully look into the genetic background of TRAMP mice, the manner with which prostate/tumors were collected and the end point(s) chosen to evaluate the efficacy. Some of the studies as shown below could be questionable in term of the conclusions. In the study by Adhami *et al* [43], TRAMP mice (C57BL/6 background) were given water containing 0.1% green tea polyphenols (GTP) starting at ages representing different stage of the disease: 6 WOA (normal prostate), 12 WOA (PIN), 18 WOA (WD) and 28 WOA (MD). Follow-up monitoring showed that the earlier the treatment started, the greater was tumor-free survival extended. The mean genitourinary weights showed the same trends. IGF-I and its downstream targets including phosphatidylinositol 3-kinase and pAkt were significantly inhibited only when GTP treatment was initiated no later than 18WOA. In another study, TRAMP mice (C57BL/6 background) starting at 4, 12, 20, and 30 WOA were fed with control or 1% silibinin supplemented diet for 8 to 15 weeks [51]. In general, silibinin feeding inhibited neoplastic progression of the prostate in TRAMP mice at various stages. For the most part, the tumor stage at onset time of treatment determined the mechanisms for silibinin's efficacy. Silibinin treatment during the early stages of prostate tumor development in TRAMP mice inhibited the progression at PIN stage *via* anti-proliferation. When the mice were burdened with higher stage lesions, silibinin significantly delayed the progression of the disease *via* both anti-proliferative and anti-angiogenesis mechanisms. Anti-angiogenesis, along with inhibition of epithelial-mesenchymal transition (EMT) *via* decreasing the expression of MMPs, snail-1, and fibronectin, as well as increasing E-cadherin expression levels might also contribute to the anti-metastatic effect of silibinin. Studies aiming to define the "stage-specific" efficacy and mechanisms of chemoprevention are very crucial for the identification of *in vivo* targets mediating the chemopreventive effect of corresponding agents. In addition, the information will be very important to select the right indications for clinical trials.

6. The concept of cancer stem cells in TRAMP model

The concept of cancer stem cells (CSC) or tumor-initiating cells assumes that cancers are mainly sustained by a small pool of neoplastic cells, which are responsible for cancer initiation and/or progression. Although currently no single protein is widely accepted as a definitive stem cell marker in the prostate, investigations using *in vitro* and *in vivo* models, especially tissue recombination strategies, reveal a multifaceted nature of stem cells for prostate cancer and highlight the importance of targeting cancer stem cells in the therapy and prevention of prostate cancer [57-59]. The role of "cancer stem cells" in TRAMP carcinogenesis has received some attention. Chiaverotti *et al* observed an increased frequency of neuroendocrine precursor lesions in TRAMP mice with FVB background as early as 4 WOA [9]. Some of these lesions exhibited properties of bi-potential stem cells as evidenced by co-expressing the transcriptional factors Foxa1 and Foxa2, and markers of epithelium (E-cadherin) and neuroendocrine (SYP). In their proposed model of two lineages of carcinogenesis [9], a pluripotent stem cell of the normal prostate is transformed by SV40 Tag expression and starts to proliferate. Initially these proliferative foci maintain a transitional epithelial/NE phenotype co-expressing E-cadherin, SYP, as well as Foxa1 and Foxa2. These bipotential cells continue to proliferate, undergo full NE differentiation with loss of E-cadherin and then progress to an overt NECa. On the other hand, luminal cells of the normal prostate proliferate and form focal areas of hyperplasia after transformed by SV40 Tag expression. These foci expand to the entire glandular lumen and end up with AHT but do not invade the surrounding stroma and do not metastasize.

Huss *et al* reported the expression and function of a breast cancer resistance protein (BCRP/ABCG2) in putative prostate stem cells and prostate tumor stem cells in several models including TRAMP mice (C57BL/6 TRAMP X FVB F1) [60]. BCRP is a member of the ATP-binding cassette (ABC) transporter family and expressed consistently by adult stem cell populations that possess pluripotentiality and long-term repopulation capability. IHC staining indicated that the BCRP+ putative tumor stem cells were localized to foci of AR- cells in glands of VP, where the greatest number of NECa would arise after castration. The AR- foci that contained the BCRP+ cells were preexisting and not induced by androgen deprivation since the frequency of BCRP+ cells was similar in intact (2.0%) and castrated (1.8%) TRAMP mice (between 1 and 14 days post-castration). In TRAMP mice, BCRP+/AR- cells behaved as label-retaining cells, a stem cell characteristic. The role of BCRP+ putative tumor stem cells as the nidus of NECa was further supported by the fact that NECa harvested from castrated TRAMP mice contained large focal areas of proliferating, BCRP+/AR-/SYP+ cells. BCRP-mediated efflux of androgen might be one of the mechanisms for maintenance of the prostate stem cell phenotype since it might be associated with their insensitivity to androgen-mediated differentiation and androgen deprivation–induced apoptotic cell death.

ADT was reported to result in a state of androgen independence with more malignant behavior in TRAMP mice [41]. Whether certain types of "cancer stem cells" were activated during or after castration awaits further investigation. Recently, Tang *et al* studied the effect of surgical castration on the expression of stem cell markers in the prostates of TRAMP mice [61]. They castrated TRAMP mice (genetic background not specified) at 12 WOA and dissected the DLP lobes at two time-points: 10 weeks (Cas-10; n=12) and 20 weeks (Cas-20; n=9) after castration. They found that stem cell markers Sca-1 (stem cell antigen-1), CD133 and c-Kit (CD117) were overexpressed in the luminal cells of the Cas-10 group, but not in the Cas-20 group. Immuno-blots showed that the expression of bcl-2 and GRP78 were significantly higher in the DLP from the Cas-10 compared to that from the Cas-20 group. Using anti-Sca-1 antibody conjugated magnetic beads, they estimated the abundance of Sca-1 positive cells in the cell suspension prepared by digesting the DLP lobes with collagenase/hyaluronidase/DNase I. They found that the abundance of Sca-1 cells was more than 3 times higher in the TRAMP Cas-10 group than in wild-type mice at 12WOA. However, it was dramatically lower in the TRAMP Cas-20 group, which was consistent with the IHC data. Although their work described the dynamic expression of certain stem cell markers during TRAMP carcinogenesis in DLP, the information is too preliminary to draw any conclusion on the effect of castration on "cancer stem cells" in TRAMP mice.

In one recently published paper [15], our group compared different treatment regimens with MSeA on TRAMP mice (C57BL/6) to investigate whether MSeA could irreversibly inhibit early events in TRAMP carcinogenesis (e.g. activation of "cancer stem cells"). MSeA exposure to TRAMP mice (C57BL/6) from 5 to 15 WOA was sufficient to elicit protective effects against the two lineages of carcinogenesis to the same extent as continuous MSeA exposure from 5 to 23 WOA [15]. Similar findings in a chemically-induced mammary carcinogenesis model was reported by Ip *et al* [62], in which selenium-enriched garlic given for 1-month duration right after a single carcinogen exposure was as effective as when it was provided throughout the 6-month post-initiation period of the study. Those data suggested a possibility that MSeA treatment during the initiation stage of carcinogenesis permanently inactivated early critical initiated ("cancer stem") cells in both lineages. The potential mechanisms of inactivation of "cancer stem cells" by MSeA might be apoptosis, which is consistent with the pro-apoptotic effect of MSeA and MSeC in TRAMP DLP reported previously [13], or another lasting epigenetic modification.

7. Conclusion

The paradigm of distinct lineages of carcinogenesis in the TRAMP model and our data with MSeA, a sulindac derivative compound and AGN extract shed new light on the utility of this preclinical model for chemoprevention studies in spite of much concern regarding of the NE nature of the resultant carcinomas and metastasis. Future data collection and analyses should incorporate this new knowledge for efficacy assessment and for molecular target validations, avoiding "apple versus orange" comparisons.

Author details

Jinhui Zhang*, Lei Wang, Yong Zhang and Junxuan Lü*
Department of Biomedical Sciences, School of Pharmacy, Texas Tech University Health Sciences Center, Amarillo, TX, USA

8. References

[1] Siegel R, Ward E, Brawley O, Jemal A. (2011) Cancer statistics, 2011: the impact of eliminating socioeconomic and racial disparities on premature cancer deaths. CA: a cancer journal for clinicians 61(4):212-236.

* Corresponding Authors

[2] Logothetis CJ, Efstathiou E, Manuguid F, Kirkpatrick P. (2011) Abiraterone acetate. Nature Reviews Drug Discovery 10(8):573-574.

[3] Jeet V, Russell PJ, Khatri A. (2010) Modeling prostate cancer: a perspective on transgenic mouse models. Cancer Metastasis Reviews 29(1):123-142.

[4] Teicher BA. (2006) Tumor models for efficacy determination. Molecular Cancer Therapeutics 5(10):2435-2443.

[5] Greenberg NM, DeMayo F, Finegold MJ, Medina D, Tilley WD, Aspinall JO, Cunha GR, Donjacour AA, Matusik RJ, Rosen JM. (1995) Prostate cancer in a transgenic mouse. Proceedings of the National Academy of Sciences of the United States of America 92(8):3439-3443.

[6] Pallas DC, Shahrik LK, Martin BL, Jaspers S, Miller TB, Brautigan DL, Roberts TM. (1990) Polyoma small and middle T antigens and SV40 small t antigen form stable complexes with protein phosphatase 2A. Cell 60(1):167-176.

[7] Frost JA, Alberts AS, Sontag E, Guan K, Mumby MC, Feramisco JR. (1994) Simian virus 40 small t antigen cooperates with mitogen-activated kinases to stimulate AP-1 activity. Molecular and Cellular Biology 14(9):6244-6252.

[8] Kaplan-Lefko PJ, Chen TM, Ittmann MM, Barrios RJ, Ayala GE, Huss WJ, Maddison LA, Foster BA, Greenberg NM. (2003) Pathobiology of autochthonous prostate cancer in a pre-clinical transgenic mouse model. Prostate 55(3):219-237.

[9] Chiaverotti T, Couto SS, Donjacour A, Mao JH, Nagase H, Cardiff RD, Cunha GR, Balmain A. (2008) Dissociation of epithelial and neuroendocrine carcinoma lineages in the transgenic adenocarcinoma of mouse prostate model of prostate cancer. The American Journal of Pathology 172(1):236-246.

[10] Huss WJ, Gray DR, Tavakoli K, Marmillion ME, Durham LE, Johnson MA, Greenberg NM, Smith GJ. (2007) Origin of androgen-insensitive poorly differentiated tumors in the transgenic adenocarcinoma of mouse prostate model. Neoplasia 9(11):938-950.

[11] Tang Y, Wang L, Goloubeva O, Khan MA, Lee D, Hussain A. (2009) The relationship of neuroendocrine carcinomas to anti-tumor therapies in TRAMP mice. Prostate 69(16):1763-1773.

[12] Gingrich JR, Barrios RJ, Foster BA, Greenberg NM. (1999) Pathologic progression of autochthonous prostate cancer in the TRAMP model. Prostate Cancer and Prostatic Diseases 2(2):70-75.

[13] Wang L, Bonorden MJ, Li GX, Lee HJ, Hu H, Zhang Y, Liao JD, Cleary MP, Lu J. (2009) Methyl-selenium compounds inhibit prostate carcinogenesis in the transgenic adenocarcinoma of mouse prostate model with survival benefit. Cancer Prevention Research 2(5):484-495.

[14] Zhang Y, Zhang J, Wang L, Quealy E, Gary BD, Reynolds RC, Piazza GA, Lu J. (2010) A novel sulindac derivative lacking cyclooxygenase-inhibitory activities suppresses carcinogenesis in the transgenic adenocarcinoma of mouse prostate model. Cancer Prevention Research 3(7):885-895.

[15] Wang L, Zhang J, Zhang Y, Nkhata K, Quealy E, Liao JD, Cleary MP, Lu J. (2011) Lobe-specific lineages of carcinogenesis in the transgenic adenocarcinoma of mouse prostate and their responses to chemopreventive selenium. Prostate 71(13):1429-1440.

[16] Zhang J, Wang L, Anderson LB, Witthuhn B, Xu Y, Lu J. (2010) Proteomic profiling of potential molecular targets of methyl-selenium compounds in the transgenic adenocarcinoma of mouse prostate model. Cancer Prevention Research 3(8):994-1006.

[17] Zhang J, Wang L, Zhang Y, Li L, Higgins L, Lu J. (2011) Lobe-specific proteome changes in the dorsal-lateral and ventral prostate of TRAMP mice versus wild-type mice. Proteomics 11(12):2542-2549.

[18] Hsu CX, Ross BD, Chrisp CE, Derrow SZ, Charles LG, Pienta KJ, Greenberg NM, Zeng Z, Sanda MG. (1998) Longitudinal cohort analysis of lethal prostate cancer progression in transgenic mice. The Journal of Urology 160(4):1500-1505.

[19] Tani Y, Suttie A, Flake GP, Nyska A, Maronpot RR. (2005) Epithelial-stromal tumor of the seminal vesicles in the transgenic adenocarcinoma mouse prostate model. Veterinary Pathology 42(3):306-314.

[20] Yeh IT, Reddick RL, Kumar AP. (2009) Malignancy arising in seminal vesicles in the transgenic adenocarcinoma of mouse prostate (TRAMP) model. Prostate 69(7):755-760.

[21] Huss WJ, Barrios RJ, Foster BA, Greenberg NM. (2003) Differential expression of specific FGF ligand and receptor isoforms during angiogenesis associated with prostate cancer progression. Prostate 54(1):8-16.

[22] Polnaszek N, Kwabi-Addo B, Peterson LE, Ozen M, Greenberg NM, Ortega S, Basilico C, Ittmann M. (2003) Fibroblast growth factor 2 promotes tumor progression in an autochthonous mouse model of prostate cancer. Cancer Research 63(18):5754-5760.

[23] Singh RP, Raina K, Sharma G, Agarwal R. (2008) Silibinin inhibits established prostate tumor growth, progression, invasion, and metastasis and suppresses tumor angiogenesis and epithelial-mesenchymal transition in transgenic adenocarcinoma of the mouse prostate model mice. Clinical Cancer Research : an official journal of the American Association for Cancer Research 14(23):7773-7780.

[24] Wang J, Eltoum IE, Lamartiniere CA. (2004) Genistein alters growth factor signaling in transgenic prostate model (TRAMP). Molecular and Cellular Endocrinology 219(1-2):171-180.

[25] Shukla S, Maclennan GT, Marengo SR, Resnick MI, Gupta S. (2005) Constitutive activation of P I3 K-Akt and NF-kappaB during prostate cancer progression in autochthonous transgenic mouse model. Prostate 64(3):224-239.

[26] Caporali A, Davalli P, Astancolle S, D'Arca D, Brausi M, Bettuzzi S, Corti A. (2004) The chemopreventive action of catechins in the TRAMP mouse model of prostate carcinogenesis is accompanied by clusterin over-expression. Carcinogenesis 25(11):2217-2224.

[27] Maddison LA, Huss WJ, Barrios RM, Greenberg NM. (2004) Differential expression of cell cycle regulatory molecules and evidence for a "cyclin switch" during progression of prostate cancer. Prostate 58(4):335-344.

[28] Morey Kinney SR, Smiraglia DJ, James SR, Moser MT, Foster BA, Karpf AR. (2008) Stage-specific alterations of DNA methyltransferase expression, DNA hypermethylation, and DNA hypomethylation during prostate cancer progression in the transgenic adenocarcinoma of mouse prostate model. Molecular Cancer Research 6(8):1365-1374.

[29] Kinney SR, Moser MT, Pascual M, Greally JM, Foster BA, Karpf AR. (2010) Opposing roles of Dnmt1 in early- and late-stage murine prostate cancer. Molecular and Cellular Biology 30(17):4159-4174.

[30] Majeed N, Blouin MJ, Kaplan-Lefko PJ, Barry-Shaw J, Greenberg NM, Gaudreau P, Bismar TA, Pollak M. (2005) A germ line mutation that delays prostate cancer progression and prolongs survival in a murine prostate cancer model. Oncogene 24(29):4736-4740.

[31] Bok RA, Hansell EJ, Nguyen TP, Greenberg NM, McKerrow JH, Shuman MA. (2003) Patterns of protease production during prostate cancer progression: proteomic evidence for cascades in a transgenic model. Prostate Cancer and Prostatic diseases 6(4):272-280.

[32] Ruddat VC, Whitman S, Klein RD, Fischer SM, Holman TR. (2005) Evidence for downregulation of calcium signaling proteins in advanced mouse adenocarcinoma. Prostate 64(2):128-138.

[33] Haram KM, Peltier HJ, Lu B, Bhasin M, Otu HH, Choy B, Regan M, Libermann TA, Latham GJ, Sanda MG *et al.* (2008) Gene expression profile of mouse prostate tumors reveals dysregulations in major biological processes and identifies potential murine targets for preclinical development of human prostate cancer therapy. Prostate 68(14):1517-1530.

[34] Morgenbesser SD, McLaren RP, Richards B, Zhang M, Akmaev VR, Winter SF, Mineva ND, Kaplan-Lefko PJ, Foster BA, Cook BP *et al.* (2007) Identification of genes potentially involved in the acquisition of androgen-independent and metastatic tumor growth in an autochthonous genetically engineered mouse prostate cancer model. Prostate 67(1):83-106.

[35] Slack-Davis JK, Hershey ED, Theodorescu D, Frierson HF, Parsons JT. (2009) Differential requirement for focal adhesion kinase signaling in cancer progression in the transgenic adenocarcinoma of mouse prostate model. Molecular Cancer Therapeutics 8(8):2470-2477.

[36] Aziz MH, Manoharan HT, Church DR, Dreckschmidt NE, Zhong W, Oberley TD, Wilding G, Verma AK. (2007) Protein kinase Cepsilon interacts with signal transducers and activators of transcription 3 (Stat3), phosphorylates Stat3Ser727, and regulates its constitutive activation in prostate cancer. Cancer Research 67(18):8828-8838.

[37] Zhang J, Nkhata K, Shaik AA, Wang L, Li L, Zhang Y, Higgins LA, Kim KH, Liao JD, Xing C *et al.* (2011) Mouse prostate proteome changes induced by oral

pentagalloylglucose treatment suggest targets for cancer chemoprevention. Current Cancer Drug Targets 11(7):787-798.

[38] Fujimoto N, Akimoto Y, Suzuki T, Kitamura S, Ohta S. (2006) Identification of prostatic-secreted proteins in mice by mass spectrometric analysis and evaluation of lobe-specific and androgen-dependent mRNA expression. The Journal of Endocrinology 190(3):793-803.

[39] Fujimoto N, Suzuki T, Ohta S, Kitamura S. (2009) Identification of rat prostatic secreted proteins using mass spectrometric analysis and androgen-dependent mRNA expression. Journal of Andrology 30(6):669-678.

[40] Berquin IM, Min Y, Wu R, Wu H, Chen YQ. (2005) Expression signature of the mouse prostate. The Journal of Biological Chemistry 280(43):36442-36451.

[41] Tang Y, Wang L, Goloubeva O, Khan MA, Zhang B, Hussain A. (2008) Divergent effects of castration on prostate cancer in TRAMP mice: possible implications for therapy. Clinical cancer research : an official journal of the American Association for Cancer Research 14(10):2936-2943.

[42] Zhang ZX, Xu QQ, Huang XB, Zhu JC, Wang XF. (2009) Early and delayed castrations confer a similar survival advantage in TRAMP mice. Asian Journal of Andrology 11(3):291-297.

[43] Adhami VM, Siddiqui IA, Sarfaraz S, Khwaja SI, Hafeez BB, Ahmad N, Mukhtar H. (2009) Effective prostate cancer chemopreventive intervention with green tea polyphenols in the TRAMP model depends on the stage of the disease. Clinical Cancer Research : an official journal of the American Association for Cancer Research 15(6):1947-1953.

[44] Gupta S, Adhami VM, Subbarayan M, MacLennan GT, Lewin JS, Hafeli UO, Fu P, Mukhtar H. (2004) Suppression of prostate carcinogenesis by dietary supplementation of celecoxib in transgenic adenocarcinoma of the mouse prostate model. Cancer Research 64(9):3334-3343.

[45] Narayanan BA, Narayanan NK, Pittman B, Reddy BS. (2004) Regression of mouse prostatic intraepithelial neoplasia by nonsteroidal anti-inflammatory drugs in the transgenic adenocarcinoma mouse prostate model. Clinical Cancer Research : an official journal of the American Association for Cancer Research 10(22):7727-7737.

[46] Raghow S, Kuliyev E, Steakley M, Greenberg N, Steiner MS. (2000) Efficacious chemoprevention of primary prostate cancer by flutamide in an autochthonous transgenic model. Cancer Research 60(15):4093-4097.

[47] Huss WJ, Lai L, Barrios RJ, Hirschi KK, Greenberg NM. (2004) Retinoic acid slows progression and promotes apoptosis of spontaneous prostate cancer. Prostate 61(2):142-152.

[48] Yin Y, Ni J, Chen M, DiMaggio MA, Guo Y, Yeh S. (2007) The therapeutic and preventive effect of RRR-alpha-vitamin E succinate on prostate cancer via induction of insulin-like growth factor binding protein-3. Clinical Cancer Research : an official journal of the American Association for Cancer Research 13(7):2271-2280.

[49] El Touny LH, Banerjee PP. (2009) Identification of a biphasic role for genistein in the regulation of prostate cancer growth and metastasis. Cancer Research 69(8):3695-3703.

[50] Harper CE, Patel BB, Wang J, Eltoum IA, Lamartiniere CA. (2007) Epigallocatechin-3-Gallate suppresses early stage, but not late stage prostate cancer in TRAMP mice: mechanisms of action. Prostate 67(14):1576-1589.

[51] Raina K, Rajamanickam S, Singh RP, Deep G, Chittezhath M, Agarwal R. (2008) Stage-specific inhibitory effects and associated mechanisms of silibinin on tumor progression and metastasis in transgenic adenocarcinoma of the mouse prostate model. Cancer Research 68(16):6822-6830.

[52] Suttie AW, Dinse GE, Nyska A, Moser GJ, Goldsworthy TL, Maronpot RR. (2005) An investigation of the effects of late-onset dietary restriction on prostate cancer development in the TRAMP mouse. Toxicologic Pathology 33(3):386-397.

[53] Gray A, de la Luz Garcia-Hernandez M, van West M, Kanodia S, Hubby B, Kast WM. (2009) Prostate cancer immunotherapy yields superior long-term survival in TRAMP mice when administered at an early stage of carcinogenesis prior to the establishment of tumor-associated immunosuppression at later stages. Vaccine 27 Suppl 6:G52-59.

[54] Liu Z, Eltoum IE, Guo B, Beck BH, Cloud GA, Lopez RD. (2008) Protective immunosurveillance and therapeutic antitumor activity of gammadelta T cells demonstrated in a mouse model of prostate cancer. Journal of Immunology 180(9):6044-6053.

[55] Lei Wang, Yong Zhang, Jinhui Zhang, Katai Nkata, Emily Quealy, Li Li, Hyo-Jeong Lee, Soo-Jin Jeong, Joshua Liao, Cheng Jiang, Sung-Hoon Kim, and Junxuan Lu. (2011) Korean Angelica gigas Nakai (AGN) and Oriental herbal cocktail ka-mi-kae-kyuk-tang (KMKKT) inhibit prostate carcinogenesis in TRAMP model. Cancer Research 71(8 (Suppl)):Abstract nr 5581.

[56] Jinhui Zhang, Li Li, Yong Zhang, Lei Wang, Cheng Jiang, Sung-Hoon kim, and Junxuan Lu. (2012) Proteomic and transcriptomic profiling of effects of Angelica gigas ethanol extract on prostate neuroendocrine carcinomas of TRAMP mice. Cancer Research 72(8 (Suppl)):Abstract nr 2587.

[57] Cheng L, Ramesh AV, Flesken-Nikitin A, Choi J, Nikitin AY. (2010) Mouse models for cancer stem cell research. Toxicologic Pathology 38(1):62-71.

[58] Taylor RA, Toivanen R, Risbridger GP. (2010) Stem cells in prostate cancer: treating the root of the problem. Endocrine-related cancer 17(4):R273-285.

[59] Miki J. (2010) Investigations of prostate epithelial stem cells and prostate cancer stem cells. International Journal of Urology : official journal of the Japanese Urological Association 17(2):139-147.

[60] Huss WJ, Gray DR, Greenberg NM, Mohler JL, Smith GJ. (2005) Breast cancer resistance protein-mediated efflux of androgen in putative benign and malignant prostate stem cells. Cancer Research 65(15):6640-6650.

[61] Tang Y, Hamburger AW, Wang L, Khan MA, Hussain A. (2009) Androgen deprivation and stem cell markers in prostate cancers. International Journal of Clinical and Experimental Pathology 3(2):128-138.

[62] Ip C, Lisk DJ, Thompson HJ. (1996) Selenium-enriched garlic inhibits the early stage but not the late stage of mammary carcinogenesis. Carcinogenesis 17(9):1979-1982.

Chapter 11

Mechanism of Urinary Bladder Carcinogenesis Induced by a Xanthine Oxidoreductase Inhibitor, in Rats

Naoki Ashizawa and Takeo Shimo

Additional information is available at the end of the chapter

http://dx.doi.org/10.5772/54971

1. Introduction

Studies on urinary bladder cancer have underpinned that the urolith is one of the key factors in the carcinogenesis process when rodents are treated with thymine, melamine [1] and uracil [2-5], all of which induce intrarenal crystal deposition/calculus formation. Fukushima et al. [2] and Cohen et al. [6-8] have investigated in detail about factors implicated in the urolith formation as well as the role of calculi in urinary bladder carcinogenesis. The crystal or calculus acts as a subsequent sustained proliferative stimulus ultimately leading to tumors. However, rodent bladder tumors cannot be directly extrapolated for humans. In fact, there is a suggestion of a weak association concerning calculi in humans as a potential risk factor for bladder cancer [9]. A major difference between rodent and human bladders, which potentially affects the carcinogenic hazard from calculi, is related to the horizontal versus vertical status. Rodents, because of their horizontal stature, have a bladder that can retain calculi in the bladder for long periods of time, without completely obstructing the urinary flow.

Xanthine oxidoreductase catalyzes the last two reactions of purine catabolism: the hydroxylation of hypoxanthine to xanthine and of xanthine to uric acid. Xanthine oxidoreductase inhibitors such as allopurinol and febuxostat are used as therapeutic agents against gout and hyperuricemia. They induce decreases in circulating uric acid and concomitant increases in blood xanthine, followed by intrarenal xanthine deposition leading to nephropathy in rodents. The xanthine crystals or calculi mediated by xanthine oxidoreductase inhibitors may repeatedly stimulate the epithelium of the renal pelvis and/or urinary bladder leading to proliferative lesions. Indeed, it has been described that carcinomas of the urinary bladder occurred in the carcinogenicity study of febuxostat [10].

However, the pathomechanism of urinary bladder carcinogenesis due to xanthine deposits remains undetermined. With the above background, the mechanism of urinary bladder carcinogenesis induced by FYX-051 [11-13], 4-(5-pyridin-4-yl-1H-[1, 2, 4]triazol-3-yl)pyridine-2-carbonitrile, a xanthine oxidoreductase inhibitor, in rats, has been investigated.

Thus far, we have performed studies of FYX-051-induced nephropathy in rats [14-17]. In this chapter, first, general aspects concerning calculi formation and its bladder carcinogenesis are described. Second, the characteristics of FYX-051-induced nephropathy are described with respect to both identification of renal deposits precipitated after FYX-051 administration and marked species difference in nephropathy. Next, our aim was to prevent xanthine deposition after FYX-051 administration in rats by simultaneous treatment with citrate, and have established the experimental model. Using the model, a mechanistic study by simultaneous treatment with citrate for 52 weeks was performed. Based on the results of the 52-week study, finally, the extrapolation of carcinogenesis in rats for humans is discussed.

2. Formation of calculi and its effects on bladder

Solid materials can be generated in the urine by administration of a variety of chemicals, which lead to the formation of calculi [18]. Urinary calculi in rats and/or mice can be produced via variety of mechanisms as described by Cohen et al. [6]. The calculi can arise from the administered chemical itself such as melamine [19, 20], or from one of its metabolites such as diethylene glycol leading to calcium oxalate [21], or from an endogenous substance that results from the administration of the chemicals such as glycine leading to orotic acid [22]. Disorders of intermediate metabolism can also result in similar effects in the kidney and lower urinary tracts, such as the formation of urate calculi following surgical portacaval shunt in rats [23].

A major consequence of a calculus in the bladder lumen is abrasion of the mucosa surface, resulting in erosion and ulceration. These cause an acute inflammatory reaction, but are always accompanied by marked regenerative hyperplasia. Urothelial cell number is markedly increased secondary to not only simple hyperplasia but papillary and nodular hyperplasia, frequently a diffuse papillomatosis. In addition, the rate of proliferation is also increased 10-100 times. This results in 1000-10000 times increase in the number of cell divisions compared with normally quiescent adult urothelium. Although the formation of proliferative lesions produced by these foreign materials are reversible as evidenced by an example of uracil [24], stimulation of the urothelium for a long period leads to papilloma followed by carcinoma.

3. Factors affecting calculus formation

Of particular importance to factors that affect the formation of calculi in the urine are species, strain and sex [7, 25-27]. Rats and mice are the most commonly used species in carcinogen bioassays and in most mechanistic studies with animal models. Of major importance for comparison to humans are the extremely high levels of protein, osmolality, and concentrations of various salts in the urine of rats and mice. There are marked variations in urinary composition and in response to treatment between rats and mice. Calculi tend to more readily form in rats than in mice [25, 28]. The proliferative response seems to be greater in rats than in mice, partly because of the reaction; primarily papillomatous response in rats, whereas there is a nodular response involving small number of cells in mice [4, 24]. As to the sex difference, male rodents are frequently affected to a greater extent than females. Several factors including potential hormonal effects and total amounts of specific types of urinary proteins have been suggested for this difference [25, 27, 29, 30, 31].

The major factor, however, related to calculus formation is the dose of the chemicals administrated [32, 33]. An adequate amount of the chemical is needed to be administered to generate a sufficiently high concentration in the urine to lead to precipitation and calculus formation. The dose effect is the greatest fundamental factor in extrapolating the results in rodents to potential carcinogenic hazards in humans. Other factors that strictly affect the formation of calculi are physical, chemical and physiological properties. Urinary pH is a particularly fundamental factor [7, 25-27]. Effects of urinary pH have been identified for a variety of chemicals, based on its effects on the solubility of various salts, for example, urate or xanthine being greater at increased pH, while calcium phosphate crystals are formed more readily by the same condition.

4. Nephropathy and identification of renal deposits precipitated after FYX-051 administration

In the long-term toxicity study of FYX-051 in rats, nephropathy with intrarenal deposits was observed. HPLC and LC-MS/MS analyses of intrarenal deposits in rats treated with FYX 051 have proven that the entity was xanthine [14]. The pathomechanism of nephropathy could be speculated as follows. Treatment with FYX-051 induced high blood xanthine levels due to its pharmacological activity, and consequently, renal xanthine deposition occurred mainly during the process of urine-condensation from distal tubules to collecting ducts. When the amount of deposited xanthine exceeds the capacity of the kidney to excrete foreign materials, renal tubules and collecting ducts (particularly remarkable in distal tubules) are occluded by these deposits, leading to secondary interstitial nephritis.

5. Species difference in nephropathy induced by FYX-051

Thirteen-week toxicity study of FYX-051 in rats and dogs demonstrated that the no observed adverse effect level (NOAEL) was estimated to be 0.3 and 10 mg/kg/day, respectively. On the other hand, no changes were seen even at 300 mg/kg/day in the case of 52-week treatment of monkeys (Table 1). It was shown that rats are very susceptible to FYX-051-induced intrarenal xanthine deposition and subsequent nephropathy. The mechanism of marked species difference on nephropathy was investigated. As a result, three factors were found to be involved in the species difference. First, urinary excretion of purine metabolites in terms of body weight as an index of the rate of purine metabolism, which is the key factor of species difference, was thirty-fold higher in rats than in monkeys (Table 2). As the second factor, urinary xanthine solubility was two- and six-fold higher in dogs and monkeys, respectively, than in rats (Table 3). The fact was mainly mediated by the higher urinary pH of the former two species than the latter, because urinary xanthine solubility is dependent on urinary pH. Third, exposure level of FYX-051 was five-fold higher in rats than in other species (Table 4). The species difference of FYX-051-induced nephropathy seems to be caused by the combined effects of the above three factors.

	NOAEL (mg/kg/day)		
	Rats	Dogs	Monkeys
13-week	0.3	10	> 100
26-week	0.2	NT	NT
52-week	NT	NT	> 300

Changes observed in rats and dogs after repeated oral treatment with FYX-051 were nephropathy. NT: Not tested.

Table 1. No observed adverse effect level (NOAEL) of FYX-051 in repeated toxicity studies using rats, dogs and monkeys

Species	(A) Body weight (kg)	(B) Urinary excretion of purine metabolites (μmol/day)	B/A (μmol/kg/day)	Ratio (to monkeys)
Rats	0.209 ± 0.023	400.7 ± 58.9	1934.7 ± 385.0	31.2
Dogs	9.8 ± 0.7	3929.2 ± 790.3	402.8 ± 74.0	6.5
Monkeys	4.51 ± 0.18	280.4 ± 123.5	62.0 ± 26.0	1.0
Humans	64.1 ± 7.5	3364.3 ± 419.3	52.8 ± 7.0	0.9

Data were cited from the references [15, 16].

Table 2. The daily urinary excretion of total purine metabolites in each species and its ratio per body weight

	Rats	Dogs	Monkeys	Humans
pH	6.7	7.8	9.0	5.5
Urinary xanthinesolubility at 37°C	ca. 150	ca. 350	ca. 950	ca. 130

Data were cited from the references [15, 16].

Table 3. Estimated urinary xanthine solubility in the control urine in each species

	Rats 3 mg/kg	Dogs 10 mg/kg	Monkeys 10 mg/kg	Humans 3 mg/kg
$AUC_{0\text{-}t}$ (μg·h/ml)	13.9	8.81	9.89	2.82
Ratio (to monkeys)	4.7	0.9	1.0	1.0

The ratio to monkey's level was calculated based on AUC of FYX-051 at 10 mg/kg estimated from those at 3 mg/kg. Data were cited from the references [15, 16].

Table 4. Exposure levels of FYX-051 in each species

6. Establishment of simultaneous treatment model with citrate for preventing nephropathy

In the carcinogenicity testing in which FYX-051 was orally given to rats for 2 years, transitional cell papilloma and carcinoma were seen in the urinary bladder of male rats, along with the xanthine calculus in the cavity at doses of 1 and 3 mg/kg. Urinary bladder tumors occurred confined to the apex, the site that easily receives physical stimulation. No bladder tumors occurred in animals that died at less than 16 months.

In order to clarify the mechanism of urinary bladder carcinogenesis observed, we tried to prevent the xanthine deposition in the urinary tract by using co-treatment with citrate. Citrate is a urine-alkalizing agent and its treatment with large amount of water causes an elevation of urinary pH and an increase in urine volume, which are attributable to rapid increase in xanthine solubility in urine. Citrate appears to act as an inhibitor of the experimental urolithiasis formation in the urine [34]. Due to its chelating effect, citrate in the urine may be expected to inhibit the formation of calcium-containing precipitates. The experimental conditions suitable for the 52-week simultaneous treatment with FYX-051 and citrate in rats were determined.

Some sodium salts, such as saccharate and ascorbate, at high doses, can lead to the formation of calcium phosphate-containing precipitate [35]. In the present study, citrate was used as a mixture of its tri-sodium salt, tri-potassium salt, and free acid in a ratio of 2:2:1, calculated as anhydrous at molar base, leading to the reduced amount of sodium salt treated.

6.1. Study on the duration of effects by citrate

Duration of effects by citrate was examined as shown in Figure 1a. Male F344 rats received a single oral dosing of FYX-051 alone at a dose of 30 mg/kg (Group 1) or FYX-051 + 2,000 mg/kg citrate (Group 2) orally at a dosing volume of 10 ml/kg. Urine just after urination was collected during 1.5 - 2 h, 3.5 - 4 h, 5.5 - 6 h, and 7.5 - 8 h after oral administration of FYX-051. Insoluble xanthine concentration in each urine sample was determined as the difference of xanthine concentration between whole urine and filtered urine through a 0.45 μm pore size filter.

Simultaneous treatment with citrate remarkably increased urinary citrate concentrations at 3.5 - 4 h (Figure 2a). In both groups, xanthine was dissolved in urine at 1.5 - 2 h after administration, since the insoluble xanthine concentration was nearly zero (Figure 2b). At 3.5 - 4 h, deposition of xanthine was observed in Group 1. Simultaneous treatment with citrate significantly prevented the xanthine deposition. Thereafter, the effects of citrate disappeared; no significant difference was observed between the two groups at 5.5 - 6 h and 7.5 - 8 h after administration. The results indicate a preventative effect of citrate on xanthine deposition in urine but also a lack of its durability.

6.2. Seven-day simultaneous treatment study with citrate

Because of the lack of durability of citrate effects, it was suggested that at least daily twice treatments of citrate are needed to prevent xanthine deposition. We carried out a 7-day simultaneous treatment study by two daily treatments to F344 rats, that is, FYX-051 (6 mg/kg) and citrate (2000 mg/kg) followed by citrate alone treatment under the conditions of selected dosing intervals, the second dose of citrate, and dosing volume. In order to establish the experimental conditions suitable for the 52-week mechanistic study, in which burdens to both animals and technicians should be reduced, the daily first treatment of citrate was done as the mixture with FYX-051, and we tried to reduce the second dose of citrate and/or dosing volume. Experimental designs are shown in Figure 1b.

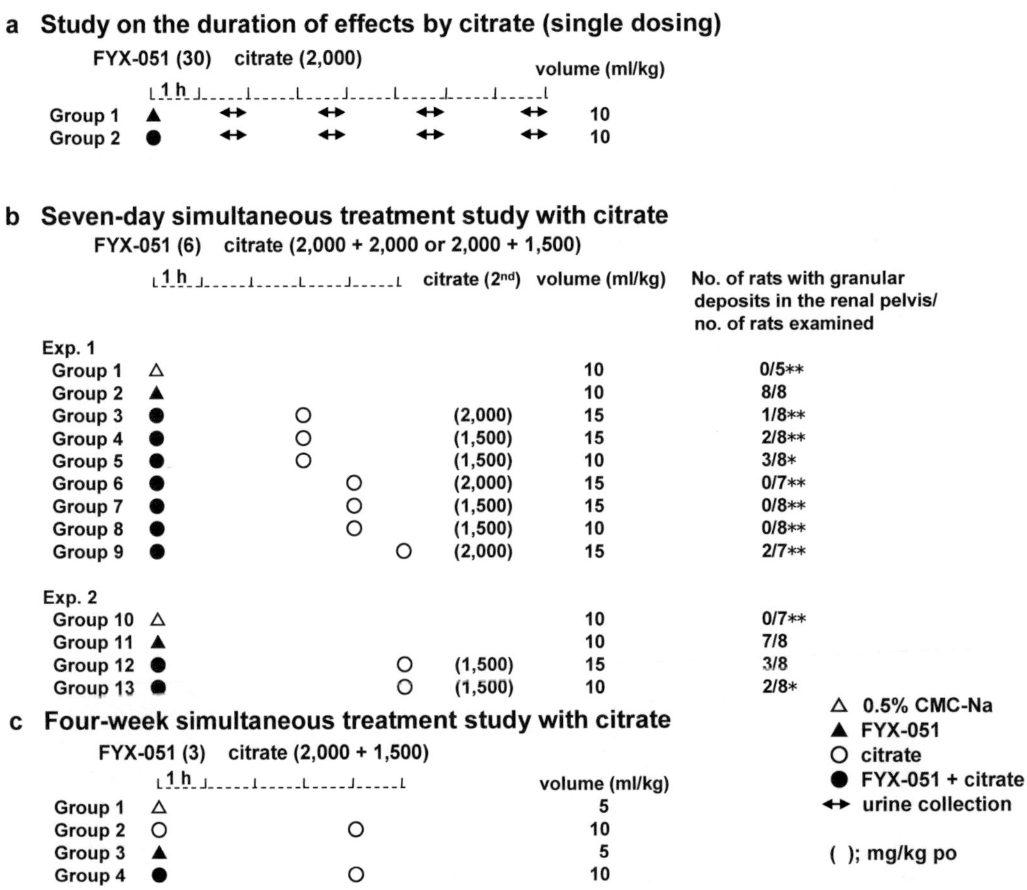

Figure 1. Experimental design (Studies a, b and c) and results (Study b) of the simultaneous treatment study with FYX-051 and citrate for the determination of experimental conditions suitable for the 52-week study. Vehicle of FYX-051 is 0.5% CMC-Na. *: P<0.05, **: P<0.01 vs. FYX-051 alone group (group 2 or group 11, by Fisher's exact probability test). Results of 'Study a' are shown in Figure 2. Results of 'Study c' are shown in Figures 3, 4 and Table 5. Figure is modified from reference [17].

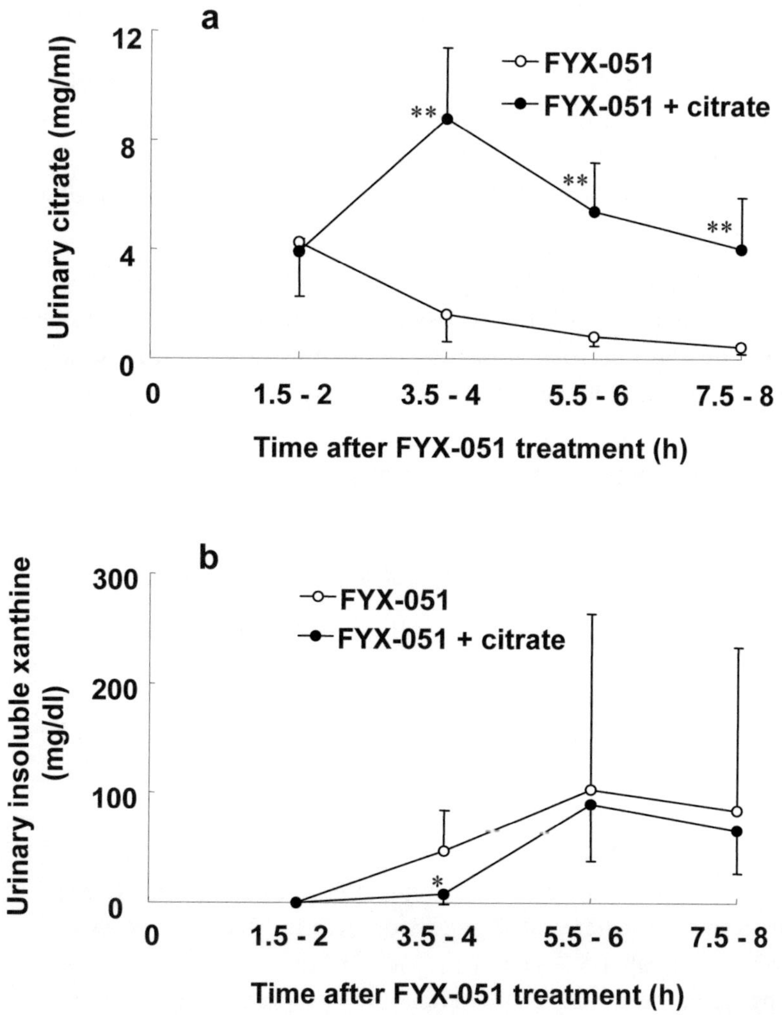

Figure 2. Changes in urinary citrate concentration (a) and insoluble xanthine concentration in urine (b) in rats receiving the single oral treatment of 30 mg/kg FYX-051 (Group 1, open circles) or 30 mg/kg FYX-051 + 2,000 mg/kg citrate (Group 2, closed circles). Each value represents the mean ± SD of 5 animals. *: P<0.05, **: p<0.01, significant difference was observed between the two groups by Student's t test. Figure is from reference [17].

Relative kidney weights and blood urea nitrogen (BUN) level significantly increased in the FYX-051 group (Group 2) compared to the controls (Group 1). Autopsy revealed yellowish-white granular deposits on the cut surface of the kidney or in the urinary bladder in all rats of Group 2. In groups treated with citrate, increased kidney weights and BUN were prevented almost completely (data not shown). Treatment of citrate, 2,000 and 2,000 mg/kg at an interval of 3 h with dosing volume of 15 ml/kg (Group 3) remarkably reduced granular deposits on the cut surface of the kidney and in the urinary bladder, although the deposition still remained in the renal pelvis in 1 out of 8 rats (Figure 1b). When the interval of citrate treatments was 5 h (Group 9), granular deposits were seen in the renal pelvis in 2 out of 7 rats. In case of 4 h (Group 6), however, no granular deposition in the renal pelvis was observed. Neither a reduction of citrate dose from 2,000 to 1,500 mg/kg (Group 7) nor decreased dosing volume from 15 to 10 ml/kg (Group 8) revealed apparent effects on the incidence of crystal deposition. Similarly, the dose of citrate and dosing volume failed to affect the granular deposition when the dosing interval was 3 h (Groups 4 and 5 vs. Group 3) or 5 h (Groups 12 and 13 vs. Group 9).

The present results indicate that the dosing interval of citrate has a great significance, and is optimal at 4 h, but not at 3 or 5 h, because this treatment completely inhibited intrarenal xanthine deposition. A decrease in dose of citrate for the second treatment or the dosing volume was well tolerated for prevention of granular deposits in the renal pelvis.

7. Effects of simultaneous treatment model with citrate on nephropathy and bladder carcinogenesis in rats

7.1. Four-week simultaneous treatment study with citrate

A 4-week study under the established conditions was carried out as shown in Figure 1c. The male F344 rats were divided into 4 groups of 8 animals each. In the simultaneous treatment group with citrate, first, animals received 3 mg/kg FYX-051 and 2000 mg/kg citrate, and 4 h later 1500 mg/kg citrate alone at a volume of 10 ml/kg, based on a 7-day study.

In the treatment group with FYX-051 alone (Group 3), laboratory investigations revealed chylous urine, granular deposits (xanthine crystals) in urinary sediments, and trends of increased serum creatinine compared with the control group (Group 1) (Table 5). Pathological examinations revealed increased relative kidney weights and gross renal findings such as focal pale changes, focal rough surface, scar, and white patch. Histopathologically, these were characterized by basophilia and dilatation of renal tubules, cell debris in tubular lumen, crystalline materials in the cortex, medulla, and papilla, calculus, fibrosis, and transitional cell hyperplasia (Figure 3a). In addition, calculus and transitional cell hyperplasia were also present in the urinary bladder in one instance each (Figure 4a, Table 5).

Citrate treatment alone (Group 2) and simultaneous treatment with FYX-051 (Group 4) apparently increased urinary pH compared with Groups 1 and 3 (Table 5). In Group 4, no noticeable changes were seen in the kidneys nor were alterations seen in the urinary bladder (Figures 3b, 4b). The serum creatinine level in the Group 4 was equivalent to the Group 1, with attaining a significant decrease compared with the Group 3. Additionally, treatment with citrate exhibited no remarkable effect on the exposure levels of FYX-051. These observations showed that FYX-051-induced nephropathy could be markedly depressed by simultaneous treatment with 3,500 mg/kg of citrate, leading to the disappearance of transitional cell hyperplasia in the urinary bladder.

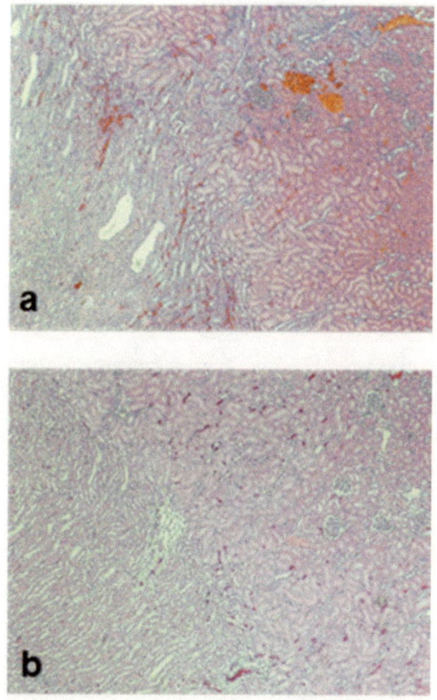

Figure 3. Photomicrographs of the kidney (cortex to outer medulla) from a male F344 rat treated orally with (a) 3 mg/kg FYX-051 (Group 3) or (b) 3 mg/kg FYX-051 + 3,500 mg/kg citrate (Group 4) for 4 weeks. Note (a) mild interstitial nephritis and (b) normal histology; magnification 100×, HE staining.

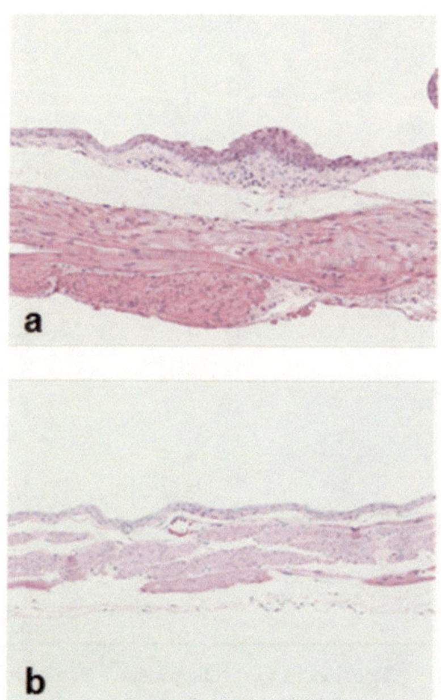

Figure 4. Photomicrographs of the urinary bladder from a male F344 rat treated orally with (a) 3 mg/kg FYX-051 (Group 3) or (b) 3 mg/kg FYX-051 + 3,500 mg/kg citrate (Group 4) for 4 weeks. Note (a) mild epithelial hyperplasia and (b) normal histology; magnification 200×, HE staining. Figures are from reference [17].

Group	1	2	3	4
No. of animals	8	8	8	8
Urinary pH				
8	1		2	
8.5	7	6	6	4
≥9		2		4
Xanthine crystals				
present	0	0	4	0
Serum creatinine (mg/dl)	0.22 ± 0.02	0.22 ± 0.03	0.26 ± 0.05	0.21 ± 0.02*
BUN (mg/dl)	20.4 ± 0.7	23.3 ± 2.3	22.5 ± 4.4	22.1 ± 1.4
Relative kidney weight (%)	0.717 ± 0.028	0.777 ± 0.016††	0.778 ± 0.070†	0.765 ± 0.022
Autopsy				
-Kidney				
pale, focal	0	0	5	0
rough surface, focal	0	0	3	0
scarred	0	0	2	1[c]
white patch	0	0	1	0
-Urinary bladder				
calculus	0	0	6	0
Histopathology				
-Kidney				
calculus	0	0	5	0
cellular infiltration	0	0	4	0
cell debris, tubular lumen	0	0	6	0
crystalline material, cortex	0	0	2	0
crystalline material,medulla	0	0	6	0
crystalline material, papilla	0	0	4	0
dilatation, tubule	0	0	7	0
tubular basophilia [a]	0	0	7	1
foreign body reaction	0	0	4	0
suppurative inflammation	0	0	1	0
pyelitis	0	0	2	0
fibrosis	0	0	5	0
hyperplasia,transitional cell	0	0	5	0
interstitial nephritis [b]	0	0	1	0
-Urinary bladder				
calculus	0	0	1	0
hyperplasia,transitional cell	0	0	1	0
Toxicokinetics				
No. of animals			6	5
$AUC_{0\text{-}24h}$ (μg·h/ml)			5.51 ± 0.75	5.03 ± 0.48

Data were expressed as the mean ± SD. [a] Regeneration [b]Diagnosis [c]No histopathological changes
*Significant difference compared with Group 3 (P<0.05, by Aspin-Welch's t test).
†Significant difference compared with Group 1 (P<0.05, by Aspin-Welch's t test).
††Significant difference compared with Group 1 (P<0.01, by Student's t test). Table is from reference [17].

Table 5. Data of urinalysis, blood chemistry, relative kidney weights, histopathology of urinary organs and toxicokinetics in male rats receiving FYX-051 alone or simultaneous treatment with citrate

7.2. Mechanistic study by simultaneous treatment with citrate for 52 weeks

The male F344 rats were divided into 4 groups of 17 males each. Treatment of FYX-051 and citrate was done in a same manner as 4 week study. As shown in Table 6, in the FYX-051 alone treatment group, the following findings were observed: a significant decrease in urinary osmolality, crystals in sediments, hematuria, significant increases of serum BUN and creatinine, pathological alterations in the kidney such as calculus, atrophy, rough

	Vehicle control (n=17)	3500 mg/kg citrate (n=16)	3 mg/kg FYX-051 (n=17)	3 mg/kg FYX-051 + 3500 mg/kg citrate (n=17)
Urinalysis Crystal in sediments	0 / 17	0 / 16	5 / 17	0 / 17
Blood biochemistry BUN (mg/dl) Creatinine (mg/dl)	 15.9 ± 1.3 0.27 ± 0.03	 22.6 ± 1.7 0.24 ± 0.02	 42.0 ± 12.8** 0.72 ± 0.19**	 21.7 ± 2.7## 0.24 ± 0.02##
Kidney weight Absolute (g) Relative (g%)	 2.27 ± 0.14 0.602 ± 0.028	 2.32 ± 0.09 0.732 ± 0.027	 2.00 ± 0.15** 0.616 ± 0.049	 2.38 ± 0.14## 0.737 ± 0.027##
Gross pathology	–	–	Kidney: atrophy (13), calculus (4), rough surfacc (5), white patch (6) Urinary bladder: calculus (16)	–
Histopathology	–	–	Kidney: interstitial nephritis (17), simple hyperplasia of transitional cell (17) Urinary bladder: simple hyperplasia (4) and papillary hyperplasia (1) of transitional cell	–

–: No remarkable change

*,** Significant difference was observed in FYX-051 alone group when compared with the vehicle control group ($p <$ 0.05. 0.01, by Student's t-test).

#,## Significant difference was observed in the simultaneous treatment group with citrate when compare with FYX-051 alone group ($p < 0.05, 0.01$, by Student's t-test).

Table 6. Data for urinalysis, blood chemistry, kidney weight, gross pathology, and histopathology in rats receiving simultaneous treatment with FYX-051 and citrate for 52 weeks

surface, interstitial nephritis, simple hyperplasia of transitional cells. In the urinary bladder, calculus, simple and papillary hyperplasia of transitional cells was observed in 16, 4 and 1/17 males in the FYX-051 alone group, respectively. Oyasu [36] has postulated that commonly, distinction between papillary hyperplasia and papilloma of transitional cells is difficult. Accordingly, papillary hyperplasia observed in this 52-week mechanistic study could be regarded as precancerous lesions for bladder carcinogenesis. Neither xanthine crystals nor lesions in any of the kidney and urinary bladder samples were observed in the simultaneous treatment group with citrate.

Thus, simple and papillary hyperplasia of transitional cells followed by papilloma and carcinoma in the urinary bladder in rats occurring after the long-term treatment of FYX-051 were secondary changes caused by xanthine crystals being deposited in the kidney, and no other causes could be implicated in these changes. Proposed histogenesis of urinary bladder carcinogenesis obtained in this study is shown in Figure 5.

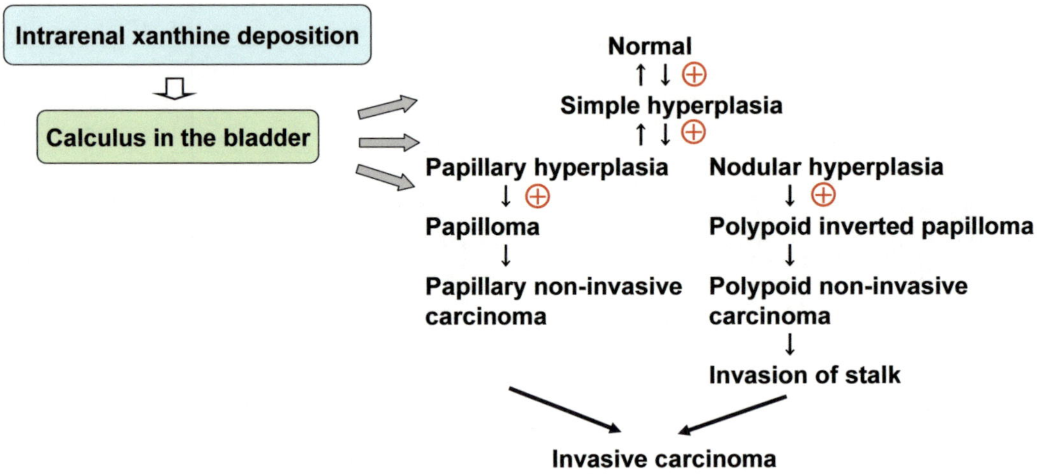

Figure 5. Proposed histogenesis of urinary bladder carcinogenesis induced by xanthine oxidoreductase inhibitors in rats

8. Extrapolation of carcinogenesis in rats for humans

The extrapolation of the results in rats into humans can be considered as follows. A marked species difference between rats and monkeys in FYX-051-induced nephropathy was suggested to be mediated by the combined effects of three factors; the rate of purine metabolism, urinary xanthine solubility and exposure level of FYX-051 as described above. A comparison of these factors relevant to species difference between monkeys and humans demonstrated that urinary xanthine solubility in the former was seven-fold higher than in the latter, without any differences in the remaining two factors. It should be emphasized that in the clinical trial of FYX-051, in which adequate hypouricemic effect was obtained, neither xanthine crystals in urine nor serious side effects have been reported, although attention must be paid in the case of Lesch-Nyhan syndrome in which hypoxanthine-guanine phosphoribosyltransferase is congenitally absent [37]. Further, small crystals or calculi can be excreted from the bladder in humans in contrast to rodents, as described in the introduction section. The outcomes of genotoxicity studies were negative, revealing that FYX-051 is a non-genotoxic compound (unpublished data). Thus, urinary bladder carcinogenesis, which would be mediated by xanthine deposition in rats after long-term treatment with FYX-051 cannot be extrapolated for humans due to extremely low occurrence of xanthine deposition in humans.

9. Conclusion

It is generally accepted that crystal or calculus in the urinary bladder of rats would ultimately cause carcinoma by acting as a proliferative stimulus. However, no direct evidence of calculus-mediated carcinogenesis was obtained in the treatment of xanthine oxidoreductase inhibitors. In this chapter, the pathomechanism of bladder carcinogenesis in rats induced by a xanthine oxidoreductase inhibitor has been clearly shown by disappearance of precancerous lesions in the case of prevention of xanthine deposition. This work will throw a light on the future studies of urinary bladder carcinogenesis in animals, since it was demonstrated that modifying experimental design that affects calculus formation produced great differences in the results of studies by long-term treatment.

Author details

Naoki Ashizawa and Takeo Shimo
Research Laboratories 2, Fuji Yakuhin Co., Ltd., Japan

10. References

[1] Okumura M, Hasegawa R, Shirai T, Ito M, Yamada S, Fukushima S. Relationship between calculus formation and carcinogenesis in the urinary bladder of rats administered the non-genotoxic agents thymine or melamine. Carcinogenesis 1992;13, 1043-1045.

[2] Fukushima S, Tanaka H, Asakawa E, Kagawa M, Yamamoto A, Shirai T. Carcinogenicity of uracil, a nongenotoxic chemical, in rats and mice and its rationale. Cancer Res 1992;52, 1675-1680.

[3] Masui T, Shirai T, Imaida K, Uwagawa S, Fukushima S. Effects of urinary crystals induced by acetazolamide, uracil, and diethylene glycol on urinary bladder carcinogenesis in N-butyl-N-(4-hydroxybutyl)nitrosamine-initiated rats. Toxicol Lett 1988;40, 119-126.

[4] Sakata T, Masui T, St. John M, Cohen SM. Uracil-induced calculi and proliferative lesions of the mouse urinary bladder. Carcinogenesis 1988;9, 1271-1276.

[5] Shirai T, Ikawa E, Fukushima S, Masui T, Ito N. Uracil-induced urolithiasis and the development of reversible papillomatosis in the urinary bladder of F344 rats. Cancer Res 1986;46, 2062-2067.

[6] Cohen SM, Lawson TA. Rodent bladder tumors do not always predict for humans. Cancer Lett 1995;93, 9-16.

[7] Cohen SM. Role of urinary physiology and chemistry in bladder carcinogenesis. Food Chem Toxicol 1995;33, 715-730.

[8] Cohen SM. Urinary bladder carcinogenesis. Toxicol Pathol 1998;26, 121-127.

[9] Burin GJ, Gibb HJ, Hill RN. Human bladder cancer: evidence for a potential irritation-induced mechanism. Food Chem Toxicol 1995;33, 785-795.

[10] European Medicines Agency. CHMP Assessment Report for Adenuric (febuxostat). 2008 Doc Ref : EMEA/258531. http://www.ema.europa.eu/docs/en_GB/document_library/EPAR_-_Public_assessment_report/human/000777/WC500021815.pdf (accessed 31 October 2012)

[11] Okamoto K, Matsumoto K, Hille R, Eger BT, Pai EF, Nishino T. The crystal structure of xanthine oxidoreductase during catalysis: Implications for reaction mechanism and enzyme inhibition. Proc Natl Acad Sci USA 2004;101, 7931-7936.

[12] Sato T, Ashizawa N, Matsumoto K, Iwanaga T, Nakamura H, Inoue T, Nagata O. Discovery of 3-(2-cyano-4-pyridyl)-5-(4-pyridyl)-1,2,4-triazole, FYX-051 - a xanthine oxidoreductase inhibitor for the treatment of hyperuricemia. Bioorg Med Chem Lett 2009;19, 6225-6229.

[13] Matsumoto K, Okamoto K, Ashizawa N, Nishino T. FYX-051: a novel and potent hybrid-type inhibitor of xanthine oxidoreductase. J Pharmacol Exp Ther 2011;336, 95-103.

[14] Shimo T, Ashizawa N, Matsumoto K, Nakazawa T, Nagata O. Simultaneous treatment with citrate prevents nephropathy induced by FYX-051, a xanthine oxidoreductase inhibitor, in rats. Toxicol Sci 2005;87, 267-76.

[15] Shimo T, Ashizawa N, Moto M, Matsumoto K, Iwanaga T, Nagata O. FYX-051, a xanthine oxidoreductase inhibitor, induces nephropathy in rats, but not in monkeys. Toxicol Pathol 2009;37, 438-445.

[16] Shimo T, Ashizawa N, Moto M, Iwanaga T, Nagata O. Study on species differences in nephropathy induced by FYX-051, a xanthine oxidoreductase inhibitor. Arch Toxicol 2011;85, 505-512.

[17] Ashizawa N, Shimo T, Matsumoto K, Taniguchi T, Moto M, Nagata O. Establishment of simultaneous treatment model with citrate for preventing nephropathy induced by FYX-051, a xanthine oxidoreductase inhibitor, in rats. Drug Chem Toxicol 2011;34, 151-161.

[18] Wolkowski-Tyl R, Chin TY, Popp JA, Heck HD. Chemically induced urolithiasis in weanling rats. Am J Pathol 1982;107, 419-421.

[19] National Toxicology Program. Carcinogenesis bioassay of melamine in F344/N rats and B6C3F1 Mice. NTP Report on Melamine, Vol. 245. NIH, US Dept. of Health and Human Services, Research Triangle Park, NC. 1983

[20] Ogasawara H, Imaida K, Ishiwata H, Toyoda K, Kawanishi T, Uneyama C, Hayashi S, Takahashi M, Hayashi Y. Urinary bladder carcinogenesis induced by melamine in F344 male rats: correlation between carcinogenicity and urolith formation. Carcinogenesis 1995;16, 2773-2777.

[21] Weil CS, Carpenter CP, Smyth HF Jr. Urinary bladder calculus and tumor response following either repeated feeding of diethylene glycol or calcium oxalate stone implantation. Ind Med Surg 1967;36, 55-57.

[22] Vasudevan S, Laconi E, Rao PM, Rajalakshmi S, Sarma DS. Incident of urinary bladder carcinogenesis by chronic administration of glycine an inducer of orotic aciduria. Proc Am Assoc Cancer Res 1986;27, 94.

[23] Engelmann U, Schramek P, Baum HP, Wertmann B, Grun M, Jacobi GH. Bladder carcinogenesis in portacaval shunt rats. Urol Int 1987;42, 165-169.

[24] Shirai T, Fukushima S, Tagawa Y, Okumura M, Ito N. Cell proliferation induced by uracil-calculi and subsequent development of reversible papillomatosis in the rat urinary bladder. Cancer Res 1989;49, 378-383.

[25] Clayson DB, Cooper EH. Cancer of the urinary tract. Adv Cancer Res 1970;13, 271-381.

[26] Clayson DB. Editorial Bladder carcinogenesis in rats and mice: possibility of artifacts. J Natl Cancer Inst 1974;52, 1685-1689.

[27] Clayson DB, Fishbein L, Cohen SM. Effect of stones and other physical factors on the induction of rodent bladder cancer. Food Chem Toxicol 1995;33, 771-784.

[28] Bryan GT. Pellet implantation studies of carcinogenic compounds. J Natl Cancer Inst 1969;43, 255-261.

[29] Fisher MJ, Sakata T, Tibbels TS, Smith RA, Patil K, Khachab M, Johansson SL, Cohen SM. Effect of sodium saccharin and calcium saccharin on urinary parameters in rats fed Prolab 3200 or AIN-76 diet. Food Chem Toxicol 1989;27, 1-9.

[30] Hard GC, Rodgers IS, Baetcke KP, Richards WL, McGaughy RE, Valcovic LR. Hazard evaluation of chemicals that cause accumulation of $\alpha_{2\mu}$-globulin, hyaline droplet nephropathy, and tubule neoplasia in the kidneys of male rats. Environ Health Perspect 1993;99, 313-349.

[31] Olson MJ, Johnson JT, Reidy CA. A comparison of male rat and human urinary proteins: implications for human resistance to hyaline droplet nephropathy. Toxicol Appl Pharmacol 1990;102, 524-536.

[32] Cohen SM., Ellwein LB. Genetic errors, cell proliferation, and carcinogenesis. Cancer Res 1991;51, 6493-6505.

[33] Cohen SM, Ellwein LB. Risk assessment based on high-dose animal exposure experiments. Chem Res Toxicol 1992;5, 742-748.

[34] Ogawa Y, Yamaguchi K, Tanaka T, Morozumi M. Effects of pyruvate salts, pyruvic acid, and bicarbonate salts in preventing experimental oxalate urolithiasis in rats. J Urol 1986;135, 1057-1060.

[35] Cohen SM. Calcium Phosphate-Containing Urinary Precipitate in Rat Urinary Bladder Carcinogenesis. World Health Organization International Agency for Research on Cancer, IARC Scientific Publications, No. 147. 1999 http://monographs.iarc.fr/ENG/Publications/pub147/IARCpub147.pdf (accessed 31 October 2012)

[36] Oyasu R. Epithelial tumours of the lower urinary tract in humans and rodents. Food Chem Toxicol 1995;33, 747-755.

[37] Brock WA, Golden J, Kaplan GW. Xanthine calculi in the Lesch-Nyhan syndrome. J Urol 1983;130, 157-159.

Section 4

Natural Products that Prevent or Treat Cancer

Chapter 12

Cancer Chemoprevention by Dietary Polyphenols

Magdy Sayed Aly and Amani Abd ElHamid Mahmoud

Additional information is available at the end of the chapter

http://dx.doi.org/10.5772/54945

1. Introduction

1.1. Chemopreventive agents

Chemoprevention is a promising and relatively new approach to cancer prevention that has precedence in cardiology, in which cholesterol lowering antihypertensive, and antiplatelet agents are administered to prevent coronary heart disease in high-risk individuals [1]. Chemoprevention can be defined as "the use of natural or synthetic chemical compounds to reverse, suppress or to prevent one or more of the biological events leading to the development of invasive cancer"

A chemopreventive strategy could potentially either prevent further DNA damage that might enhance carcinogenesis or suppress the appearance of the cancer phenotype [2]. Chemopreventive agents inhibit or reverse cellular events associated with tumor initiation, promotion, and/or progression. The mechanism of chemoprotective activities might correlate and balance between phase I + phase II enzymes levels, and influence cellular macromolecules, transporters, release of carcinogens, or DNA adducts and DNA repair [3].

More than 1000 potential chemopreventive agents have been identified in dietary sources, and many are being tested *in vitro* and *in vivo* systems with a variety of cancer types. Identification and testing of a successful chemopreventive agent is a long process, requiring *in vitro* studies, animal efficacy and toxicity studies, and eventually lengthy human clinical trials [4].

1.2. Mechanisms of action of chemopreventive agents

Broadly defined on the basis of their mechanisms of action, chemopreventive agents can be grouped into two general classes: blocking agents and suppressing agents. Blocking agents (e.g., flavonoids, oltipraz, indoles, and isothiocyanates) prevent carcinogenic compounds from reaching or reacting with critical target sites by preventing the metabolic activation of carcinogens or tumor promoters via enhancing detoxification systems and by trapping reactive carcinogens [5]. Suppressing agents (e.g., vitamin D and related compounds, nonsteroidal anti-inflammatory drugs [NSAIDS], vitamin A and retinoids, DFMO (2-difluoromethylornithine), monoterpenes and calcium) prevent the evolution of the neoplastic process in cells that would otherwise become malignant. Mechanisms of action for suppressing agents are not well understood. Some produce differentiation, some counteract the consequences of genotoxic events such as oncogene activation, some inhibit cell proliferation, and some have undefined mechanisms [5].

An ideal chemopreventive agent should have 1. Little or no toxic effects 2. High efficacy against multiple sites 3. Capability of oral administration 4. a known mechanism of action 5. Human acceptance [6]. A chemopreventive program identifies and accesses specific chemical substances, many naturally occurring in foods, with the potential to prevent cancer initiation and to either slow or reverse the progression of premalignant lesions to invasive cancer.

1.3. Types of chemopreventive agents:

Promising chemopreventive agents being investigated include micronutrients (e.g. vitamin A, C and E, β-carotene, molybdenum, and calcium), phytochemicals (e.g. indoles, polyphenols, isothiocyanates, flavonoids, monoterpenes, and organosulfides), and synthetics (e.g. vitamin A derivatives, piroxicam, tamoxifen, 2-difluoromethylornithine [DFMO] and oltipraz). More than 40 promising agents and agent combinations are being evaluated clinically as chemopreventive drugs for major cancer targets [7].

1.3.1. Synthetic chemopreventive agents (Non-Steroidal-anti-inflammatory drugs):

Several studies have reported a 40-50% decrease in the relative risk of colorectal cancer in persons who are continuous users of aspirin or other non steroidal anti-inflammatory drugs (NSAIDS) [8], suggesting that these drugs can serve as effective cancer chemopreventive agents. Hixson *et al.,* [9] showed that the synthesis of prostaglandins is limited by cyclooxygenase. NSAIDS reversibly interrupted prostaglandin synthesis by inhibiting cyclooxygenase. NSAIDS can prevent tumor formation by their actions on prostaglandins, which can have an immune modulating effect. High levels of prostaglandin E2 can suppress the immune system, which keeps malignant cells in check.

Other mechanisms that can explain the antiproliferative antitumor effects of NSAIDS include: interference with membrane-associated processes, such as G-protein signal transduction and transmembrane calcium influx, and inhibition of other enzymes, such as phospho-diesterase, folate-dependant enzymes, and cyclic adenosine-5`-monophosphatase-dependent protein kinase, as well as enhancement of immunologic responses and cellular apoptosis [10].

At a macroscopic level, NSAIDS prevent incident neoplasia (adenomas and carcinomas), and suppress the growth of carcinomas. Therefore, NSAIDS are effective when given "early" (proceeding adenoma-formation), as well as "late" (following the emergence of adenomas) [11]. An alternative explanation for the efficacy of NSAIDS in the prevention of colorectal cancer is their ability to scavenge reactive oxygen species [12].

1.3.2. Naturally-occurring chemopreventive agents:

Frequent consumption of fruits and vegetables has been associated with lower incidence of cancers at different organ sites. Several factors can contribute to this association, first, the nutrients in fruits and vegetables, notably vitamin C, vitamin E, folic acid, provitamin A, selenium and zinc, are essential for normal cellular functions, a deficiency in these nutrients can enhance the susceptibility of an individual to cancer, second, some nutrients, such as vitamin C, vitamin E, selenium and β-carotene, at levels above nutritional needs, can display inhibitory activities against carcinogenesis. A third factor is that non-nutritive constituents, such as polyphenols, organosulfur compounds, and indoles have anticarcinogen activities. Finally, fruits and vegetables contribute fibers and bulkiness to the diet. Persons who consume large amounts of fruits and vegetables can eat smaller amounts of meat and other animal products that can contribute to higher cancer incidence in the western countries. Supplementation with these antioxidant nutrients apparently produces a protective effect against cancer.

Comprehensive reviews of case-control and prospective cohort studies found that the relationship between high vegetable and fruit intake and reduced cancer risk appears to be strongest for cancers of the alimentary and respiratory tracts (cancers of the colon, esophagus, oral cavity and lung) and weakest for hormone related cancers (cancers of the breast, ovary, cervix, endometrium and prostate) [13-15]. Reduced cancer risk has been linked primarily to consumption of raw vegetables and fresh fruits (citrus, carrots, green leaf vegetables, cruciferous vegetables, soy products, and whole grain wheat products) [13-15]. The beneficial effect of vegetables, fruits and whole grains can be due to either individual or combined effects of their constituents, including, fiber, micronutrients and phytochemicals.

2. Dietary polyphenols and cancer chemoprevention

Polyphenols constitute one of the largest and ubiquitous groups of phytochemicals. One of the primary functions of these plant-derived polyphenols is to protect plants from photosynthetic stress, reactive oxygen species, and consumption by herbivores. Polyphenols are also an essential part of the human diet, with flavonoids and phenolic acids being the most common ones in food. Not surprisingly, there is a growing realization that lower incidence of cancer in certain populations can probably be due to consumption of certain nutrients, and especially polyphenol rich diets. Consequently, a systematic dissection of the chemopreventive potential of polyphenolic compounds in the recent years has clearly supported their health benefits, including anti-cancer properties. Given the challenges of cancer therapy, 'chemoprevention'-which uses pharmacological or natural agents to impede, arrest or reverse carcinogenesis at its earliest stages' remains the most practical and promising approach for the management of cancer patients [16].

Till date, A substantial number of studies in cultured cells, animal models and human clinical trials have illustrated a protective role of dietary polyphenols against different types of cancers [17–20]. Polyphenols are present in fruits, vegetables, and other dietary botanicals. Some estimates suggest that more than 8000 different dietary polyphenols exist, and these can be divided into ten different general classes based on their chemical structure [21]. Phenolic acids, flavonoids, stilbenes and lignans are the most abundantly occurring polyphenols that are also an integral part of everyday nutrition in populations worldwide. Some of the common examples of the most studied and promising cancer chemopreventive polyphenols include EGCG (from green tea), curcumin (from curry) and resveratrol (from grapes and berries). Significant gains have been made in understanding the molecular mechanisms underpinning the chemopreventive effects of polyphenols, and consequently, a wide range of mechanisms and gene targets have been identified for individual compounds. Various mechanistic explanations for their chemopreventive efficacy include their ability to interrupt or reverse the carcinogenesis process by acting on intracellular signaling network molecules involved in the initiation and/or promotion of cancer, or their potential to arrest or reverse the promotion stage of cancer [22; 23]. Polyphenolic compounds can also trigger apoptosis in cancer cells through the modulation of a number of key elements in cellular signal transduction pathways linked to apoptosis (caspases, *bcl-2* genes) [17; 22; 23]. Several elegant reviews have described in detail specific genetic and signaling mechanisms that are targeted by different polyphenols, and this is beyond the scope of this review article [24–26]. However, recent research has suggested that some of the chemopreventive potential of dietary polyphenols can in part be due to their ability to modulate epigenetic alterations in cancer cells. This is of interest; as epigenetic modifications occur early and are potentially reversible, making dietary polyphenol-induced chemoprevention of various human cancers an attractive possibility from a clinical standpoint. However, the mechanism of how flavonoids do regulate and effect various epigenetic modifications in cancer cells is a topic that is still in its infancy. Nevertheless, increasing number of reports has repeatedly shown the promise of epigenetic prevention and possibly therapy by dietary polyphenols.

2.1. Tea

Tea (*Camellia sinensis*), next to water, is the most popular beverage consumed by over two thirds of the world's population. The Chinese used tea as a medical drink as early as 3000 BC, and by the end of the sixth century as a beverage. Tea essentially signifies two or three leaves and the terminal apical buds of the shrubs *C. sinensis*, *Camellis asamica* and other southern varieties. The cultivation area of the tea has gradually expanded in the world, especially in tropical countries, and the total cultivation area has expanded to 2,300,000 ha with a total amount of production of 2,600,000 t [27].

An estimated 2.5 million metric tons of dried tea are manufactured annually. Of this amount about 20% is green tea, mainly consumed in Asian countries where tea is a major beverage. About 78% is black tea mainly consumed in the western nations and some Asian countries and about 2% is oolong tea mainly produced and consumed in South Eastern China.

2.1.1. Chemistry and mechanism of action of tea polyphenols:

Manufacture of black tea takes place by crushing the leaves causing polyphenol oxidase-dependent oxidative polymerization that leads to the formation of theaflavins, thearubigins and other oligomers in a process known as fermentation. Theaflavins (about 1% - 2% of the total dry matter of black tea) including theaflavin, theaflavin-3-O-gallate, theaflavin-3/-O-gallate and theaflavin-3-3/-O-digallate, possess benzotropolone rings with dihydroxy or trihydroxy substitution systems which give the characteristic color and taste of black tea. About 10 - 20% of the dry weight of black tea is due to thearubigens, which are even more extensively oxidized and polymerized, have a wide range of molecular weights and are less well characterized.

Oolong tea, a partially fermented tea, contains monomeric catechins, theaflavins and thearubigins. Some characteristic components, such as epigallocatechin esters, theasinensins, dimeric catechins and dimeric proanthocyanidins are also found in oolong tea.

Commercial green tea is made by steaming or drying fresh tea leaves at elevated temperature. Its chemical composition is similar to that of fresh tea leaves. Green tea contains polyphenols that include flavanols, flavandiols, flavonoids and phenolic acids. These compounds can account for up to 30% of the dry weight. Most of the green tea polyphenols are flavonols commonly known as catechin. Some major green tea catechins are epigallocatechin-3-gallate (EGCG), (-) - epigallocatechin (EGC), epicatechin-3-gallate (ECG), - (-) -epicatechin (EC), (+) -gallocatechin and (+)-catechin (Figure 1). Caffeine, theobromine and theophylline the principal alkaloids account for about 4% of the dry weight.

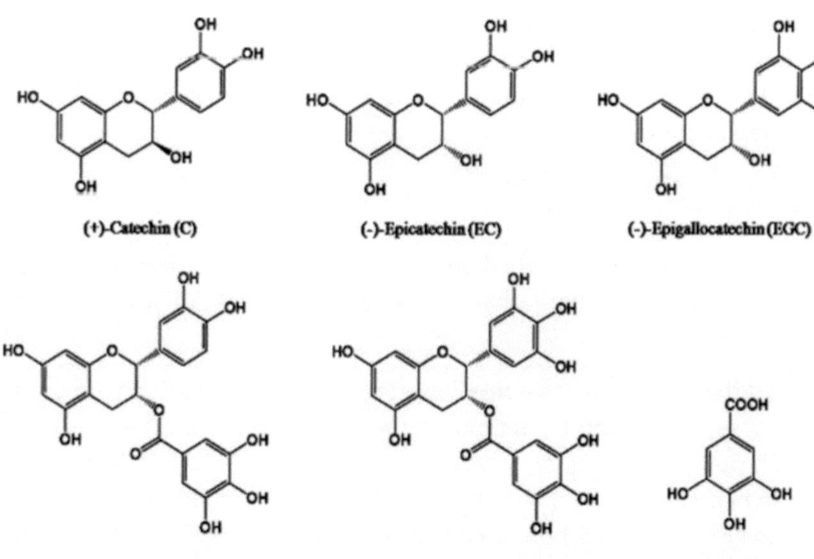

Figure 1. Components of green tea

It has been stated that a cup (200 ml) of green tea contains about 142 mg EGCG, 65 mg EGC, 17 mg EcC and 76 mg caffeine. The most important chemicals present in tea, which are of considerable pharmacological significance, are the polyphenols and caffeine [28]. Polyphenols are present to the extent of 30-35% in the dry tea leaf and determine the quality of the beverage. The amount of polyphenols depends on the genetic make up of tea and environmental factors such as climate, light, rainfall, temperature, nutrient availability and leaf age [27].

Because the mechanisms of antimutagenesis and anticarcinogenesis by tea polyphenols vary for different cancers and for the same cancer in different population, tea consumption can affect carcinogenesis only in selected situations. Many laboratory studies have demonstrated inhibitory effects of tea preparation and tea polyphenols against tumor formation and growth. This inhibitory effect is believed to be mainly due to the antioxidative and possible antiproliferative effects of polyphenolic compounds in green and black tea. These polyphenolics can also inhibit carcinogenesis by blocking the endogenous formation of N-nitroso compounds, suppressing the activation of carcinogen and trapping of genotoxic agents. Yang and Wang [28] showed that tea polyphenols also have high complexation affinity to metals, alkaloids and biologic macromolecules such as lipids, carbohydrates, proteins and nucleic acids.

Work of Kuroda and Hara [27] illustrates that the polyphenols in tea have a strong radical scavenging and reducing activity. They capture and detoxify radicals of various promoters of carcinogenesis and radicals produced in the process of exposure to radiation and light. Since tea polyphenols inactivate enzyme and virus activity, they could be effective against carcinogenesis caused by some viruses. Tea polyphenols exert their inhibitory actions via various mechanisms at different stages of mutagenesis, carcinogenesis, invasion and metastasis of tumor cells; they act extracellularly as desmutagens and intracellularly as bio-antimutagens. Tea polyphenols modulate metabolism, block, suppress, or affect DNA replication and repair effects.

2.1.2. The health effects of green tea

Green tea has been extensively studied in people, animals, and laboratory experiments. Results from these studies suggest that green tea can be useful for the several health conditions.

It has been found that green tea consumption is significantly associated with a lower risk of mortality due to stroke [29] and pneumonia [30] and imparts a lower risk of cognitive impairment [31], depression [32], and psychological distress [33]. These results have been confirmed by other researchers [34–37]. In addition, other epidemiologic studies have indicated that green tea consumption is associated with a lower risk of osteoporosis [38, 39], and randomized placebo-controlled trials have indicated that green tea is effective in lowering cardiovascular risk factors [40, 41]. Because all of the above conditions are major causes of functional disability [42–44], it is expected that green tea consumption would contribute to disability prevention. Green tea consumption is associated with a lower risk of developing functional disability.

Atherosclerosis

Population-based clinical studies indicate that the antioxidant properties of green tea can help prevent atherosclerosis, particularly coronary artery disease. (Population-based studies mean studies that follow large groups of people over time or studies that are comparing groups of people living in different cultures or with different dietary habits.) Researchers are not sure why green tea reduces the risk of heart disease by lowering cholesterol and triglyceride levels. Studies show that black tea has similar beneficial effects. In fact, researchers estimate that the rate of heart attack decreases by 11% with consumption of 3 cups of tea per day [45].

High cholesterol and cardiovascular Disease

Research shows that green tea lowers total cholesterol and raises HDL ("good") cholesterol in both animals and people. One population-based clinical study found that men who drink green tea are more likely to have lower total cholesterol than those who do not drink green tea. Results from one animal study suggest that polyphenols in green tea can block the intestinal absorption of cholesterol and promote its excretion from the body. In another small study of male smokers, researchers found that green tea significantly reduced blood levels of harmful LDL cholesterol.

Substantial evidence from *in vitro* and animal studies indicates that green tea (GT) preparations inhibit cardiovascular disease (CVD) processes [46-49]. In a previous observational study, it has been shown that GT consumption was associated with a significantly lower risk of mortality due to CVD among middle-aged adults [50]. The study also indicated that GT consumption was associated with reduced mortality from cerebral infarction but not with mortality from cerebral hemorrhage. These associations were consistent with those reported in another observational study [51].

Obesity

Obesity and its related metabolic abnormalities, including insulin resistance, alterations in the insulin-like growth factor-1 (IGF-1)/IGF-1 receptor (IGF-1R) axis, and the state of chronic inflammation, increase the risk of colorectal cancer (CRC) and hepatocellular carcinoma (HCC). However, these findings also indicate that the metabolic disorders caused by obesity might be effective targets to prevent the development of CRC and HCC in obese individuals. Green tea catechins (GTCs) possess anticancer and chemopreventive properties against cancer in various organs, including the colorectal and liver. GTCs have also been known to exert anti-obesity, antidiabetic, and anti-inflammatory effects, indicating that GTCs might be useful for the prevention of obesity-associated colorectal and liver carcinogenesis. Further, branched-chain amino acids (BCAA), which improve protein malnutrition and prevent progressive hepatic failure in patients with chronic liver diseases, might be also effective for the suppression of obesity-related carcinogenesis because oral supplementation with BCAA reduces the risk of HCC in obese cirrhotic patients. BCAA shows these beneficial effects because they can improve insulin resistance. Here, we review the detailed relationship between metabolic abnormalities and the development of CRC and

HCC. We also review evidence, especially that based on our basic and clinical research using GTCs and BCAA, which indicates that targeting metabolic abnormalities by either pharmaceutical or nutritional intervention can be an effective strategy to prevent the development of CRC and HCC in obese individuals [52].

Diabetes

Several studies have reported a protective effect for tea consumption on incident diabetes, and the results of a recent meta-analysis indicated that drinking more than 3–4 cups of tea (black, green or oolong) per day decreases the risk of Diabetes Mellitus by 20% [53]. Despite very high intake of black tea, no significant association for black tea consumption was observed, but an inverse correlation was found between green tea drinking and diabetes prevalence. Several animal and human studies have shown an antidiabetic effect for green tea polyphenols, specifically epigallocatechin gallate (EGCG) [54-57]. EGCG induces its antidiabetic effects mostly through reduced hepatic glucose production and enhanced pancreatic function [56]. Green tea has been shown to improve glucose tolerance and has been suggested as a prophylactic agent against diabetes [55].

Weight loss

Clinical studies suggest that green tea extract can boost metabolism and help burn fat. One study confirmed that the combination of green tea and caffeine improved weight loss and maintenance in overweight and moderately obese individuals. Some researchers speculate that substances in green tea known as polyphenols, specifically the catechins, are responsible for the herb's fat-burning effect.

Cancer

Many studies suggest an inverse relationship between green tea intake and the risk of a variety of cancers, although other studies have found no association. Clinical trials have been small and heterogenous with contradictory results. Dietary, environmental, and population differences can account for these inconsistencies [58].

Several population-based clinical studies have shown that both green and black teas help protect against cancer. For example, cancer rates tend to be low in countries such as Japan where people regularly consume green tea. However, it is not possible to determine from these population-based studies whether green tea actually prevents cancer in people. Emerging clinical studies suggest that the polyphenols in tea, especially green tea, can play an important role in the prevention of cancer [59].

Bladder Cancer. Only a few clinical studies have examined the relationship between bladder cancer and tea consumption. In one study that compared people with and without bladder cancer, researchers found that women who drank black tea and powdered green tea were less likely to develop bladder cancer. A follow-up clinical study by the same group of researchers revealed that bladder cancer patients (particularly men) who drank green tea had a substantially better 5-year survival rate than those who did not. Other study has demonstrated the anti-oxidant properties of green tea extract (GTE) against human bladder uroepithelial cells. The data demonstrate that under *in vitro* conditions, green tea extract can afford both normal and tumorigenic human bladder urothelial cells protection (i.e., prevent apoptosis) to various degrees after chemical insult with H_2O_2 [60].

Breast Cancer. Although tea has been extensively investigated in *in vitro* and *in vivo* studies, few epidemiologic studies have evaluated the relationship between green tea and breast cancer risk. The results from these studies are inconsistent [61-63]. In general, the cohort studies, all based in Japan, report no significant association [61] and the case-control studies [62, 63], based on Asian-American or Chinese populations, all report an inverse relationship between green tea and breast cancer risk [62]. Previous studies have not evaluated the relationship between green tea consumption and pre- and postmenopausal breast cancer.

The most recent meta-analysis included 7 (2 cohort, 1 nested case–control and 4 case–control) epidemiological studies of green tea and breast cancer that were published as of December 2008 [64]. An inverse association between green tea and breast cancer risk was reported from case–control data, while no association was observed from cohort data [64]. The nested case–control study reported no association [65], so even if it had been included as a cohort study in the pooled analyses, the overall finding would have remained the same.

In summary, green tea could exert beneficial effects on breast carcinogenesis through inhibition of estrogen's pro-carcinogenic activity either alone by itself or in combination with other estrogen-inhibiting factors. Black tea does not appear to have protective effects on breast cancer incidence, and can increase risk of hormone-dependent tumors. Future research is needed to elucidate the interactive role of tea catechins and other dietary cancer-inhibitory compounds in mammary carcinogenesis in humans.

Ovarian Cancer. In a clinical study conducted on ovarian cancer patients in China, researchers found that women who drank at least one cup of green tea per day survived longer with the disease than those who did not drink green tea. In fact, those who drank green tea lived the longest. Other studies found no beneficial effects [66, 67]. In view of the variations in rates of breast cancer and tea-drinking practices, one case–control study was conducted in Southeast China to evaluate the association between breast cancer and tea consumption measured by type, duration, frequency and quantity of tea and the interactions between tea consumption and other lifestyle factors.

Esophageal Cancer. In the Indian studies [68-70], some results indicated that tea (presumably black tea) consumption could be responsible for the development of esophageal cancer. The authors indicated that this result could be due to drinking hot tea, which was shown to occur a couple of decades before in a Chinese cohort. The other possibility could be that Indians drink their black tea with milk, which was shown before to counteract positive effects of tea.

The higher content of tea catechins present in green tea than in black tea can explain the more consistent inverse association between tea and esophageal cancer risk in studies conducted in China and Japan than in European and American countries. The putative protective effect of tea consumption, if any, on esophageal cancer development could be confounded and/or overshadowed by the thermal effect of tea beverages, if consumed at high temperature, as well as cigarette smoking or alcohol intake. Future prospective cohort studies are required to collect detailed information on tea temperature and histories of tobacco and alcohol use that can then be adjusted for when evaluating the protective effect of tea on esophageal cancer.

Prostate Cancer. Among all cancers, prostate cancer is an ideal candidate disease for chemoprevention because it is typically diagnosed in men ages >50 years and has a high latency period [71, 72]. Therefore, even a slight delay in the progression of this disease by chemopreventive intervention could result in a substantial reduction in the incidence of the disease and, more importantly, improve the quality of life of the patients [71, 72]. Evidences collected from geographic, epidemiologic, and migration studies suggest that frequent consumption of green tea is associated with lower frequencies of prostate cancer in Asian populations in general compared with those in western societies [73-77]. Laboratory and preclinical animal studies also indicate a protective role of green tea against prostate cancer [78-82].

In summary, observational studies do not provide strong evidence for a protective effect of green tea or black tea intake against the development of prostate cancer. There is some suggestive evidence that green tea intake can reduce the risk of advanced prostate cancer. The phase II clinical trials have provided encouraging evidence in the development of green tea catechins as a chemopreventive agent against prostate carcinogenesis.

Skin Cancer. There has been considerable interest in the use of naturally occurring plant products, including polyphenols, for the prevention of UV-induced skin photodamage primarily including the risk of skin cancer. Polyphenols, specifically dietary, possessing anti-inflammatory, immunomodulatory and anti-oxidant properties are among the most promising group of compounds that can be exploited as ideal chemopreventive agents for a variety of skin disorders in general and skin cancer in particular. In this respect, chemoprevention offers a realistic strategy for controlling the risk of cancers. Furthermore, a chemopreventive approach appears to have practical implications in reducing skin cancer risk because, unlike the carcinogenic environmental factors that are difficult to control, individuals can modify their dietary habits and lifestyle in combination with a careful use of skin care products to prevent the photodamaging effects in the skin. Studies from our laboratory have shown the efficacy of naturally occurring polyphenols, such as green tea polyphenols (GTPs), silymarin from milk thistle and proanthocyanidins from grape seeds (GSPs), against UV radiation-induced inflammation, oxidative stress, DNA damage and suppression of immune responses [83].

Stomach cancer. Recently, Myung et al. conducted a meta-analysis investigating the quantitative association between the consumption of green tea and the risk of stomach cancer in humans [84]. The analysis included 13 (5 cohort and 8 case–control) studies, all conducted in Japanese or Chinese populations. An inverse association was seen in case–control studies only, but not in cohort studies. However, in a recent pooled analysis of 6 cohort studies that included more than 218,000 Japanese men and women aged 40 years or older and more than 3500 incident stomach cancer cases found a statistically significant, inverse association between green tea consumption and stomach cancer risk in women, but not in men [85]. Compared with those drinking <1 cup/day, women with the consumption of ≥5 cups/day green tea had an approximately 20% decreased risk of stomach cancer. This protective effect was primarily seen among female nonsmokers [85].

In the study by Kinlen et al., the positive association between black tea consumption and stomach cancer death could be, at least partly, due to the effects of smoking and social class [86]. Whereas in the cohort analysis by Khan et al. that included approximately 3100 Japanese men and women, black tea consumption was associated with a statistically significantly increased risk of stomach cancer for women [87]. Given the small sample size and low intake of black tea in a population that usually consumed green tea, this positive association could be a chance finding.

Both case–control and cohort studies demonstrated an inverse association between green tea consumption and risk of stomach cancer. The protection can be stronger for women than men since the former are less likely to smoke cigarettes or drink alcoholic beverages. There is lack of evidence in support of a protective role of black tea consumption against the development of stomach cancer.

Cervical Cancer. Cancer of the cervix is the third most common malignancy worldwide in women, and the most common gynecologic cancer in the developing world. In developed countries, prevention of cervical cancer achieved by the widespread and systematic use of cervical cytologic screening, has contributed to the successful decrease in the incidence of invasive cervical carcinomas. In the developing world, cervical cancer remains a common malignancy impacting the lives of women during their period of highest productivity. Especially in low-resource settings, an inexpensive dietary chemo-preventive intervention would be an attractive adjunct to existing cervical cancer prevention programs It is well-known that the regular consumption of fruits and vegetables is highly associated with the reduced epidemiologic risk of different types of cancer [88-91] and green tea consumption is associated with lowering certain cancer incidences including cervical cancer [92].

Lung Cancer. Numerous epidemiological studies examined the association between green tea or black tea consumption and risk of lung cancer. A systematic review was conducted to evaluate the association between the consumption of green tea or black tea and lung cancer risk among 19 studies (13 case–control, 6 prospective cohort) that were published prior to September 2007 [93]. Among the 8 studies examining green tea and lung cancer risk, 3 reported a significantly lower risk while one reported a significantly increased risk of lung cancer with high green tea consumption. The remaining 4 studies reported no association [93]. More recently, Tang et al. conducted a similar meta-analysis for green tea or black tea consumption with lung cancer risk [94]. This analysis included 22 studies published from 1966 to November 2008 and 12 of them also were included in the analysis by Arts [93]. Twelve studies examined the association between green tea and lung cancer risk. A statistically significant 18% decreased risk of lung cancer was associated with every 2 cups/day of green tea consumption. This inverse green tea-lung cancer association was slightly stronger for prospective cohort studies than retrospective case–control studies. The protective effect of green tea consumption on lung cancer risk was confined to nonsmokers [94].

In the same review by Arts [93], 11 of the 19 studies included examined the association between black tea consumption and lung cancer risk. Among them, two reported a statistically significantly reduced risk while one reported an increased risk for lung cancer associated with black tea intake. The remaining 8 studies reported a null association [93]. In a more recent meta-analysis by Tang et al., no statistically significant association was observed between black tea consumption and lung cancer risk based on 14 studies included [94]. Not included in the meta-analyses was a case–control study in Los Angeles, CA with 558 cases and 837 controls. The results showed that high consumption of dietary epicatechin, mainly from black tea, was associated with significantly reduced risk of lung cancer, especially among smokers [95].

One potential mechanism for the chemopreventive effect of tea on carcinogenesis is the strong antioxidant effect of tea polyphenols. Hakim et al. conducted a phase II randomized controlled tea intervention trial to evaluate the efficacy of regular green tea drinking in reducing DNA damage as measured by urinary 8-hydroxydeoxyguanosine among heavy smokers [96]. After consuming 4 cups/day of decaffeinated green tea for 4 months, smokers showed a statistically significant 31% decrease in urinary 8-hydroxydeoxyguanosine compared with the baseline value. In the same study, no change in urinary 8-hydroxydeoxyguanosine was seen among smokers assigned to the black tea group [96]. These findings support that tea catechins, with highest levels in green tea, exert their antioxidative role in reducing the formation of 8-hydroxydeoxyguanosine. However, a lack of inverse association between green tea consumption and lung cancer risk in smokers suggest that the antioxidation mechanism plays a limited role in reducing the risk of lung cancer development. Furthermore, the protective effect of tea consumption on lung cancer development for nonsmokers, especially among women, indicates an alternative cancer-preventive mechanism of tea that is not driven by antioxidation. Additional experimental studies that utilize animal models to elucidate the cancer-preventive mechanisms of tea catechins on lung carcinogenesis are needed.

Pancreatic Cancer. Similar to other gastrointestinal organs, epidemiological studies have provided mixed results on the association between tea consumption and risk of pancreatic cancer. There are a limited number of studies that examined the association between green tea consumption and pancreatic cancer. From an early hospital-based case–control study in Japan (124 cases and 124 matched controls), no association was observed for pancreatic cancer risk with green tea drinking [97]. In contrast, analyses from a population based case–control study conducted in Shanghai, China (451 cases and 1552 controls) demonstrated a statistically significant inverse association with increased green tea consumption and pancreatic cancer risk [98]. A prospective cohort study in Japan involved more than 100,000 Japanese adults with up to 11 years of follow-up and 233 incidents of pancreatic cancer cases did not find an association between green tea intake and pancreatic cancer risk [99]. In another prospective cohort study with up to 13 years of follow-up and 292 incident pancreatic cancer cases in Japan, Lin et al. reported a higher percentage of dying from pancreatic cancer for subjects who consumed ≥7 cups/day of green tea compared with those <1 cup/day [100].

Available epidemiological data are insufficient to conclude that either green tea or black tea can protect against the development of pancreatic cancer. Given the short survival and rapid progression of pancreatic cancer, the low participation rates of pancreatic cancer patients in retrospective case–control studies or the use of proxy respondents in interview for collection of information on tea consumption and other risk factors could bias the results of case–control studies. Prospective cohort studies offer methodological advantages over case–control studies. Additional data from well-designed and well-executed prospective cohort studies are required before any conclusion on the protective effect of green tea and/or black tea against the development of pancreatic cancer can be reached.

Oral cavity and pharynx Although numerous epidemiological studies examined the association between dietary factors and risk of oral and pharyngeal cancers [101], there are limited data on the effect of tea consumption on these malignancies. Combining a series of case–control studies in Italy with a total of 119 patients with cancer of the oral cavity and 6147 hospital controls, La Vecchia et al. reported a reduced, but statistically non-significant, risk of oral cancer with black tea consumption [102]. Using a similar approach, Tavani et al. combined datasets of two hospital-based case–control studies conducted in Italy and Switzerland, respectively, and reported no association between black tea consumption and oral cancer risk [103]. Recently, Ren et al. examined the association between black tea consumption and the risk of developing oral and pharyngeal cancers in the National Institutes of Health (NIH)-American Association of Retired Persons (AARP) Diet and Health Study [104].

The NIH-AARP cohort study enrolled 481,563 AARP members aged 51–71 years who resided in eight states of the United States in 1995–1996. After up to 8 years of follow-up, 392 study participants developed oral cancer and 178 developed pharyngeal cancer. The study demonstrated a statistically significant positive relationship between consumption of hot tea and risk of pharyngeal cancer. There was a suggestive positive relationship between hot tea intake and risk of oral cancer [104]. Consumption of iced tea was not associated with risk of oral or pharyngeal cancer.

There was one prospective cohort study that examined the association between green tea consumption and risk of oral cancer in the Japan Collaborative Cohort Study. The cohort consisted of 50,221 Japanese men and women aged 40–79 years at baseline and identified 37 incident oral cancer cases after 10.3 years of follow-up. The inverse association was slightly stronger for women than for men [105]. The inverse relation did not reach statistical significance due to the relatively small number of cancer cases included in the analysis.

A randomized, placebo-controlled, phase II clinical trial was conducted to examine the effect of green tea extract on the oral mucosa leukoplakia, a well established precancerous lesion of oral cancer [106]. Fifty-nine patients were randomly assigned to either the treatment group, who were given 3 g/day of a mixed green tea product composed of dried water extract, polyphenols and pigments, or the placebo group. After 6 months, 37.9% patients in the green tea treatment arm showed reduced size of oral lesions whereas 3.4% patients had increased lesion size. In contrast, 6.7% patients in the placebo group had decreased and 10% patients had increased size of oral mucosa leukoplakia. The differences in the changes of lesion sizes between the treatment and placebo arms are statistically significant [106]. Recently, Tsao et al. completed another randomized, placebo-controlled phase II trial to evaluate the oral cancer prevention potential of green tea extract [107]. Forty-two patients with one or more histologically confirmed, bidimentionally measurable oral premalignant lesions with high-risk features of malignant transformation that could be sampled by biopsy were randomly assigned to receive 500, 750, or 1000 mg/m2 of green tea extract per day or placebo orally. The efficacy was determined by the disappearance of all lesions (a complete response) or 50% or greater decrease in the sum of products of diameters of all measured lesions (a partial response). At 12 weeks after the initiation of the treatment, 39 patients who completed the trial were evaluated; 14 (50%) of the 28 patients in the three combined green tea extract groups had a favorable response whereas only 2 (18.2%) of the 11 patients in the placebo group showed the similar response. A dose-dependent effect was observed; the favorable response rates were 58% in patients given 750 or 1000 mg/m2 green tea extract and 36.4% in those given 500 mg/m2, but only 18.2% in those assigned to the placebo arm [107].

Although limited, data from the prospective cohort study suggest a moderate protective effect of green tea consumption against the development of oral cancer. Both phase II clinical trials further support a protective role of green tea extract against the progression of precancerous lesions in the oral cavity towards malignant transformation. Phase III clinical trials with large number of patients are required to confirm the efficacy of green tea extract against the formation of oral cancer in humans. Data on the effect of black tea consumption against the development of oral cancer are too limited to draw any conclusion. One prospective study showed a statistically significant inverse association between black tea consumption and risk of pharyngeal cancer, more epidemiological studies are warranted to evaluate the potential protective effect of either green tea or black tea on the development of pharyngeal cancer in humans.

Large bowel. Numerous epidemiological studies have examined the association between tea consumption and colorectal cancer. Sun et al. conducted a meta-analysis that included 25 epidemiological studies evaluating tea consumption and risk of colorectal cancer in 11 countries [108]. The inverse association between green tea intake and colon cancer risk was mainly observed in 4 case–control studies, but not in 4 cohort studies. There was no relationship between green tea intake and rectal cancer risk in 6 case–control or cohort studies.

Following the meta-analysis, several studies examined and published the results on the green tea consumption and colorectal cancer risk. After analyzing the database of the Singapore Chinese Health Study, a prospective cohort study of diet and cancer involved over 60,000 Chinese men and women aged 45–74 years, Sun et al. found that subjects who drank green tea daily had a statistically non-significant increased risk for colorectal cancer relative to nondrinkers of green tea. This association was confined to men and was stronger for colon cancer than rectal cancer, especially for the advanced stage of colon cancer [109].

These data suggest that substances in green tea can exert an adverse, late-stage effect on the development of colorectal cancer.

Yang et al. prospectively evaluated the association between green tea consumption and colorectal cancer risk in a cohort of 69,710 Chinese women aged 40–70 years, most of which were Lifelong nonsmokers (97.3%) or nondrinkers of alcoholic beverages (97.7%). Information on tea consumption was assessed through inperson interviews at baseline and reassessed 2–3 years later in a follow-up survey. During the first 6 years of follow-up, 256 incident cases of colorectal cancer were identified. Regular tea drinkers had significantly reduced risk of colorectal cancer compared with nondrinkers. The reduction in risk was most evident among those who consistently reported to drink tea regularly at both the baseline and follow-up surveys [110].

There were two recent prospective studies on green tea consumption and colorectal cancer incidence and mortality in Japan [111, 112]. The first consisted of 96,162 Japanese men and women, and 1163 incident cases of colorectal cancer [111]. There was no statistically significant association between green tea consumption and incidence of colon and rectal cancers combined or separately in either men or women or both. The second cohort consisted of 14,001 Japanese men and women. After up to 6 years of follow-up, 43 subjects died from colorectal cancer. Given the small number of cases, the results should be interpreted with caution. Using validated biomarkers of specific tea polyphenols, Yuan et al. prospectively examined the urinary levels of specific tea catechins and their metabolites and the risk of developing colorectal cancer in the Shanghai Cohort Study as described above [113]. EGC, 4_-O-methyl-epigallocatechin (4_-MeEGC) and EC, and their metabolites in baseline urine samples were measured in 162 incident colorectal cancer cases (83 colon and 79 rectal cancer cases) and 806 matched controls. Individuals with high prediagnostic urinary catechin levels had a lower risk of colon cancer. There was no association between urinary green tea catechins or their metabolites and risk of rectal cancer. This study provided a direct evidence for the chemopreventive effect of tea catechins against the development of colon cancer in humans [113].

In terms of black tea, the meta-analysis by Sun et al. [108] included 20 studies that examined black tea consumption and colorectal cancer risk and found no association. No association was found separately in case–control studies or prospective cohort studies. In our analysis of the Singapore Chinese Health Study, we did not find any association between black tea consumption and risk of colon cancer and rectal cancer combined or separately [109]. More recently, Zhang et al. conducted a pooled analysis for black tea intake and colon cancer risk on the combined dataset of 13 cohort studies conducted in North America or Western Europe. The analysis included 731,441 subjects and 5604 incident colon cancer cases [114]. Compared with nondrinkers, consumption of 900 g/day tea (approximately four 8-oz cups/day) was associated with a modest, but statistically significantly increased risk of colon cancer. This increased risk for colon cancer was only in women, but not in men.

Epidemiological studies provided suggestive evidence to support a protective role of green tea consumption, especially in high amount and long-term duration of consumption, in reducing the risk of colon cancer. This effect of green tea on colon carcinogenesis can depend on the time of exposure, where late exposure can promote the growth of colon tumor cells. Current epidemiological data suggest that black tea consumption can increase, instead of decrease, the risk of colorectal cancer.

Kidney. Several epidemiological studies examined the relationship between tea consumption and kidney cancer risk. Mellemgaard et al. conducted a population-based case–control study that enrolled 368 renal cell cancer cases and 396 matched controls living in Denmark [115]. The study did not find an association between black tea consumption and renal cell cancer risk. Bianchi et al. conducted a population-based case–control study of renal cell cancer in Iowa (406 cases and 2434 controls), and found no association [116].

Similarly, a more recent case–control study of renal cell cancer in Italy including 767 cases and 1534 controls did not find any association between tea consumption and risk of renal cell cancer [117]. Lee et al. analyzed datasets of the Nurses' Health Study and the Health Professionals Follow-up Study and found that consumption of >1 cup/day tea was associated with statistically non-significantly reduced risk of renal cell cancer relative to <1 cup/month [118]. In a pooled analysis, Lee et al. combined data of 13 prospective cohorts including more than 774,000 men and women and 1478 incident renal cell cancer cases. Compared with nondrinkers, individuals who consumed ≥1 cups/day of tea had a statistically borderline significant 15% risk reduction in renal cell cancer after adjustment for body mass index, cigarette smoking, hypertension and other potential confounders [119]. All these studies were conducted in North America and West Europe and examined the effect of presumably black tea on renal cell cancer risk. These findings do not support a protective role of black tea on kidney cancer. Additional prospective epidemiological studies are warranted to examine the association between green tea consumption and kidney cancer risk.

Glioma. Regular intake of tea was not associated with risk of adult glioma in a case–control study [120]. Recently Holick et al. examined the association between coffee, black tea and caffeine intake and risk of adult glioma in three prospective cohort studies in the United States. The analysis included 335 incident glioma cases. Compared with nondrinkers, there was a statistically non-significant, approximately 30% decreased risk of glioma incidence for those consuming 4 cups/week of black tea [121]. More data are warranted to draw any conclusion on the association between tea consumption and adult glioma risk.

Lymphoma. Thompson et al. examined the association between black tea consumption and risk of non-Hodgkin's lymphoma in the Iowa Women's Health Study. The analysis included 415 incident lymphoma cases during the 20 years of follow-up following baseline interview. No association was found between black tea consumption and risk of non-Hodgkin's lymphoma [122].

Leukemia. A hospital-based case–control study involving 107 adults with leukemia and 110 orthopaedic controls in China found that green tea consumption was associated with a statistically significant 50% decreased risk of leukemia. The inverse association was dose dependent with number of cups of tea per day, number of years of tea consumption, and the amount of dry tea leaves consumed [123]. A similar case–control study enrolled 252 leukemia patients aged 0–29 years and 637 sex- and age matched control subjects in Taiwan. Compared with nondrinkers, high intake of total tea catechins was associated with approximately 50% reduced risk. This inverse association was stronger in older (16–29 years) than in the younger (0–15 years) group [124]. Given the limitations of small study size and hospital-based study design, further studies are warranted to confirm these results.

2.1.3. Possible active tea components and their tissue levels

Plasma EGCG, EGC and EC exist in free and conjugated (glucuronide and sulfate) forms. The plasma tea polyphenol levels in rats and mice in some anticarcinogenesis experiments were comparable to the peak levels in humans after consuming two or three cups of tea [125]. In a preliminary experiment, after administration of regular green tea in drinking fluid to rats, the EGCG was detected in the esophagus (410 ng/g) but not in the lung, the EGCG, EGC and EC levels in the small intestine and intestinal contents were rather high (1.5 - 5.5 mg/g) due to the unabsorbed and biliary excreted glucuronides of polyphenols in the intestine. High EGC and EC levels were also observed in the colon tissues (1.8 and 0.3 mg/g respectively). Due to possible glucuronidase and esterase activities in the colon, most of the EGC and EC were found in the free form and EGCG was found at lower levels. EGCG has been usually considered the active anticarcinogenic components in tea because it is the most abundant polyphenol in tea.

Hackett *et al.*, [126] reported that three human volunteers were given 2 g of (+)- catechin and the metabolic changes in it were then examined by looking at their blood and urine. About 55% of the labeled catechin was excreted in urine within 2 h after its uptake. The metabolites in urine were (+) - catechin, and glucuronic and sulfate compounds of 3-O-methye- (+)-catechin. These metabolites were about ¾ of the catechin uptake.

Matsumoto *et al.*, [127] determined the amount of tea polyphenols in organs and tissues to examine the fate of catechin in the digestive canal, such as the stomach; small and large intestines of rats. EGCG given orally was transferred from the stomach to the small intestine within several hours and moved to the large intestine after 8 hours. Most of the amount of catechins taken in orally moved into the digestive tract and were excreted in the feces. Some part of the catechins was metabolized by intraintestinal bacteria and about 20% of the catechin can have been absorbed by the digestive organs.

Tea catechins and crude extracts, however, have some beneficial effects on human health, such as suppression of high blood pressure [128], reduction of blood glucose levels [129] suppression of cholesterol and prevention of fat increase [130]. Tea drinking can also induce higher levels of glutathione [131], so that detoxification of reactive forms of carcinogens can occur more efficiently, other biochemical mechanisms have been hypothesized for the anticancer properties of tea e.g. induction of DNA repair, binding with activated carcinogens. Moderate tea consumption (5 cups / day an extract of about 11 g of tea) can be readily curable in some types of human cancer [132]. In other studies on the inhibitory effects of tea catechins, black tea extract and oolong tea extract and EC, EGC, ECG, EGCG and other tea extracts (0.05 or 0.1%) showed a significant decrease in the number and area of preneoplastic glutathione S-transferase placental form (GSTP)-positive foci in the liver of rats [133].

2.1.4. *Antioxidative function of tea polyphenols*

The most noteworthy properties of tea polyphenols and other flavonoids are their antioxidative activities. Reactive oxygen species may play important roles in carcinogenesis through damaging DNA, altering gene expression, or affecting cell growth and differentiation. The anticarcinogenic activities of tea polyphenols are believed to be closely related to their antioxidative properties. The findings that green tea preparations inhibited 12-0-tetradecanoylphorbol- 1 3-acetate-induced hydrogen peroxide formation in mouse epidermis and NNK-induced 8-hydroxydeoxyguanosine formation in mouse lung are consistent with this concept. Inhibition of tumor promotion-related enzymes such as ornithine decarboxylase, protein kinase C, lipoxygenase, and cyclooxygenase by tea preparations has also been reported. Although inhibition of carcinogen activation by tea or green tea polyphenol fractions could be demonstrated *in vitro* and, in certain cases, *in vivo* [134], this mechanism was not demonstrated for NNK bioactivation *in vivo*. Oral administration of tea preparations to animals has been reported to moderately enhance the activities of glutathione peroxidase, catalase, glutathione S-transferase, NADPH-quinone oxidoreductase, uridine diphosphate-glucuronosyltransferase, and methoxyresorufin O-dealkylase. The effects of a mild induction of these enzymes on carcinogenesis are not clear. Mechanisms relating to the quenching of activated carcinogens, antiviral activity, and enhancing immune functions have also been suggested, but their relevance to carcinogenesis remains to be determined. Inhibition of nitrosation by tea preparations has been demonstrated *in vitro* and in humans [135]; this may be an important factor in preventing certain cancers, e.g., gastric cancer, if the endogenously formed N-nitroso compounds are causative factors. Other results suggest that the antiproliferative effect of tea is important for the anticarcinogenic activity. One may speculate that tea polyphenols inhibit growth-related signal transduction pathways [136].

2.1.5. *Effects of tea on mutation and genotoxicty*

As to the genotoxic profile of tea catechins when tested alone, Chang *et al.* [137] have shown that there is minimal genotoxic concern with a decaffeinated green tea catechin mixture (Polyphenon E) that contains about 50% epigallocatechin gallate and 30% other catechins. Isbrucker *et al.* [138] have also found no genotoxic concern with a epigallocatechin gallate (GTE) preparation, Teavigo. On the other hand, many studies have demonstrated that tea catechins could suppress the genotoxic activity of various carcinogens with both *in vitro* and *in vivo* systems.

a. *In vivo* studies

Imanishi *et al.,* [139] reported that when green tea or black tea polyphenols was administered orally 6, 12 or 18 hours before an intraperitoneal injection of mitomycin C resulted in a statistically significant decrease of micronucleus formation in mouse bone marrow, although, post-treatment administration had no effect.

Hot water extracts of green tea effectively suppressed AFB1 (aflatoxin B1) induced chromosome aberrations in bone marrow cells in rats when given green tea extract 24 h before injection with AFB1 [140]. Rats administered green tea extract 2 h before or after the AFB1 injection showed no suppressive effect. The suppressive effect of green tea extracts on AFB1 induced chromosome aberration was directly related to the dose of green tea extract (in the range of 0.1 to 2 g/kg). Black tea or coffee given 24 or 2 h before the AFB1 injection produced no suppressive effect.

De boer, [141] showed that the mutagenic potency of several chemicals including the dietary heterocyclic amine 2-amino-1-methyl-6-phenyl-imidazo(4,5-b) pyridine (PhIP)(the environmentally important aromatic hydrocarbon benzo(a)pyrene) and the food contaminant aflatoxin B1 can be modulated by dietary compounds including green tea in lacI transgenic rodent.

Green tea effectively inhibited oxidative DNA damage and cell proliferation in liver of 2-nitropropane (2NP) treated rats [142]. It was suggested that pyrogallol-related compounds of green tea such as EGCG, ECG and EGC are antimutagenic factors in the *Escherichia coli* B/R Wp2 assay system [143-146].

Significant inhibition activity of the tea catechins ECG and EGCG, against the mutagenicity of Trp-P-2 and N-OH-Trp-P-2 has been found by [143] using *Salmonella typhimurium*, TA98 and TA100 with and without rat liver S9 mix. EGCG has also an inhibitory effect against the mutagenicity of benzo[a]pyrene (B[a]P) diol epoxide in TA100 strain without S9 mix. Green tea has potent suppressive effects against gene expression of the SOS response in *salmonella typhimurium* TA1535/psk 1002 induced by four nitroarenes [147].

A study performed by [148] reported that EGCG suppressed the direct-acting mutagenicity of 3-hydroxyamino-1-methyl-5H-pyrido-(4,3 b) indole (Trp-p-2(NHOH)) and 2-hydroxyamino-6-methyldipyrido(1,2-a:3,2-d) imidazole (Glu-p-1(NHOH)) in the Ames *salmonella* test. furthermore, they added that EGCE has also a suppressive effect in the *in vivo* Drosophila mutation assays, i.e., the wing spot test, and the DNA repair test, on several carcinogens.

Kada *et al.*, [144] showed that a homogenate of Japanese green tea gave high bioantimutagenic activity against spontaneous mutations resulting from altered DNA-polymerase III in strain NIG 1125 of *Bacillus subtilis*. They identified chemically the active principles and they obtained 0.85 g EC, 1.44 g EGC, 1.24 g ECG and 4.87 g EGCG from 12 g of a crude extract of green tea powder.

Green tea extract reduced the levels of ischemia/reperfusion induced hydrogen peroxide, lipid peroxidation and oxidative DNA damage (formation of 8-hydroxydeoxyguanosine) by pretreatment of 0.5 or 2% green tea water extract for 3 weeks, respectively in Mongolian gerbils. Moreover, green tea also reduced the number of ischemia/reperfusion- induced apoptotic cells and locomotors activity [149].

Li *et al.*, [150] indicated that green tea, tea pigments, and mixed tea could effectively inhibit DMBA (7,12-dimethyl-benz(a)anthracene) induced oral carcinogenesis in hamster. Protection from DNA damage and suppression of cell proliferation could be important mechanisms of anticarcinogenic effects of the tea preparations. Another study reported that green tea consumption inhibited the formation of micronuclei in peripheral blood lymphocytes in smokers [151].

Katiyar *et al.*, [152] demonstrated that green tea polyphenols (GTP) prevent ultraviolet (UV)-B-induced cyclobutane pyrimidine dimers (CPD), which are considered to be mediators of UVB induced immune suppression and DNA damage on human skin. It has been also demonstrated that standardized green tea extract protects against psoralen plus ultraviolet A-induced phototoxicity to human skin by inhibiting DNA damage and diminishing the inflammatory effects of this modality.

Binding of AFB1 to hepatic nuclear DNA was inhibited in rats given 0.5% instant green tea for 2 or 4 weeks before a single injection of AFB1 [153].

The oral administration of 0.2% green tea or 0.1% black tea for 28 days decreased the extent of chromosome damages (micronuclei) in the peripheral blood of mice subsequently treated with B[a]P [154].

The level of one of the two lung DNA adducts produced by the lung carcinogen NNK (4(methylnitrosamino)-1-(3-pyridyl)-1-butanone) during and after carcinogen treatment was reduced in mice given 2% green tea as their sole source of drinking water [155]. Green tea suppressed 8-OH-2'deoxyguanosine or 8-OH-guanosine, but not ^{6}O-methylguanine levels, in lung DNA.

Recently, it has been demonstrated that the administration of green tea extract 24 hr before the dimethylnitrosoamine (DMN) injection significantly suppressed DMN-induced chromosomal aberrations and sister chromatid exchanges. The suppression was observed 18 hr, 24 hr and 48 hr after the DMN treatment but no suppressive effect was observed at the early period (6 hr and 12 hr) after the DMN treatment. Furthermore, the suppression was observed for all doses of DMN investigated. Mice given green tea 2 hr before the DMN injection displayed no suppressive effect. Mice that were given 2% green tea extract as the sole source of drinking water for four days before sacrifice displayed significantly suppressed DMN-induced chromosomal aberrations and sister chromatid exchanges [156]. They conclude that the suppression of DMN-induced chromosomal aberrations and sister chromatid exchanges should be considered as a green tea exerting a preventive action.

b. *In vitro* studies

Studies with cell lines had demonstrated that tea polyphenols affect signal transduction pathways, inhibit cell proliferation and induce apoptosis, but the effective concentrations are usually much higher than those observed in blood and tissue [157].

Islami *et al.*, [158] described a novel observation that EGCG displayed strong inhibitory effects on the proliferation and viability of HTB-94 human chondrosarcoma cells in a dose-dependent manner and induced apoptosis. The induction of apoptosis by EGCG via activation of caspase-3/cpp32 - like proteases can provide a mechanistic explanation for its antitumor effects.

Supplementation with green tea extract significantly decreased malondialdehyde production and DNA damage after Fe(+2) oxidative treatment in jurkat T-cell line [159]. EGCE was effective in reducing the mutagenecity of Trp-p-2(NHOH) in mouse FM3A cells in culture. EGCE was also effective in inhibiting DNA single strand breaks *in vitro* caused by Glu-p-1(NHOH) [160].

Jain *et al.*, [161] found that the extract of green tea leaves decreased the mutagenic activity of N-methyl-N′-nitro-N-nitrosoguanidine (MNNG) to E.coli Wp2 *in vitro* in a desmutagenic manner.

In cultured mammalian cells, the frequencies of mitomycin C or ultraviolet light-induced sister-chromatid exchanges and chromosomal aberrations were suppressed by subsequent treatment with tea polyphenols in the presence of liver-metabolizing enzymes (S9 fraction). In the absence of such enzymes, however, the tea extracts suppressed sister chromatid exchanges and chromosomal aberrations at low concentrations but enhanced them at high concentration [162].

It was shown that EGCG and EGC rather than ECG and EC were found to induce apoptosis in lovo cells. Moreover, EGCG, EGC and ECG caused the arrest at the G1-phase of the cell cycle, whereas EC induced the S-phase arrest [163].

Zhao *et al.*, [164] illustrated that after HL-60 cells were treated by tea polyphenols (250 micro g/ml) for 5h, DNA extracted from HL-60 cells showed a typical internucleosomal DNA degradation i.e. DNA ladder and apoptotic vehicles were observed.

Ahmed *et al.*, [165] studied the effect of green tea polyphenols and the major constituent epigallocatechin-3-gallate on the induction of apoptosis and regulation of cell cycle in human and mouse carcinoma cells and found that treatment of A431 cells with green tea polyphenols and its components epigallocatechin-3-gallate, epigallocatechin and epicatechin-3-gallate resulted in the formation of internucleosomal DNA fragments, a characteristic of apoptosis. Treatment with epigallocatechin-3-gallate also resulted in apoptosis in HaCaT, L5178Y, and Du145 cells. The DNA cell cycle analysis showed that in A431 cells, epigallocatechin-3-gallate treatment resulted in arrest in the G0/G1 phase of cell cycle and a dose-dependent apoptosis. The G0/G1 arrest shown by epigallocatechin-3-gallate, therefore suggested that this agent might slow down the growth of cancer cells by artificially imposing the cell cycle checkpoint. The loss of cell cycle checkpoint results in the selection of cells that have a growth advantage and a predisposition for acquiring more chromosomal aberrations.

2.2. Coffee polyphenols

Caffeic acid and chlorogenic acid are catechol-containing coffee polyphenols that, in a similar way to the tea polyphenols, have shown to be demethylating agents. Lee et al., studied the modulating effects of these two compounds on the *in vitro* methylation of synthetic DNA substrates and also on the methylation status of the promoter region of *RARβ* in two human breast cancer cells lines [166]. The presence of caffeic acid or chlorogenic acid inhibited in a concentration-dependent manner the DNA methylation catalyzed by DNMT1, predominantly through a non-competitive mechanism. This inhibition, similar to other dietary polyphenols, was largely due to the increased formation of SAH. Treatment of MCF-7 and MAD-MB-231 human breast cancer cells with these two compounds partially inhibited the methylation of the promoter region of *RARβ*.

Caffeic acid phenethyl ester (CAPE), which also is a chatechol, kills various types of cancer cells but is innocuous to normal cells. There are several studies reporting the *in vitro* and *in vivo* inhibitory ef1fects of CAPE in multiple cancer models, such as colon cancer [167], lung cancer [168], melanoma [169], glioma [170], pancreatic cancer [171], gastric cancer [172], cholangiocarcinoma [173], hepatocellular carcinoma [174], and breast cancer [175, 176].

2.3. Sulforaphane

Sulforaphane, a dietary phytochemical obtained from broccoli, has been implicated in several physiological processes consistent with anticarcinogenic activity, including enhanced xenobiotic metabolism, cell cycle arrest, and apoptosis. Although the effect of sulforaphane as a demethylating agent has not been specifically studied, this compound was found to down regulate DNMT1 in CaCo-2 colon cancer cells [177].

2.4. Isothiocyanates

Isothiocyanates comprise another class of dietary compounds known to affect the epigenome. Isothiocyanates are metabolites of glucosinolates present in a wide variety of cruciferous vegetables and demonstrated to have anticancer properties. Treatment of prostate cancer cells with phenethyl isothiocyanate, a metabolite of gluconasturtin from watercress, was shown to lead to demethylation and re-expression of *GSTP1* [178]. On the other hand, treatment with different isothiocyanates prevented the esophageous tumorigenesis induced by the methylating agent *N*-nitrosomethylbenzylamine (NMBA) in male rats [179].

2.5. Curcumin

Curcumin is a polyphenolic compound derived from the dietary spice turmeric and possesses diverse pharmacological effects including antioxidant, anti-inflammatory, anti-proliferative, and anti-angiogenic activities. Curcumin has been used for centuries in Asia, both in traditional medicine and in cooking where curcumin gives natural yellow color to the food. It has been well known that curcumin possesses potent antiinflammatory activity because of its inhibitory effects on cyclooxygenases 1, 2 (COX-1, COX-2), lipoxygenase (LOX), TNF-α, interferon γ (IFN-γ), inducible nitric oxide synthase (iNOS), and NF-κB [180, 181]. Importantly, experimental evidences suggest that curcumin could exert its inhibitory effects on cancer development and progression. The mechanisms implicated in the inhibition of tumorigenesis by curcumin are unclear but could involve a combination of anti-oxidant, anti-proliferation, pro-apoptotic, and anti-angiogenic properties through the regulation of genes and molecules that are involved in multiple signaling pathways. Moreover, preclinical animal experiments and phase I clinical trials have demonstrated minimal toxicity of curcumin even at relatively high doses (12 g/day) [182]. However, curcumin exhibits poor bioavailability because of poor absorption and rapid metabolism [182]. To improve the bioavailability of curcumin, liposomal curcumin, nanoparticle curcumin, and structural analogs of curcumin have been synthesized and investigated to determine the absorption and anti-cancer activity [183, 184]. The results are promising, which further suggest that curcumin or its novel structural analogs could serve as potent agents for the prevention and/or treatment of human malignancies, and thus requires more phase II and III clinical trials.

2.6. Rosmarinic acid

Rosmarinic acid is a natural polyphenol antioxidant carboxylic acid found in many *Lamiaceae* herbs used commonly as culinary herbs such as lemon balm, rosemary, oregano, sage, thyme and peppermint. Rosmarinic acid has been recently shown to be a potent inhibitor of DNMT1 activity in nuclear extracts from MCF7 breast cancer cells and decrease the protein levels of DNMT1. However, this compound was unable to demethylate and reactivate known hypermethylated genes such as *RASSF1A, GSTP1* and *HIN-1* in this cell line (185).

2.7. Resveratrol

Resveratrol, a phytoalexin made naturally by several plants, has been produced by chemical synthesis because of its potential anti-cancer, anti-inflammatory, blood-sugar-lowering and other beneficial cardiovascular effects. There is limited evidence about the potential demethylating activity of this compound. Resveratrol has shown to be a weak DNMT activity inhibitor in nuclear extracts from MCF7 cells, and as rosmarinic acid, was unable to reverse the methylation of several tumor suppressor genes [185]. In MCF-7 cells, resveratrol improved the action of adenosine analogues to inhibit methylation and to increase expression of RARβ2, although without significant effect on its own [186].

3. Summary and conclusions

There is traditional and widespread use of dietary polyphenols all around the world. While the anecdotal epidemiological evidence has historically supported the idea of different diet and good health, experimental evidence accumulated in the recent years from various preclinical and clinical studies clearly support the idea that dietary polyphenols have potentially beneficial effects on multitude of health conditions, including cancer. Although the health effects of dietary polyphenols in humans are generally considered promising, there are definite challenges and limitations of the current data in better understanding the molecular mechanisms responsible for this effect, together with the possible interactions between different polyphenols and other dietary constituents. While *in vitro* models have enormously contributed to the understanding of polyphenols mediated regulation of the epigenetic network, there is still a paucity of *in vivo* data for the majority of these dietary compounds. Therefore, until sufficient preclinical and clinical data has been gathered on the epigenetic changes induced by some of the dietary polyphenols, one should be cautious while interpreting and extrapolating the significance of current *in vitro* evidence. Once such evidence is established, the next and more important step would be to determine the most effective doses of these 'dietary nutraceuticals' in order to obtain various beneficial effects in human subjects.

Additional clinical work is required to examine the safety profile of various doses of dietary polyphenols, and more basic science studies are needed to improve our understanding of the molecular mechanisms underlying the chemopreventive effect of various dietary polyphenols. It is really exciting to witness that we have at least begun to explore the molecular mechanistic underpinnings of the "goodness" of certain diets and diet-related factors, which have been in existence for centuries.

The mere fact that currently hundreds of dietary polyphenols are being characterized from an "epigenomic" perspective clearly reflects our enthusiasm and trust we pose in the concept of safe and natural agents for cancer chemoprevention. Of course, the current evidence is thin and it is a long and treacherous road ahead of us; nonetheless, given the promise and potential of these polyphenols it is realistic to fathom that some of these compounds can become integral for the cancer chemoprevention in future.

Author details

Magdy Sayed Aly
Faculty of Science, Beni-Suef University, Egypt,
Faculty of Science, Jazan Univeristy, Jazan, Saudi Arabia

Amani Abd ElHamid Mahmoud
Faculty of Science, Jazan Univeristy, Jazan, Saudi Arabia

4. References

[1] Kelloff GJ, Boone CW, Crowell JA, Steele VE, Lubet R, Sigman CC (1994) Chemopreventive drug development: perspectives and progress. Cancer Epidemiol Biomarkers Prev. 3(1):85-98.

[2] Sporn MB (1996) The war on cancer. Lancet. 18;347(9012):1377-81.

[3] Prochaska HJ, Santamaria AB, and Talalay P (1992). Rapid detection of inducers of enzymes that protect against carcinogens. Proc Natl Acad Sci U S A. 15; 89(6): 2394–2398.

[4] Garewal HS, Meyskens FL Jr. (1991) 1. Chemoprevention of cancer. Hematol Oncol Clin North Am. 5(1):69-77.
[5] Wattenberg LW. (1996) Chemoprevention of cancer. Prev Med. (1):44-5. Review. No abstract available
[6] Mukhtar H, Agarwal R. (1996) Skin Cancer Chemoprevention. J Investig Dermatol Symp Proc. 1(2):209-14.
[7] Kelloff GJ, Sigman CC, Greenwald P. (1999) Cancer chemoprevention: progress and promise. Eur J Cancer. 35(14):2031-8.
[8] Smalley WE, DuBois RN.(1997) Colorectal cancer and nonsteroidal anti-inflammatory drugs. Adv Pharmacol. 1997;39:1-20.
[9] Hixson LJ, Alberts DS, Krutzsch M, Einsphar J, Brendel K, Gross PH, Paranka NS, Baier M, Emerson S, Pamukcu R, et al. (1994) Antiproliferative effect of nonsteroidal antiinflammatory drugs against human colon cancer cells. Cancer Epidemiol Biomarkers Prev. 3(5):433-8.
[10] Earnest DL, Hixson LJ, Alberts DS. (1992) Piroxicam and other cyclooxygenase inhibitors: potential for cancer chemoprevention. J Cell Biochem Suppl. 16I:156-66.
[11] Decensi A, Costa A. (2000) Recent advances in cancer chemoprevention, with emphasis on breast and colorectal cancer. Eur J Cancer. Apr; 36(6):694-709.
[12] Vainio H. (1999) Chemoprevention of cancer: a controversial and instructive story. Br Med Bull.; 55(3):593-9.
[13] Steinmetz KA, Potter JD. (1991) Vegetables, fruit, and cancer. II. Mechanisms. Cancer Causes Control. 2(6):427-42
[14] Block G, Patterson B, Subar A. (1992) Fruit, vegetables, and cancer prevention: a review of the epidemiological evidence. Nutr Cancer. 18(1):1-29.
[15] Negri E, La Vecchia C, Franceschi S, D'Avanzo B, Parazzini F. (1991) Vegetable and fruit consumption and cancer risk. Int J Cancer. 30;48(3):350-4.
[16] Sporn MB, Suh N. (2002) Chemoprevention: an essential approach to controlling cancer. Nat Rev Cancer. 2(7):537–543.
[17] Yang CS, Landau JM, Huang MT, Newmark HL. (2001) Inhibition of carcinogenesis by dietary polyphenolic compounds. Annu Rev Nutr. 21:381–406.
[18] Singh UP, Singh N, Singh B, Hofseth LJ, Price BL, Nagarkatti M, et al. (2009) Resveratrol (trans-3, 5, 4'-trihydroxystilbene) induces SIRT1 and down-regulates NF-{kappa}B activation to abrogate DSS induced colitis. J Pharmacol Exp Ther. 30.
[19] Cui X, Jin Y, Hofseth AB, Pena E, Habiger J, Chumanevich A, et al. (2010) Resveratrol suppresses colitis and colon cancer associated with colitis. Cancer Prev Res (Phila Pa). 3(4):549–559.
[20] Singh UP, Singh NP, Singh B, Hofseth LJ, Price RL, Nagarkatti M, et al. (2010) Resveratrol (trans-3,5,4'-trihydroxystilbene) induces silent mating type information regulation-1 and down-regulates nuclear transcription factor-kappaB activation to abrogate dextran sulfate sodium-induced colitis. J Pharmacol Exp Ther. 332(3):829–839.
[21] Bravo L. (1998) Polyphenols: chemistry, dietary sources, metabolism, and nutritional significance. Nutr Rev. 56(11):317–333.

[22] Manson MM. (2003) Cancer prevention -- the potential for diet to modulate molecular signalling. Trends Mol Med. 9(1):11–18.
[23] Surh YJ. (2003) Cancer chemoprevention with dietary phytochemicals. Nat Rev Cancer. 3(10): 768–780.
[24] Aggarwal BB, Shishodia S. (2006) Molecular targets of dietary agents for prevention and therapy of cancer. Biochem Pharmacol. 14; 71(10):1397–1421.
[25] Shishodia S, Chaturvedi MM, Aggarwal BB. (2007) Role of curcumin in cancer therapy. Curr Probl Cancer. 31(4):243–305.
[26] Russo GL. (2007) Ins and outs of dietary phytochemicals in cancer chemoprevention. Biochem Pharmacol. 15; 74(4):533–544.
[27] Kuroda Y, Hara Y. (1999) Antimutagenic and anticarcinogenic activity of tea polyphenols. Mutat Res. 436(1):69-97
[28] Yang CS, Wang ZY. (1993) Tea and cancer. J Natl Cancer Inst. Jul 7;85(13):1038-49.
[29] Kuriyama S, Shimazu T, Ohmori K, Kikuchi N, Nakaya N, Nishino Y, Tsubono Y, Tsuji I. (2006) Green tea consumption and mortality due to cardiovascular disease, cancer, and all causes in Japan: the Ohsaki study. JAMA; 296:1255–65.
[30] Watanabe I, Kuriyama S, Kakizaki M, Sone T, Ohmori-Matsuda K,Nakaya N, Hozawa A, Tsuji I. (2009) Green tea and death from pneumonia in Japan: the Ohsaki cohort study. Am J Clin Nutr;90:672–9.
[31] Kuriyama S, Hozawa A, Ohmori K, Shimazu T, Matsui T, Ebihara S,Awata S, Nagatomi R, Arai H, Tsuji I. (2006) Green tea consumption and cognitive function: a cross-sectional study from the Tsurugaya Project1. Am J Clin Nutr 83:355–61.
[32] Niu K, Hozawa A, Kuriyama S, Ebihara S, Guo H, Nakaya N, Ohmori-Matsuda K, Takahashi H, Masamune Y, Asada M, et al. (2009) Green tea consumption is associated with depressive symptoms in the elderly. Am J Clin Nutr 90:1615–22.
[33] Hozawa A, Kuriyama S, Nakaya N, Ohmori-Matsuda K, Kakizaki M, Sone T, Nagai M, Sugawara Y, Nitta A, Tomata Y, et al. (2009) Green tea consumption is associated with lower psychological distress in a general population: the Ohsaki Cohort 2006 Study. Am J Clin Nutr 90:1390–6.
[34] Arab L, Liu W, Elashoff D. (2009) Green and black tea consumption and risk of stroke: a meta-analysis. Stroke 40:1786–92.
[35] Mineharu Y, Koizumi A,Wada Y, Iso H,Watanabe Y, Date C, Yamamoto A, Kikuchi S, Inaba Y, Toyoshima H, et al. (2011) Coffee, green tea, black tea and oolong tea consumption and risk of mortality from cardiovascular disease in Japanese men and women. J Epidemiol Community Health 65:230–40.
[36] Tanabe N, Suzuki H, Aizawa Y, Seki N. (2008) Consumption of green and roasted teas and the risk of stroke incidence: results from the Tokamachi-Nakasato cohort study in Japan. Int J Epidemiol 37: 1030–40.
[37] Ng TP, Feng L, Niti M, Kua EH, Yap KB. (2008) Tea consumption and cognitive impairment and decline in older Chinese adults. Am J Clin Nutr 88:224–31.
[38] Wu CH, Yang YC, Yao WJ, Lu FH, Wu JS, Chang CJ. (2002) Epidemiological evidence of increased bone mineral density in habitual tea drinkers. Arch Intern Med 162:1001–6.

[39] Muraki S, Yamamoto S, Ishibashi H, Oka H, Yoshimura N, Kawaguchi H, Nakamura K. (2007) Diet and lifestyle associated with increased bone mineral density: cross-sectional study of Japanese elderly women at an osteoporosis outpatient clinic. J Orthop Sci 12:317–20.

[40] Nantz MP, Rowe CA, Bukowski JF, Percival SS. (2009) Standardized capsule of Camellia sinensis lowers cardiovascular risk factors in a randomized, double-blind, placebo-controlled study. Nutrition 25: 147–54.

[41] Hooper L, Kroon PA, Rimm EB, Cohn JS, Harvey I, Le Cornu KA, Ryder JJ, Hall WL, Cassidy A. (2008) Flavonoids, flavonoid-rich foods, and cardiovascular risk: a meta-analysis of randomized controlled trials. Am J Clin Nutr 88:38–50.

[42] Sousa RM, Ferri CP, Acosta D, Albanese E, Guerra M, Huang Y, Jacob KS, Jotheeswaran AT, Rodriguez JJ, Pichardo GR, et al. (2009) Contribution of chronic diseases to disability in elderly people in countries with low and middle incomes: a 10/66 Dementia Research Group population-based survey. Lancet 374:1821–30.

[43] Spiers NA,Matthews RJ, Jagger C,Matthews FE, Boult C, Robinson TG, Brayne C. (2005) Diseases and impairments as risk factors for onset of disability in the older population in England and Wales: findings from the Medical Research Council Cognitive Function and Ageing Study. J Gerontol A Biol Sci Med Sci 60:248–54.

[44] Wolff JL, Boult C, Boyd C, Anderson G. (2005) Newly reported chronic conditions and onset of functional dependency. J Am Geriatr Soc 53(5):851-5.

[45] Lee W, Min WK, Chun S, Lee YW, Park H, Lee do H, Lee YK, Son JE.(2005) Long-term effects of green tea ingestion on atherosclerotic biological markers in smokers. *Clin Biochem*. Jan 1,;38(1):84-87.

[46] Basu A, Lucas EA. (2007) Mechanisms and effects of green tea on cardiovascular health. Nutr Rev; 65: 361-75.

[47] Zaveri NT. (2006) Green tea and its polyphenolic catechins: medicinal uses in cancer and noncancer applications. Life Sci; 78:2073-80.

[48] Cooper R, Morre′ DJ, Morre′ DM. (2005) Medicinal benefits of green tea: part I. Review of noncancer health benefits. J Altern Complement Med; 11: 521 0-8

[49] Frei B, Higdon JV. (2003) Antioxidant activity of tea polyphenols *in vivo*: evidence from animal studies. J Nutr; 133: 3275S-84S.

[50] Kuriyama S, Shimazu T, Ohmori K, Kikuchi N, Nakaya N, Nishino Y, et al. (2006) Green tea consumption and mortality due to cardiovascular disease, cancer, and all causes in Japan: the Ohsaki study. JAMA; 296: 1255-65.

[51] Larsson SC, Ma¨nnisto¨ S, Virtanen MJ, Kontto J, Albanes D, Virtamo J. (2008) Coffee and tea consumption and risk of stroke subtypes in male smokers. Stroke; 39: 1681-7.

[52] Schimizu M, Kubota M, Tanaka T and Moriwaki H. (2012) Nutraceutical Approach for Preventing Obesity-Related Colorectal and Liver Carcinogenesis. *Int. J. Mol. Sci., 13,* 579-595; doi: 10.3390/ijms13010579.

[53] Huxley R, Lee CM, Barzi F, Timmermeister L, Czernichow S, et al. (2009). Coffee, decaffeinated coffee, and tea consumption in relation to incident type 2 diabetes mellitus: A systematic review with meta-analysis. Arch Intern Med 169(22): 2053–2063.

[54] Tsuneki H, Ishizuka M, Terasawa M, Wu JB, Sasaoka T, et al. (2004) Effect of green tea on blood glucose levels and serum proteomic patterns in diabetic (db/db) mice and on glucose metabolism in healthy humans. BMC Pharmacol 4: 18.

[55] Venables MC, Hulston CJ, Cox HR, Jeukendrup AE (2008) Green tea extract ingestion, fat oxidation, and glucose tolerance in healthy humans. Am J Clin Nutr 87(3): 778–784.

[56] Wolfram S, Raederstorff D, Preller M, Wang Y, Teixeira SR, et al. (2006) Epigallocatechin gallate supplementation alleviates diabetes in rodents. J Nutr 136(10): 2512–2518.

[57] Sabu MC, Smitha K, Kuttan R (2002) Anti-diabetic activity of green tea polyphenols and their role in reducing oxidative stress in experimental diabetes. J Ethnopharmacol 83(1–2): 109–116.

[58] Craig Schneider, Tiffany Segre. (2009) Green Tea: Potential Health Benefits Am Fam Physician.; 79(7):591-594.

[59] Bushman JL. (1998) Green tea and cancer in humans: a review of the literature. *Nutr Cancer.*; 31(3):151-159.

[60] Coyle CH, Philips BJ, Morrisroe SN, Chancellor MB, and Yoshimura N (2008) Antioxidant Effects of Green Tea and Its Polyphenols on Bladder Cells. *Life Sci.* July 4; 83(1-2): 12–18.

[61] Suzuki Y, Tsubono Y, Nakaya N, Suzuki Y, Koizumi Y, Tsuji I. (2004) Green tea and the risk of breast cancer: pooled analysis of two prospective studies in Japan. *Br J Cancer.* Apr 5; 90(7)1361-1363.

[62] Yuan JM, Koh WP, Sun CL, Lee HP, Yu MC. (2005) Green tea intake, ACE gene polymorphism and breast cancer risk among Chinese women in Singapore. Carcinogenesis. 26:1389–94.

[63] Zhang M, Holman CD, Huang JP, Xie X. (2007) Green tea and the prevention of breast cancer: a case-control study in Southeast China. Carcinogenesis; 28:1074–8.

[64] Ogunleye AA, Xue F, Michels KB. (2010) Green tea consumption and breast cancer risk or recurrence: a meta-analysis. Breast Cancer Res Treat; 119:477–84.

[65] Inoue M, Robien K, Wang R, Van Den Berg DJ, Koh WP, Yu MC. (2008) Green tea intake, mthfr/tyms genotype and breast cancer risk: the Singapore Chinese health study. Carcinogenesis; 29:1967–72.

[66] Zhang M, Lee AH, Binns CW, Xie X. (2004) Green tea consumption enhances survival of epithelial ovarian cancer. *Int J Cancer* Nov 10; 112(3):465-469.

[67] Zhou B, Yang L, Wang L, Shi Y, Zhu H, Tang N, Wang B. (2007) The association of tea consumption with ovarian cancer risk: a meta-analysis. *Am J Obstet Gynecol.*; 197(6):594.e1-6.

[68] Islami F, Boffetta P, Ren JS, Pedoeim L, Khatib D, Kamangar F.(2009) High temperature beverages foods esophageal cancer risk – a systematic review. Int J Cancer; 125:491–524.

[69] Ren JS, Freedman ND, Kamangar F, Dawsey SM, Hollenbeck AR, Schatzkin A, et al. (2010) Tea, coffee, carbonated soft drinks and upper gastrointestinal tract cancer risk in a large United States prospective cohort study. Eur J Cancer; 46:1873–81.

[70] Ganesh B, Talole SD, Dikshit R. (2009) Tobacco, alcohol and tea drinking as risk factors for esophageal cancer: a case–control study from Mumbai, India. Cancer Epidemiol; 33:431–4.
[71] Syed DN, Khan N, Afaq F, Mukhtar H. (2007) Chemoprevention of prostate cancer through dietary agents: progress and promise. Cancer Epidemiol Biomarkers Prev; 16:2193-203.
[72] Adhami VM, Mukhtar H. (2007) Anti-oxidants from green tea and pomegranate for chemoprevention of prostate cancer. Mo l Biotechnol; 37:52-7.
[73] Boyle P, Severi G. (1999) Epidemiology of prostate cancer chemoprevention. Eur Urol; 35:370-6.
[74] Hsing AW,Tsao L , Devesa SS. (2000) International trends and patterns of prostate cancer incidence and mortality. Int J Cancer; 85:60-7.
[75] Peto J. (2001) Cancer epidemiology in the last century and the next decade. Nature; 411:390- 5.
[76] Angwafo FF. (1998) Migration and prostate cancer: an international perspective. J Natl Med Assoc; 90:S720-3.
[77] Jian L, Xie LP, Lee AH, Binns CW. (2004) Protective effect of green tea against prostate cancer: a case-control study in southeast China. Int J Cancer; 108:130 - 5.
[78] Khan N, Mukhtar H. (2007) Tea polyphenols for health promotion. Life Sci; 81:519-33.
[79] Siddiqui IA, Afaq F, Adhami VM, Mukhtar H.(2008) Prevention of prostate cancer through custom tailoring of chemopreventive regimen. Chem Biol Interact; 171:122- 32.
[80] Adhami VM, Afaq F, Mukhtar H. (2006) Insulin-like growth factor-I axis as a pathway for cancer chemoprevention. Clin Cancer Res; 12:5611- 4.
[81] Khan N, Afaq F, Saleem M, Ahmad N, Mukhtar H. (2006) Targeting multiple signaling pathways by green tea polyphenol (-)-epigallocatechin-3-gallate. Cancer Res; 66:2500-5.
[82] Siddiqui IA, Afaq F, Adhami VM, Ahmad N, Mukhtar H. (2004) Antioxidants of the beverage tea in promotion of human health. Antioxid Redox Signal; 6:571- 82.
[83] Nichols JA and Katiyar SK (2010) Skin photoprotection by natural polyphenols: Anti-inflammatory, anti-oxidant and DNA repair mechanisms. *Arch Dermatol Res*. March; 302(2): 71. doi:10.1007/s00403-009-1001-3.
[84] Myung SK, Bae WK, Oh SM, Kim Y, Ju W, Sung J, et al. (2009) Green tea consumption and risk of stomach cancer: a meta-analysis of epidemiological studies. Int J Cancer; 124:670–7.
[85] Inoue M, Sasazuki S, Wakai K, Suzuki T, Matsuo K, Shimazu T, et al. (2009) Green tea consumption and gastric cancer in Japanese: a pooled analysis of six cohort studies. Gut; 58:1323–32.
[86] Kinlen LJ, Willows AN, Goldblatt P, Yudkin J. (1988) Tea consumption and cancer. Br J Cancer; 58:397–401.
[87] Khan MM, Goto R, Kobayashi K, Suzumura S, Nagata Y, Sonoda T, et al. (2004) Dietary habits and cancer mortality among middle aged and older Japanese living in Hokkaido, Japan by cancer site and sex. Asian Pac J Cancer Prev; 5:58–65.
[88] Doll R. (1990) An overview of the epidemiological evidence linking diet and cancer. Proc Nutr Soc; 49(2):119–131.

[89] Ames BN, Gold LS. (1998)The prevention of cancer. Drug Metab Rev; 30(2):201–223.

[90] Ames BN, Gold LS. (1998) The causes and prevention of cancer: the role of environment. Biotherapy; 11(2–3):205–220.

[91] Block G, Patterson B, Subar A. (1992) Fruit, vegetables, and cancer prevention: a review of the epidemiological evidence. Nutr Cancer; 18(1):1–29.

[92] Zou C, Liu H, Feugang J. M., Hao Z, Chow H-H S, and Garcia F. (2010) Green Tea Compound in Chemoprevention of Cervical Cancer. Int J Gynecol Cancer. Can; 20(4): 617– 624. doi:10.1111/IGC.0b013e3181c7ca5c.

[93] Arts IC. (2008) A review of the epidemiological evidence on tea, flavonoids, and lung cancer. J Nutr; 138:1561S–6S.

[94] Tang N, Wu Y, Zhou B, Wang B, Yu R. (2009) Green tea, black tea consumption and risk of lung cancer: a meta-analysis. Lung Cancer; 65:274–83.

[95] Cui Y, Morgenstern H, Greenland S, Tashkin DP, Mao JT, Cai L, et al. (2008) Dietary flavonoid intake and lung cancer – a population-based case–control study. Cancer; 112:2241– 8.

[96] Hakim IA, Harris RB, Brown S, Chow HH, Wiseman S, Agarwal S, et al. (2003) Effect of increased tea consumption on oxidative DNA damage among smokers: a randomized controlled study. J Nutr; 133:3303S–9S.

[97] Mizuno S, Watanabe S, Nakamura K, Omata M, Oguchi H, Ohashi K, et al. (1992) A multi- institute case–control study on the risk factors of developing pancreatic cancer. Jpn J Clin Oncol; 22:286–91.

[98] Ji BT, Chow WH, Hsing AW, McLaughlin JK, Dai Q, Gao YT, et al. (1997) Green tea consumption and the risk of pancreatic and colorectal cancers. Int J Cancer; 70:255–8.

[99] Luo J, Inoue M, Iwasaki M, Sasazuki S, Otani T, Ye W, et al. (2007) Green tea and coffee intake and risk of pancreatic cancer in a large-scale, population-based cohort study in Japan (JPHC study). Eur J Cancer Prev; 16:542–8.

[100] Lin Y, Kikuchi S, Tamakoshi A, Yagyu K, Obata Y, Kurosawa M, et al.(2008) Green tea consumption and the risk of pancreatic cancer in Japanese adults. Pancreas; 37:25–30.

[101] World Cancer Research Fund, American Institute for Cancer Research. Food, nutrition, physical activity, and the prevention of cancer, a global perspective. Washington, DC: American Institute for Cancer Research;(2007).

[102] La Vecchia C, Negri E, Franceschi S, D'Avanzo B, Boyle P. (1992) Tea consumption and cancer risk. Nutr Cancer; 17:27–31.

[103] Tavani A, Bertuzzi M, Talamini R, Gallus S, Parpinel M, Franceschi S, et al. (2003) Coffee and tea intake and risk of oral, pharyngeal and esophageal cancer. Oral Oncol; 39:695–700.

[104] Ren JS, Freedman ND, Kamangar F, Dawsey SM, Hollenbeck AR, Schatzkin A, et al. (2010) Tea, coffee, carbonated soft drinks and upper gastrointestinal tract cancer risk in a large United States prospective cohort study. Eur J Cancer; 46:1873–81.

[105] Ide R, Fujino Y, Hoshiyama Y, Mizoue T, Kubo T, Pham TM, et al. (2007) A prospective study of green tea consumption and oral cancer incidence in Japan. Ann Epidemiol; 17:821–6.

[106] Li N, Sun Z, Han C, Chen J. (1999) The chemopreventive effects of tea on human oral precancerous mucosa lesions. Proc Soc Exp Biol Med; 220: 218–24.

[107] Tsao AS, Liu D, Martin J, Tang XM, Lee JJ, El-Naggar AK, et al. (2009) Phase ii randomized, placebo-controlled trial of green tea extract in patients with high-risk oral premalignant lesions. Cancer Prev Res; 2:931–41.

[108] Sun CL, Yuan JM, Koh WP, Yu MC. (2006) Green tea, black tea and colorectal cancer risk: a meta-analysis of epidemiological studies. Carcinogenesis; 27:1301–9.

[109] Sun CL, Yuan JM, Koh WP, Lee HP, Yu MC. (2007) Green tea and black tea consumption in relation to colorectal cancer risk: the Singapore Chinese health study. Carcinogenesis; 28:2143–8.

[110] Yang G, Shu XO, Li H, Chow WH, Ji BT, Zhang X, et al. (2007) Prospective cohort study of green tea consumption and colorectal cancer risk in women. Cancer Epidemiol Biomarkers Prev; 16:1219–23.

[111] Lee KJ, Inoue M, Otani T, Iwasaki M, Sasazuki S, Tsugane S. (2007) Coffee consumption and risk of colorectal cancer in a population-based prospective cohort of Japanese men and women. Int J Cancer; 121:1312–8.

[112] Suzuki E, Yorifuji T, Takao S, Komatsu H, Sugiyama M, Ohta T, et al. (2009) Green tea consumption and mortality among Japanese elderly people: the prospective Shizuoka elderly cohort. Ann Epidemiol; 19:732–9.

[113] Yuan JM, Gao YT, Yang CS, Yu MC. (2007) Urinary biomarkers of tea polyphenols and risk of colorectal cancer in the shanghai cohort study. Int J Cancer; 120:1344–50.

[114] Zhang X, Albanes D, Beeson WL, van den Brandt PA, Buring JE, Flood A, et al. (2010) Risk of colon cancer and coffee, tea, and sugar-sweetened soft drink intake: pooled analysis of prospective cohort studies. J Natl Cancer Inst; 102:771–83.

[115] Bianchi GD, Cerhan JR, Parker AS, Putnam SD, See WA, Lynch CF, et al. (2000) Tea consumption and risk of bladder and kidney cancers in a population-based case–control study. Am J Epidemiol; 151:377–83.

[116] Mellemgaard A, Engholm G, McLaughlin JK, Olsen JH. (1994) Risk factors for renal cell carcinoma in Denmark. I. Role of socioeconomic status, tobacco use, beverages, and family history. Cancer Causes Control; 5:105–13.

[117] Montella M, Tramacere I, Tavani A, Gallus S, Crispo A, Talamini R, et al. (2009) Coffee, decaffeinated coffee, tea intake, and risk of renal cell cancer. Nutr Cancer;61:76–80.

[118] Lee JE, Giovannucci E, Smith-Warner SA, Spiegelman D, Willett WC, Curhan GC. (2006) Total fluid intake and use of individual beverages and risk of renal cell cancer in two large cohorts. Cancer Epidemiol Biomarkers Prev; 15:1204–11.

[119] Lee JE, Hunter DJ, Spiegelman D, Adami HO, Bernstein L, van den Brandt PA, et al. (2007) Intakes of coffee, tea, milk, soda and juice and renal cell cancer in a pooled analysis of 13 prospective studies. Int J Cancer; 121: 2246–53.

[120] Burch JD, Craib KJ, Choi BC, Miller AB, Risch HA, Howe GR. (1987) An exploratory case– control study of brain tumors in adults. J Natl Cancer Inst; 78:601–9.

[121] Holick CN, Smith SG, Giovannucci E, Michaud DS. (2010) Coffee, tea, caffeine intake, and risk of adult glioma in three prospective cohort studies. Cancer Epidemiol Biomarkers Prev; 19:39–47.

[122] Thompson CA, Habermann TM, Wang AH, Vierkant RA, Folsom AR, Ross JA, et al. (2010) Antioxidant intake from fruits, vegetables and other sources and risk of non-hodgkin's lymphoma: the Iowa women's health study. Int J Cancer; 126:992–1003.

[123]] Zhang M, Zhao X, Zhang X, Holman CD. (2008) Possible protective effect of green tea intake on risk of adult leukaemia. Br J Cancer; 98:168–70.

[124]] Kuo YC, Yu CL, Liu CY, Wang SF, Pan PC, Wu MT, et al. (2009) A population-based, case–control study of green tea consumption and leukemia risk in Southwestern Taiwan. Cancer Causes Control; 20:57–65.

[125] Katiyar SK, Mukhtar H. (1996) Tea in chemoprevention of cancer: Epidemiologic and experimental studies (Review). Int J Oncol; 8: 221–38.

[126] Hackett A.; Criffiths L.A.; Broillct A. and Werrneille M. (l983) The metabolism and excretion of (+) - [^{14}C] cyanidanol-3 111 man following oral administration. Xenobiotica. 13: 279-286.

[127] Matsumoto N.; Tono-Oka F.; Ishigaki A.; Okas1lio K and Hara Y. (1991) The fate of (-)-EGCG in the digestive tract of rats. Proc. In Syrup. Tea Sci. 253-257.

[128] Taniguchi S.; Miyasbita Y.; Ueyama T.; Haze K; Hirase J.; Takemoto T.; Arihara S. and Yoshikawa K. (1988) A hypotensive constituents in hot water extracts of green tea, Yakugaku Zasshi (1. Pharmaceut. Soc. Japan). 08: 77-81.

[129] Tanaka N. and Okamura H. (1989) Effects oftannin (Polyphenols) in a black tea solution on a.-amylase activity in Saliva, Nippon Kase Gakkaishi. (J. Home. Been. Japan). 7: 587-592.

[130] Muramatsu K.; Fukuyo M. and Hara Y. (1986) Effect of green tea catechins on plasma cholesterol level in cholesterol-fed rats. .J. Nutr. Sci. Vitaminol. 32: 613-622.

[131] Prestera; Zhang T. Y.; Spencer S.R; \Vilczal CA. and Talalay P. (1993) The electrophile Counterattack response: protection against neoplasia and toxicity. Adv. Enzyme Regul, 33: 281-296.

[132] Apostolides Z.; Balentine D.A.; Harbowy M.E. and Weisburger J.H. (1996) Inhibition of 2- amino-l-methyl-6-phenylimidazo [4,5-6] pyridine (PhIP) mutagenicity by black and green tea extracts and polyphenols. Mutat. Res. 359: 159-163.

[133] Matsumoto N.; Kohri T.; Okushio K. and Hara Y. (1996) Inhibitory effects of tea catechins, black tea extract and oolong tea extract on hepatocarcinogenesis in rat. Japan .T. Cancer Res. 87: 1034-1038.

[134] Chen J-S. The effects of Chinese tea on the occurrence of esophageal tumors induced by N- nitrosomethylbenzylamine in rats. Prev Med 21:385-391 (1992).

[135] Stich HF. Teas and tea components as inhibitors of carcinogen formation in model systems and man. Prev Med 21:377-384 (1992).

[136] Yang G-Y, Wang Z-Y, Kim S, Liao J, Seril D, Chen X, Smith TJ, Yang CS. Characterization of early pulmonary hyperproliferation, tumor progression and their inhibition by black tea in a 4-(methylnitrosamino)-1-(3-pyridyl)-1-butanone (NNK)-

induced lung tumorigenesis model with A/J mice. Cancer Res 1997 May 15;57(10):1889-94.

[137] Chang PY, Mirsalis J, Riccio ES, Bakke JP, Lee PS, Shimon J, Phillips S, Fairchild D, Hara Y, Crowell JA. (2003) Genotoxicity and toxicity of the potential cancer-preventive agent polyphenon E. Environmental and Molecular Mutagenesis; 41: 43–54.

[138] Isbrucker RA, Bausch J, Edwards JA, Wolz E. (2006) Safety studies on epigallocatechin gallate (EGCG) preparations Part 1: Genotoxicity. Food Chem Toxicol; 44: 626–35.

[139] Imanishi H, Sasaki YF, Ohta T, Watanabe M, Kato T, Shirasu Y. (1991) Tea tannin components modify the induction of sister-chromatid exchanges and chromosome aberrations in mutagen-treated cultured mammalian cells and mice. Mutat Res. Jan; 259(1):79-87.

[140] Ito Y, Ohnishi S, Fujie K. (1989) Chromosome aberrations induced by aflatoxin B1 in rat bone marrow cells *in vivo* and their suppression by green tea. Mutat Res; 222: 253–61.

[141] de Boer JG. (2001) Protection by dietary compounds against mutation in a transgenic rodent. J Nutr. Nov; 131(11 Suppl):3082S-6S.

[142] Sai K, Kai S, Umemura T, Tanimura A, Hasegawa R, Inoue T, Kurokawa Y. (1998) Protective effects of green tea on hepatotoxicity, oxidative DNA damage and cell proliferatio in the rat liver induced by repeated oral administration of 2-nitropropane. Food Chem Toxicol. Dec; 36(12):1043-51.

[143] Okuda T, Mori K, Hayatsu H. (1984) Inhibitory effect of tannins on direct-acting mutagens. Chem Pharm Bull (Tokyo). Sep; 32(9):3755-8.

[144] Kada T, Kaneko K, Matsuzaki S, Matsuzaki T, Hara Y. (1985) Detection and chemical identification of natural bio-antimutagens. A case of the green tea factor. Mutat Res. Jun-Jul; 150(1-2):127-32.

[145] Shimoi K, Nakamura Y, Tomita I, Hara Y, Kada T. (1986) The pyrogallol related compounds reduce UV-induced mutations in Escherichia coli B/r WP2. Mutat Res. Apr;173(4):239-44.

[146] Jain AK, Shimoi K, Nakamura Y, Kada T, Hara Y, Tomita I. (1989) Crude tea extracts decrease the mutagenic activity of N-methyl-N0-nitro-N-nitrosoguanidine *in vitro* and in intragastric tract of rats. Mutat Res; 210. 1–8.

[147] Ohe T, Marutani K, Nakase S. (2001) Catechins are not major components responsible for anti-genotoxic effects of tea extracts against nitroarenes. Mutat Res. Sep 20; 496(1-2):75-81.

[148] Hayatsu H, Inada N, Kakutani T, Arimoto S, Negishi T, Mori K, Okuda T, Sakata I. (1992) Suppression of genotoxicity of carcinogens by epigallocatechin gallate. Prev Med; 21: 370– 76.

[149] Hong J.T.; Ryu S.R.; Kim H.J.; Lee J.K.; Lee S.H.; Yun Y.P.; Lee B.M. and Kim P.Y. (2001) Protective effect of green tea extract on ischemia reperfusion induced brain injury in Mongolian gerbils. Brain Res. 888 : 11-18.

[150] Li N, Han C, Chen J. (1999) Tea preparations protect against DMBA-induced oral carcinogenesis in hamsters. Nutr Cancer; 35(1):73-9.

[151] Xue XX, Wang S., Ma C.J.; Zhou P.; Wu P.Q.; Zhang R.F.; Xu Z.; Chen W.S. and Wang Y.Q. (1992) Micronucleus formation in peripheral blood lymphocytes from smokers and the influence of alcohol and tea drinking habits. Int. 1. Cancer.50: 702-705.
[152] Katiyar S.K. and Mukhtar H. (1996) Tea in chemoprevention of cancer : epidemiological and experimental studies. Review. Int. J. Oneal. 8: 221-238.
[153] Qiu G.; Gopalan-Kriczky P.; Su J.; Ning Y. and Lotliker P.D. (1997) Inhibition of aflatoxin B l-induced inhibition of hepatocarcinogenesis in the rats by green tea. Cancer Lett. 1[2: 149- 154.
[154] Sasaki Y.F.; Yamada H.j Shimoi K: Kator K and Kinae N. (1993) The clastogen-suppressing effects of green tea, PO-Lei tea and Rooibos tea in CHO cells and mice. Mutat. Res. 286: 221 - 232.
[155] Xu Y.; Ho C-T.; Amin S.C.; Ran C. and Chung F-L. (1992) Inhibition of tobacco-specific nitrosamine induced lung tumorigenesis in All mice by green tea and its major polyphenol as antioxidants. Cancer Res. 52: 3875-3879.
[156] Al-Fify ZI and Aly MS. (2010) Protective effect of green tea against Dimethylnitrosamine induced genotoxicity in mice bone marrow cells. The Open Cancer Journal, 3:16-21.
[157] Yang C.S.; Chung J.Y.; Yang G.; Chhabra S. and Lee M.J. (2000) Tea and tea polyphenols in cancer prevention. 1. Nutr. 130: 472S-478S.
[158] Islam S.; Islam N.; Kerrnode T.; Johnstone B.; Mukhtar N.; Moskowitz R.W.; Coldberg V.M.; Malernud Ci.I, and Haqqi T.M. (2000) Involvement of caspase-3 III epigallocatechin-3- gallate mediated apoptosis of human chondrosarcoma cells. Biochem. Biophys. Res. Cornrnun. 270: 793-797.
[159] Erba D.; Riso P.; Colombo A. and Tcstolin G. (1999) Supplementation of jurkat I-cells with green tea extracts decreases oxidative damage due to iron treatment. J. Nutr. 129: 2130-2134.
[160] Hayatsu H.; Inada N.; Kakutani T.; Arimoto S.; Negisbi T.; Mori K.; Okuda T. and Sakata I. (1992) Suppression of genotoxicity of carcinogens by (-) epigallocatechin gallate. Prevo Med. 21: 370 - 376.
[161] Jain N.K.; Shimoi K.; Nakamura Y.; Kada T.; Hara Y. and Tomita I. (1989) Crude tea extracts decrease the mutagenic activity of N-methyl-N'-nitro-N-nitrosoguanidine *in vitro* and in intragastric tract of rats. Murat. Res. 210: 1-8.
[162] Imanishi H.; Sasaki Y.F.; Ohta T.; Watanabe M.; Kato T. and Shirasu Y. (1991) Tea tannin components modify the induction of sister-chromatid exchanges and chromosome aberrations in mutagen-treated cultured mammalian cells and mice. Mutat. Res. 259:79-87
[163] Tan X.; Hu D.; Li S.; Han Y.; Zhang Y. and Zbou, D. (2000) Differences of four catechins in cell cycle arrest and induction of apoptosis in Lovo cells. Cancer Lett. 29; 158: 1-6.
[164] Zhao Y.; Cao J.; Ma H. and Lill J. (1997) Apoptosis induced by tea polyphenols inHL-60 cells. Cancer Lett. 121: 163-167.

[165] Ahmed N.; Feyes D.K.; Nieminen A.L.; Agarwal R. and Mukhtar H. (1997) Green tea constituent Epigallocatechin-3-Gallate and induction of apoptosis and cell cycle arrest in human carcinoma cells. J. Natl. Cancer Inst. 89: 1881-1886.

[166] Lee WJ, Zhu BT. (2006) Inhibition of DNA methylation by caffeic acid and chlorogenic acid, two common catechol-containing coffee polyphenols. Carcinogenesis. Feb; 27(2):269–277.

[167] Xiang D., Wang D., He Y., Xie J., Zhong Z., Li Z., Xie J. (2006) Caffeic acid phenethyl ester induces growth arrest and apoptosis of colon cancer cells via the beta-catenin/T-cell factor signaling, Anti Cancer Drugs 17(7): 753–762.

[168] Chen M.F., Wu C.T. Chen Y.J., Keng P.C., Chen W.C. (2004) Cell killing and radiosensitization by caffeic acid phenethyl ester (CAPE) in lung cancer cells, J. Radiat. Res. 45 (2): 253– 260.

[169] Kudugunti S.K., Vad N.M., Ekogbo E., Moridani M.Y. (2011) Efficacy of caffeic acid phenethyl ester (CAPE) in skin B16-F0 melanoma tumor bearing C57BL/6 mice, Invest. New Drugs 29: 52–62. doi:10.1007/s10637-009-9334-5.

[170] Kuo H.S., Kuo W.H., Lee Y.J., Lin W.L., Chou F.P., Tseng T.H. (2006) Inhibitory effect of caffeic acid phenethyl ester on the growth of C6 glioma cells in vitro and in vivo, Cancer Lett. 234(2): 199–208.

[171] Chen M.J., Chang W.H., Lin C.C., Liu C.Y., Wang T.E., Chu C.H., Shih S.C., Chen Y.J. (2008) Caffeic acid phenethyl ester induces apoptosis of human pancreatic cancer cells involving caspase and mitochondrial dysfunction, Pancreatology 8 (6) 566–576.

[172] Wu C.S., Chen M.F., Lee I.L., Tung S.Y. (2007) Predictive role of nuclear factor-kappa B activity in gastric cancer: a promising adjuvant approach with caffeic acid phenethyl ester, J. Clin. Gastroenterol. 41(10): 871–873.

[173] Onori P., DeMorrow S., Gaudio E., Franchitto A., Mancinelli R., Venter J., Kopriva S., Ueno Y., Alvaro D., Savage J., Alpini G., Francis H. (2009) Caffeic acid phenethyl ester decreases cholangiocarcinoma growth by inhibition of NF-kappa B and induction of apoptosis, Int. J. Cancer 125(3): 565–576.

[174] Lee K.W., Kang N.J., Kim J.H., Lee K.M., Lee D.E., Hur H.J., Lee H.J. (2008) Caffeic acid phenethyl ester inhibits invasion and expression of matrix metalloproteinase in SK-Hep1 human hepatocellular carcinoma cells by targeting nuclear factor kappa B, Genes Nutr. 2(4): 319–322.

[175] Omene C., Mu J., Frenkel K. (2012) Caffeic Acid Phenethyl Ester (CAPE) derived from propolis, a honeybee product, inhibits growth of breast cancer stem cells, Invest. New Drugs 30(4):1279-88. doi:10.1007/s10637-011-9667-8.

[176] [176 Wu J, Omene C, Karkoszka J, Bosland M, Eckard J, Klein CB, Frenkel K. (2011) Caffeic acid phenethyl ester (CAPE), derived from a honeybee product propolis, exhibits a diversity of anti-tumor effects in pre-clinical models of human breast cancer. Cancer Letters 308 43–53

[177] Traka M, Gasper AV, Smith JA, Hawkey CJ, Bao Y, Mithen RF. (2005) Transcriptome analysis of human colon Caco-2 cells exposed to sulforaphane. J Nutr. Aug; 135(8):1865–1872.

[178] Wang LC, Beklemisheva A, Liu XM, Ferrari AC, Feng J, Chiao JW. (2007) Dual action on promoter demethylation and chromatin by an isothiocyanate restored GSTP1 silenced in prostate cancer. Mol Carcinog. Jan; 46(1):24–31.

[179] Wilkinson JT, Morse MA, Kresty LA, Stoner GD. (1995) Effect of alkyl chain length on inhibition of Nnitrosomethylbenzylamine-induced esophageal tumorigenesis and DNA methylation by isothiocyanates. Carcinogenesis. Can; 16(5):1011–1015.

[180] Kunnumakkara AB, Anand P, Aggarwal B.B. (2008) Curcumin inhibits proliferation, invasion, angiogenesis and metastasis of different cancers through interaction with multiple cell signaling proteins. Cancer Lett. 269:199–225.

[181] Surh YJ, Chun KS, Cha HH, Han SS, Keum YS, Park KK, et al. (2001) Molecular mechanisms underlying chemopreventive activities of anti-inflammatory phytochemicals: down-regulation of COX-2 and iNOS through suppression of NF-kappa B activation. Mutat Res. 480– 481:243–268.

[182] Anand P, Kunnumakkara AB, Newman RA, Aggarwal BB. (2007) Bioavailability of curcumin: problems and promises. Mol Pharm. 4:807–818.

[183] Anand P, Nair HB, Sung B, Kunnumakkara AB, Yadav VR, Tekmal RR, Aggarwal BB. (2010) Design of curcumin-loaded PLGA nanoparticles formulation with enhanced cellular uptake, and increased bioactivity *in vitro* and superior bioavailability *in vivo*. Biochem Pharmacol. 1;79(3):330-8. doi: 10.1016/j.bcp

[184] Wang D, Veena MS, Stevenson K, Tang C, Ho B, Suh JD, et al. (2008) Liposome-encapsulated curcumin suppresses growth of head and neck squamous cell carcinoma *in vitro* and in xenografts through the inhibition of nuclear factor kappaB by an AKT-independent pathway. Clin Cancer Res. 14:6228–6236.

[185] Paluszczak J, Krajka-Kuzniak V, Baer-Dubowska W. (2010) The effect of dietary polyphenols on the epigenetic regulation of gene expression in MCF7 breast cancer cells. Toxicol Lett. 1;192(2):119-25. doi: 10.1016/j.toxlet.2009 .

[186] Stefanska B, Rudnicka K, Bednarek A, Fabianowska-Majewska K. (2010) Hypomethylation and induction of retinoic acid receptor beta 2 by concurrent action of adenosine analogues and natural compounds in breast cancer cells. Eur J Pharmacol. 25; 638(1–3):47–53.

Chapter 13

Kuguacin J, a Triterpenoid from *Momordica charantia* Linn: A Comprehensive Review of Anticarcinogenic Properties

Pornngarm Limtrakul, Pornsiri Pitchakarn and Shugo Suzuki

Additional information is available at the end of the chapter

http://dx.doi.org/10.5772/55532

1. Introduction

Momordica charantia (MC) L. belongs to a short-fruited group of the Cucurbitaceae family and has been widely cultivated as a vegetable crop in many tropical and subtropical countries. The fruit, vines, leaves and roots of this plant have been used as a traditional medicine for the treatment of toothaches, diarrhea, furuncle, and diabetes [1-3]. Its fruit, referred to as kugua in the Chinese language, Mara Kee Nok in Thai and bitter melon in English, has been used in Chinese, Indian and Thai Cooking. Bitter melon, also known as bitter gourd, is cylindrical shaped and 4 to 12 inches in length and 1 and a half to 3 inches in diameter and contains large seeds inside. It tastes very bitter and is considered a blood purifier. It can be cut into rings and deep-fried for a snack. It is also often stir fried with meat, shrimp or fish.

In view of the popularity of bitter melon in the Asian tropics and the fact that the results of using bitter melon as a remedy for diabetes has yielded conflicting results [2,4,5], more research needs to be done on its hypoglycemic activity. In addition, several compounds from bitter melon have shown interesting pharmacological activities, including antitumor, immunotoxic and anti-HIV properties, which merit further research, and may have strong potential in the development of future medicines [2,6-9]. Although different types of synthetic drugs are available for the treatment of chronic diseases, such as diabetes and cancer, the synthetic agents in use can produce serious side effects and toxicity. Hence there is a demand for safer and more effective agents. In many parts of the world, an Ayurvedic (traditional Indian) approach has been used for the treatment of a number of diseases, including diabetes and cancer and therein exists a hidden wealth of potential for useful natural products in the control of diseases. The World Health Organization (WHO) has recommended that this area warrants further evaluation that might reveal effective dietary adjuncts, either for the treatment or prevention of specific diseases [10]. With traditional use supported by modern scientific evidence of the beneficial function of MC, it is one of the most promising plants for drug development. However, its phytochemicals and mechanism of action are poorly understood. Extensive research has studied the isolation of several classes of active components, including cucurbitane-type triterpenoids and the potential biological and pharmacological activities of natural products in MC [7,11]. The aim of this chapter is to review the cucurbitane type triterpenoids, particularly kuguacin J, in MC with the goal of encouraging future studies.

1.1. Geographic distribution and monograph

MC is an herbaceous, tendril-bearing vine growing up to 5 m in length. It bears simple, alternate leaves, with 3-7 deeply separated lobes. Each plant bears separate yellow male and female flowers [12]. Fruit 2.5-25 cm long, oblong, pendulous, fusiform, usually pointed or beaked, ribbed and bearing numerous triangular tubercles, 3 valves are present at the apex when mature. MC are perennial climbers cultivated throughout India and in Southern China and is now found naturalized in almost all tropical and subtropical regions. It is an important vegetable in India, Sri Lanka, Vietnam, Thailand, Malaysia, the Philippines and Southern China. It is also cultivated on a small scale in tropical America. MC is grown mainly for the production of immature fruit, although the young leaves are edible as a vegetable [3]. The young fruit is emerald green, but turns to orange-yellow when ripe. At maturity, the fruit splits into irregular valves that curl backwards and release numerous brown or white seeds encased in scarlet arils (Figure 1). All parts of the plant, including the fruit, taste bitter. It has been used extensively in traditional medicine as a remedy for diabetes.

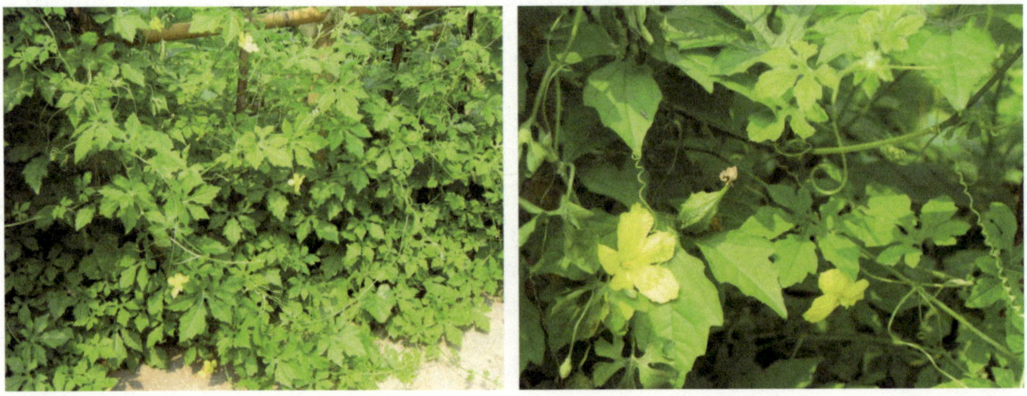

Figure 1. Flowers, immature fruit and young leaves of *Momordica charantia* (MC) at a home garden in Chiang Mai, Thailand (the picture was taken in March, 2012).

1.2. Pharmacological activities

Previous investigations have shown that water extracts of the leaf and fruit of MC exhibited high antioxidant activity and that bitter melon fractions are rich in phenolics and have a strong antioxidant activity [13]. The role of free radicals and active oxygen in treating chronic diseases including cancer, aging and atheroscerosis has been recognized [14]. Therefore, much attention has been focused on the use of antioxidants in protecting against the threat of damage of free radicals. The active fractions from the fruit of MC have been reported to have significant hypoglycemic and antidiabetic effects [1,5]. Its active compounds were reported to be saponins [15,16] and peptides [17,18]. Charantin, an antidiabetic compound, is a typical cucurbitane-type triterpenoid in MC and is a potential and promising substance for the treatment of diabetes [19]. A number of studies have reported the effects of MC unrelated to diabetes. MC has some interesting biological and pharmacological activities. Extracts of MC have been reported to possess antitumor activity, such as the inhibition of mouse spontaneous mammary tumourigenesis [20] and benzo(a)pyrene-induced mouse forestomach tumourigenesis [21]. Besides, antioxidant activities [22], the antiviral [9], antidiabetic and immunomodulating properties [23] of this plant have also been explored.

1.3. Ethnomedical uses

The fruit, leaves and roots of MC have been used in Ayurveda in the treatment of a number of diseases. They have been used as a bitter stomachic, a laxative and an anthelmintic [24]. The whole extract of the fruit is also advocated in the treatment of diseases of the spleen, liver, and in rheumatism and gout [25]. An active ingredient from this plant has been used in diabetes mellitus [6,11,26]. In KwaZulu-Natal, the Zulus drink a concoction of the root or leaf for the treatment of boils and take an infusion of the runner as a sedative for an irritable stomach [27]. It has also been reported that it has been used as a remedy for hypertension and is reported to have antidiabetic properties. The leaf is used by the Chagga as an earache remedy [28] and in tropical Africa, the leaf is used to treat roundworm [29]. In Uganda, an infusion of the leaf and roots is used as an abortifacient and ecbolic [28] and in Tanzania the fruit pulp is regarded as being poisonous to weevils, moths and ants and is used as a repellant [30]. In the Philippines, the leaves are often used for children's coughs. It is used in the treatment of skin diseases, sterility in women, as a parasiticide, as an antipyretic, and as a purgative. MC is also known as the Ampalaya tree, which is a vegetable grown throughout the Phillipines [31] and Ampalaya tea is a bitter brew made from the fruit or leaves. Ayurveda knowledge has claimed that Amapalaya stimulates digestion, helping those with dyspepsia or constipation. The tea seems to help people with diabetes mellitus control the disease, and it may provide some antimalarial benefits. Ampalaya has been traditionally regarded by Asians, as well as Panamanians and Columbians, as being useful in the prevention and treatment of malaria. Laboratory studies have confirmed that various species of the bitter fruit have anti-malarial activity, although human studies have not yet been published. In the Philippines, the effect of MC capsule preparation on glycemic control in type 2 diabetes mellitus has been studied [32]. However, there was no significant effect on mean fasting blood sugar, total cholesterol, and weight or on serum creatinine, ALT, AST, sodium and potassium in 40 outpatients who received treatment at the Phillippine General Hospital.

1.1. Phytochemicals and cucurbitane triterpenoids

Since the early 1960's the constituents of bitter melon have been investigated and several classes of primary and secondary metabolites have been isolated from MC fruits, seeds and whole plants. It contains biologically active chemicals that include crude fat, crude protein, soluble dietary fiber, minerals, essential oil, flavonoids, phenolic acids, glycosides and triterpenes. The young fruit is a good source of vitamin C and vitamin A [33-35]. A steroid saponin called charantin has been isolated from the fruits and leaves. It also contains a polypeptide named gurmarin, which is similar to insulin in composition.

Among the secondary metabolites of MC, cucurbitane-type triterpinoids are one of the main bioactive constituents. The terpenoids, referered to as isoprenoids, are a class of natural products and the related compounds have been formally derived from five-carbon isoprene units. Terpenoids of different sizes and composition are found in all classes of living things and are the largest groups of naturally occurring chemicals. This class has been subdivided according to the number of carbon atoms. The triterpenoids are terpenoids with a C30 skeleton. These C30 constituents are isolated and characterized from various sources in nature, particularly in resins and may occur as either esters or glycosides [36,37]. More extensive backbone rearrangement of the protostane cation affords the curcubitane skeleton. The cucurbitacins are a typical group of cucurbitane-type triterpenoids found in plants and belong to the cucumber family (Cucurbitaceae). The natural cucurbitracins are well-known for their bitterness and toxicity [38]. The cucurbitane-type triterpenoids and their aglycones have shown some biological effects beneficial in treating diabetes and obesity, and possess anticancer, anti-HIV and antifeedant properties [7,39]. More than fifty cucurbitacins and cucurbitane glycosides from the fruits, seeds, leaves, vines and stems have been reported [40-48]. Recently, Chen et al (2008, 2009) isolated and structured elucidation of nineteen cucurbitacins named kuguacins A-E from the roots of MC [49] and kuguacins F-S [50] from the vines and leaves of MC. They claimed that some of them are artifacts formed during the extraction process. The kuguacin C and E showed moderate anti-HIV-1 activity with EC_{50} values of 8.45 and 25.62 μg/ml. The kuguacins F-S exhibited weak anti-HIV activities *in vitro*.

Recently, several triterpenoids from various plants have been reported to feature anti-proliferative [51-53] and anti-invasive [54,55] bioactive components. More than 50 triterpenoids have been isolated from bitter melon, but their biological activities have yet to be explored in detail. However, it has been shown that Cucurbitacin B (cucB), a triterpenoid from Cucurbitaceae vegetables also found in bitter melon seeds, has caused cell cycle arrest and apoptosis induction in human colon adenocarcinoma cancer cells [53]. Moreover, 2 flavonoids and 4 phenolic acids, including rutin, naringin, gentistic acid, benzoic acid, *o*-coumaric acid, and *t*-cinnamic acid, are present in bitter melon leaves [35]. Rutin, a flavonoid glycoside, has been reported to successfully show growth inhibition of leukemia and ovarian carcinomas, with anti-invasive effects on melanoma [35,56-58]. Triterpenoids and flavoniods included in bitter melon leaf extract (BMLE) might be promising components with critical roles against cancer cell progression, but the active compound(s) remain to be identified.

This review presents previously published and current information regarding a cucurbitane type triterpenoid, kuguacin J, and provides new insights into the underlying potential of the chemical isolation and biological activities of kuguacin J in MC. Molecular mechanisms of kuguacin J, as a promising anticancer agent, will be discussed in detail.

1.5. Isolation and purification of kuguacin J from MC leaf

Our previous study [59] has compared the effects of the ethanolic extracts from leaves, fruits and tendrils of MC on drug accumulation and P-gp activity *in vitro*. The leaf extract (BMLE) showed a concentration-dependent effect on P-gp-mediated vinblastine accumulation and efflux in drug resistant KB-V1 cells, but had no effect in drug-sensitive KB-3-1 cells, which lack P-gp, while there was no change in drug accumulation and efflux in KB-V1 cells in the presence of the fruit and tendril extracts [59]. These firstly inspired us to further identify the active component(s) of BMLE, which modulate the function of P-gp and the multidrug-resistant (MDR) phenotype in multidrug-resistant human cervical carcinoma KB-V1 cells using Bioassay-guided fractionation.

In the next study [60], the ethanolic fraction, BMLE, was subsequently extracted with solvents increasing in polarity (i.e., ethanol, hexane, diethyl ether, chloroform and ethyl acetate). These extraction samples were tested for their abilities to modulate the function of P-gp in the multidrug-resistant human cervical carcinoma KB-V1 cells in comparison with wild type drug sensitive KB-3-1 cells. Among the extracts tested, the hexane and diethyl ether fractions had the most effective MDR reversing properties, and increased intracellular [^{3}H]-vinblastine accumulation and decreased the [^{3}H]-vinblastine efflux in KB-V1 cells. The percent yield of the diethyl ether fraction was higher than the hexane fraction. Moreover, in another of our studies, the growth inhibitory effects on LNCaP cells showed that the diethyl ether fraction (DEF) of BMLE displayed the strongest inhibitory effect on the cell growth [61]. So, we therefore purified the active component using the diethyl ether fraction as a principle material. Bioassay-guided fractionation led us to isolate a purified white crystal. The IR, NMR and MS data of the compound was compared with previous reports [62] and it was identified as kuguacin J (3,7,23-trihydroxycucurbita-5,24-dien-19-al), (Figure 2). We further characterized the anticancer properties of BMLE (*in vitro* and *in vivo*) and kuguacin J (*in vitro*) and these will be further discussed in the following sections.

2. Bitter melon and cancer

Cancer is a disease in which the cell presents itself with uncontrolled proliferative potential. The transition of normal cells towards the cancerous phenotype occurs at various stages [63]. Since these defects are mostly due to aberrant signaling cascades involving numerous molecular players, targeting them by chemopreventive agents at any stage could be a rationalized approach in achieving the control of cancer.

Carcinogenesis is generally a complex and multi-step process in which distinct molecular and cellular alterations occur. In order to simplify the understanding of the different possible options for chemoprevention and chemotherapy in cancer development and progression, the following stages have been described: (i) initiation, when cells are exposed to a carcinogenic agent, (ii) promotion, when abnormal cells persist and initiate a preneoplastic stage (iii) progression, final phase of the tumorigenesis, when uncontrolled cell growth is resistant to anticancer drugs (Multidrug Resistance; MDR), and aggressiveness or metastasis occur. A cancer chemopreventive agent could be effective at any of the classically defined stages of carcinogenesis: initiation, promotion, and/or progression [64,65]. As discussed earlier, extracts of bitter melon have been reported to possess anti-tumor activity [20,21] and the following sections detail the signaling cascades that are targeted.

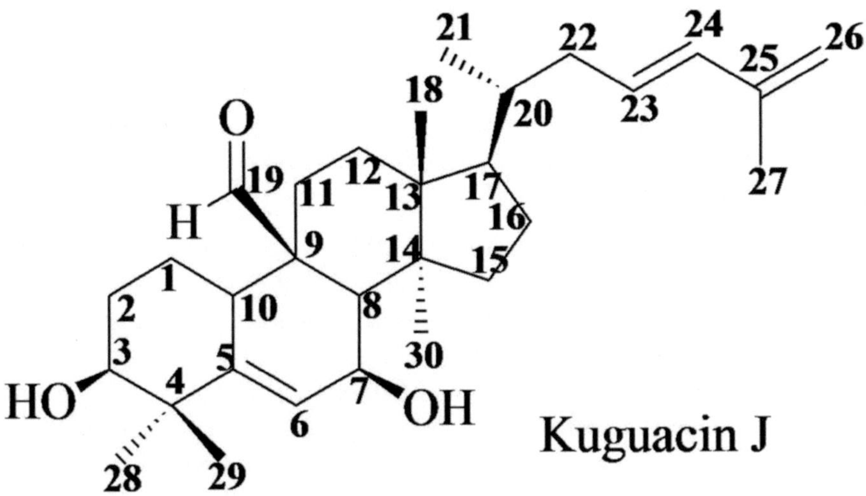

Figure 2. Chemical structure of kuguacin J isolated from MC.

2.1. Anticancer *in vitro* studies

Prevention by the use of naturally occurring dietary substances is considered a practical approach in reducing the increasing incidence of cancer. The intervention of multi-stage carcinogenesis by modulating intracellular signaling pathways may provide the molecular basis of chemoprevention with a wide variety of dietary phytochemicals [66,67].

Anticancer activities of MC against numerous cancers have revealed that it contains active compounds that provide anticancer potential to inhibit cell growth and proliferation, as well as to induce apoptotic cell death in several cancer cell lines [68-71]. Our studies [60,61,72,73] found that kuguacin J, one of the active compounds contained in MC extracts, exerts anticancer properties in various experimental models, which will be discussed further in the following sections.

2.1.1. *Antiproliferative and antiapoptotic activities*

Generally, deregulation of cell growth and resistance to apoptosis are the major defects in uncontrolled cancer cell growth, hinting that development of approaches that induce cell cycle arrest and apoptotic machineries in cancer cells could be effective measures against their proliferation. Recently, dietary phytochemicals are considered promising chemopreventive or chemotherapeutic agents [67,74]. Thus, the induction of cell cycle arrest or apoptosis using dietary chemopreventive compounds might be an excellent approach to inhibit the promotion and progression of carcinogenesis and to remove genetically deregulated, premalignant and malignant cells from the body. We have investigated the growth inhibitory effect of BMLE and kuguacin J on androgen-dependent and androgen-independent prostate cancer models [61,72,73].

Our study [61] found that BMLE exerted significant growth inhibitory effects on LNCaP via the induction of G1 arrest and apoptosis cell death and the alteration of cyclin D1, PCNA, Bcl-2/Bax, caspase-3 and cleaved caspase-3 protein levels. The data prompted us to characterize the active compound(s) in the extract, which could be valuable in the prevention and intervention of cancers. It was found that kuguacin J exerted a marked decrease of LNCaP cell proliferation and viability, suggesting that kuguacin J is at least one of the active components in BMLE that plays a critical role in the growth inhibition of LNCaP.

The treatment of androgen-sensitive (LNCaP) cells with kuguacin J resulted in a significant G1-phase arrest of cell cycle progression [61], which indicates that one of the mechanisms by which kuguacin J may act to inhibit the proliferation of cancer cells is the regulation of cell cycle progression. We next examined the effect of kuguacin J on cell cycle regulatory molecules operative in the G1 phase of the cell cycle. The reduction of cyclinD1, cyclinE, Cdk2 and Cdk4 in LNCaP cells by kuguacin J suggests the disruption of the uncontrolled cell cycle progression of these cells and that the kuguacin J-induced G1 arrest is mediated through the up-regulation of p21 and p27 proteins, which enhances the formation of heterotrimeric complexes with the G1-S Cdks and cyclins, thereby inhibiting their activity. Additionally, kuguacin J also dramatically suppressed the expression of a proliferation marker, PCNA, which is expressed late in the G1 phase and early in the S phase [75]. The inhibition of cell proliferation or the induction of cell death in LNCaP by kuguacin J might be associated with the G1 arrest machinery.

G1-phase arrest of cell cycle progression provides an opportunity for cells to either undergo repair mechanisms or follow the apoptotic pathway. Apoptosis plays a crucial role in that it functions as an essential mechanism of tissue homeostasis, eliminating the mutated neoplastic and hyperproliferating neoplastic cells from the system. Acquired resistance toward apoptosis is a hallmark of most, and perhaps all, types of cancer. Cancer cells become resistant to apoptosis and do not respond to the cytotoxic effects of the chemotherapeutic agents [76]. Therefore induction of apoptosis is considered a protective mechanism against cancer progression. We thus determined the effect of kuguacin J on the induction of apoptosis in LNCaP cells [61]. Kuguacin J treatment caused significant induction of apoptosis. Hence, kuguacin J seems to be a potent chemotherapeutic agent for prostate cancer inhibition. Moreover, kuguacin J treatment reduced the protein level of surviving, which might be associated with kuguacin J-induced cell cycle arrest and apoptosis in LNCaP. Kuguacin J treatment could alter the protein levels of key members of the Bcl-2 family in a manner that favors an increase in the ratio of Bax/Bcl-2 and Bad/Bcl-xL and increases the activation of caspase-3 and cleavage of PARP. This may represent the mechanism by which cancer cells are susceptibility to kuguacin J mediated apoptosis.

LNCaP is an androgen-dependent, androgen receptor (AR)-positive prostate cancer cell line. AR is known to play a critical role in the development and progression of prostate cancer [77]. The ability of AR to cross-talk with several growth factor signaling cascades toward the regulation of cell cycle, apoptosis, and differentiation outcomes in prostate cancer cells has been reported [77]. Inhibition of AR activity could be the major therapeutic goal to delay prostate cancer progression. Kuguacin J decreased the expression of AR followed by the reduction of the protein level of PSA [61], which is one major AR-dependent target gene. The diminishment of PSA represents the effective inhibition of AR activity by kuguacin J treatments. The decrease of AR might be involved in the kuguacin J-caused growth inhibition of LNCaP through the induction of G1 arrest and apoptosis.

The tumor suppressor p53 protein is a regulator of genotoxic stress that plays an important role in DNA damage response, DNA repair, cell cycle regulation, and in triggering apoptosis after cell injury [78]. Induction of apoptosis is considered to be central to the tumor-suppressive function of p53 [79]. Kuguacin J-treated LNCaP cells markedly increased the expression of the p53 protein [61]. We further investigated whether kuguacin J-induced cell cycle arrest and apoptosis of LNCaP cells are p53-dependent using p53 RNA interference. We found that kuguacin J induced p53-mediated partly cell cycle arrest, and mainly apoptosis, which led to the inhibition of cell growth and may be related to the activation of p53 signaling pathway [61].

Treatment of androgen-independent prostate cancer cells (PC3) with kuguacin J caused a significant G1-phase arrest along with a reduction of survivin, cyclinD1, cyclinE, Cdk2 and Cdk4 [73]. Kuguacin J also dramatically suppressed the expression of a proliferation marker, PCNA, that is expressed in both late G1 phase and early S phase [61,73] .

Kuguacin J appears to inhibit the growth of the androgen-dependent LNCaP cells to a greater degree compared to the androgen-independent PC3 cell line [61,73]. A number of differences between PC3 and LNCaP cells may account for this difference in sensitivity. PC3 is a more aggressively growing cell line and is null for both p53 and the AR. LNCaP is a much less aggressive cell line and possesses wild-type p53 and an AR, which although mutated, is responsive to androgen. Our study revealed that kuguacin J markedly decreased AR expression and induced p53 levels in LNCaP cells. We also found that p53 played a critical role in the kuguacin J-mediated induction of apoptosis by LNCaP cells. The data could explain the lower induction of apoptosis in PC3 cells compared to LNCaP. The induction of G1 arrest by kuguacin J, however, was similar in AR-dependent LNCaP cells and AR-independent PC3 cells, suggesting that the AR might not be a critical component in mediating the growth-arresting properties of kuguacin J.

The sensitivity of the human normal prostatic epithelial cell line PNT1A to the cytotoxic effects of kuguacin J was much lower than that of the prostate cancer cell lines (LNCaP and PC3) [61]. Thus, kuguacin J could be an effective chemopreventive and chemotherapeutic agent against prostate cancer, which might have no or a low side effect on normal cells and tissues.

Our studies [61,73] provide the evidence that shows the significant inhibitory effects on carcinogenic progression of LNCaP and PC3 cells via inhibition of cell growth and proliferation by kuguacin J. Thus, kuguacin J is able to induce apoptosis/cell cycle arrest in pre-initiated/initiated tumor cells, while in more advanced tumors kuguacin J is still able to induce apoptosis/cell cycle arrest. Taken together, kuguacin J might be a promising candidate as a new chemopreventive agent for both androgen-dependent and androgen-independent prostate cancer and could be developed as an alternative treatment option in cancer therapy. The *in vivo* study and growth inhibitory effects of kuguacin J on other cancers has to be further investigated.

Because kuguacin J is a purified compound from BMLE, the differences of the anti-tumor effects between kuguacin J and BMLE were investigated. The growth inhibition effects of kuguacin J on LNCaP are similar to BMLE with the phenomena of cell cycle arrest and apoptosis induction and alteration of the expression of cell cycle- and apoptosis-regulators. However, kuguacin J is included as only 1.6% of the BMLE, and the effective concentration to inhibit cancer cell growth of kuguacin J was 10 times lower than that of BMLE [60,61,73]. Therefore, BMLE may include other compounds, which also have anti-tumor function towards LNCaP cells.

2.1.2. Multidrug resistance reversing properties via modulation of P-glycoprotein function

The development and strategic use of anticancer drugs has become one of the most important ways of controlling malignant diseases. However, the emergence of drug resistance has made many of the currently available chemotherapeutic agents ineffective. Efforts to reverse the drug resistance of tumor cells have been largely unsuccessful [80]. In recent years, considerable research has been directed toward understanding the underlying mechanisms that confer drug resistance. Many studies using tumor cell lines as model systems have demonstrated that the exposure of cells to one drug often results in cross-resistance to many other structurally, chemically, and functionally distinct agents. This phenomenon is broadly known as the MDR phenotype [81-84]. The mechanism of MDR has now shown that some of the ATP-binding cassette (ABC) transporter proteins, especially ABCB1, or as it is more commonly referred to in literature, P-glycoprotein (P-gp), which is normally expressed in tumors derived from epithelial tissues including cancers of the kidney, liver, colon, and brain, has been associated with the intrinsic drug resistance of these cancers [85]. Some other tumors (for example breast, ovarian and small cell lung cancers) exhibit generally low levels of P-gp expression at diagnosis. However, the P-gp expression can be induced during the course of treatment, causing the cancer to become resistant to anticancer drugs [85]. At present, due in part to the disappointing results associated with the many side effects of P-gp modulators that have been used in clinical trials, current research efforts have been directed towards the identification of novel compounds with an attention toward dietary natural products or dietary herbs. The advantage is that these dietary herbs exhibit little or virtually no side effects and do not further increase the patient's medication burden.

Our study investigated the effects of bitter melon extracts from leaves, fruits and tendrils on drug accumulation and P-gp activity *in vitro* [59]. We found that the leaf extract showed the greatest efficacy on P-gp-mediated vinblastine accumulation and effux in drug resistant KB-V1 cells, but had no effect in drug-sensitive KB-3-1 cells, which lack P-gp. There was no change in drug accumulation and effux in KB-V1 cells in the presence of fruit and tendril extracts. The protein expression level of P-gp in KB-V1 cells was not altered by BMLE. Therefore, BMLE possibly modulates intracellular drug levels by inhibiting P-gp activity. We next identified the active component(s) in BMLE that act to modulate the function of P-gp and the MDR phenotype in multidrug-resistant human cervical carcinoma using Bioassay-guided fractionation and led us to isolate a purified white crystal that was further identified as kuguacin J [60].

Kuguacin J increased the sensitivity of KB-V1 cells to vinblastine and paclitaxel, but did not have this effect on KB-3-1 cells [60]. Moreover, the treatment of KB-V1 and KB-3-1 cells with kuguacin J yielded a marked increase in C-AM and Rh123 accumulation in a concentration-dependent manner in KB-V1 cells, but had no effect on KB-3-1 cells. C-AM and Rh123 are known to be good substrates for P-gp, indicating that kuguacin J modulates intracellular drug levels by inhibiting P-gp activity. The inhibitory effect of kuguacin J on P-gp function by [^{3}H]-vinblastine transportation assays showed that kuguacin J also increased [^{3}H]-vinblastine accumulation in KB-V1 cells and decreased [^{3}H]-vinblastine efflux from KB-V1 cells. As our previous study showed, P-gp expression in KB-V1 cells was not affected by treating the cells with BMLE [59]. Our data suggests that kuguacin J inhibits P-gp activity, but does not inhibit its expression.

The photoaffinity labeled transport substrate of P-gp, [^{125}I]-IAAP, has been used extensively to study the interaction of the modulators at the substrate-binding site of P-gp [86]. It is also known that P-gp can be specifically labeled with [^{125}I]-IAAP, and the drug-substrates of P-gp can inhibit the photocrosslinking of [^{125}I]-IAAP to P-gp [87]. Kuguacin J inhibited the photocrosslinking of [^{125}I]-IAAP to P-gp in a concentration-dependent manner. This is direct evidence that kuguacin J interacts with the substrate-binding site of P-gp. We further verified the interaction of kuguacin J with P-gp using an ATPase assay, which is another useful assay in the study of the interaction of transport-substrates with P-gp, as ATP hydrolysis is coupled with the transport function of this transporter [88]. Although kuguacin J had a negligible effect on the basal ATPase activity of P-gp, a low concentration of kuguacin J slightly stimulated P-gp-mediated ATP hydrolysis. This finding also implies that kuguacin J interacts with the substrate-binding site of P-gp. We next investigated the effect of kuguacin-J on verapamil-stimulated ATPase activity to further characterize the nature of the interactions of kuguacin J. Kuguacin J indeed inhibited the verapamil-stimulated ATPase activity of P-gp. Furthermore, the kinetic analyses clearly showed that kuguacin J competes with verapamil for the substrate-binding site of P-gp. Taken together, the biochemical data suggest that kuguacin J inhibits the transport function of P-gp by interacting with the substrate-binding site of P-gp where verapamil also binds.

These results demonstrate that kuguacin J, an active compound isolated from BMLE, is an effective inhibitor of P-gp activity, and could be a candidate molecule for treating cancers exhibiting P-gp-mediated MDR. Investigations in animal experiments to determine whether kuguacin J has potential as an effective chemosensitizer that could be used in combination with conventional chemotherapy, needs to be explored.

2.1.3. Modulation potential on cancer cell metastasis

Metastasis, the spreading of malignant cells from the primary site to form a tumor mass at distant organs of the body, is the major cause of death in cancer patients. One of the critical characteristics of a metastatic cell is its invasion or ability to penetrate and invade the extracellular matrix and surrounding tissue. Invasion itself is a multistep process, requiring the coordination of various events, including the alteration of cell adhesion, promotion of cell migration, and degradation of the extracellular matrix barrier. Specifically, metastatic cells adhere to the basement membrane, secrete matrix-degrading enzymes such as matrix metalloproteinases (MMPs) to degrade the extracellular matrix barrier, and migrate from its original site. Therefore, the inhibition of these steps might be an effective approach in the prevention of cancer metastasis. The agents used in cancer metastasis therapy have been cytotoxic, with serious side effects that can diminish the quality of life of the cancer patients [89]. Recently, many efforts have therefore been made to search for non- or low-cytotoxic agents, which can reduce the spread of malignant tumors. One focus is to target cell invasion using substances found in medicinal plants [90,91].

We have provided clear evidence that BMLE can exert inhibitory potential against the metastatic properties of PLS10 cells *in vitro* [72]. Our results pointed to the beneficial effects at non-toxic levels. BMLE might thus afford an advantageous anti-cancer progression agent especially for tumor metastasis therapy. Non-cytotoxic BMLE treatment dramatically reduced migration and invasion properties and reduced, not only secretion, but also expression of MMP-2 and MMP-9 in androgen-independent rat prostate cancer cells. Additionally, uPA, which is an upstream enzyme of MMPs also implicated in tumor cell invasion, survival, and metastasis [92,93], was similarly reduced by BMLE treatment. Since TIMPs have the ability to form tight 1:1 complexes with the active MMP enzymes, changes in TIMP levels directly affect MMP activity [94,95]. BMLE treatment induced the expression of TIMP-2 that may be involved in the inhibition of tumor cell invasion. In addition, BMLE slightly reduced the proteolytic activity of collagenase type IV. Therefore, BMLE might mainly reduce the activity of MMPs by suppression of u-PA and induction of TIMP-2, and also may partially inhibit MMP activity through direct action.

The exact nature of the active components of BMLE, which exerts anti-invasion effects, now needs to be explored along with further elucidation of the underlying molecular mechanisms. Kuguacin J, which already has been investigated for its effects to inhibit P-gp function and reverse MDR in cervical carcinoma [60] and to induce G1 arrest and apoptosis in human prostate cancer cell lines [61,73], could be a candidate for a purified compound with inhibitory activities against cancer cell invasion and metastasis.

Our study showed that non-cytotoxic levels of kuguacin J dramatically reduced the migration and invasion of androgen-independent human prostate cancer PC3 cells [73]. Kuguacin J treatment reduced the secretion of active MMP-2, but did not reduce mRNA expression. Importantly, kuguacin J treatment also reduced the expression of MT1-MMP. Besides, kuguacin J inhibited the secretion of active MMP-9 and uPA. MMP-9 expression also appeared to be reduced by kuguacin J, but the reduction was not significant. The activity of purified collagenase type IV was not directly modulated by kuguacin J, indicating that kuguacin J-mediated the inhibition of the PC3 MMP enzymes, but was not affected by the direct inhibition of their collagenase activities.

BMLE and kuguacin J exert inhibitory effects *in vitro* on the progression of androgen-independent rat and human prostate cancer cells, respectively, by suppressing cancer cell invasion and metastasis [72,73]. These provide a basis for the use of BMLE as a dietary supplement and kuguacin J as a broader antineoplastic agent for cancer progression. Further studies are underway to explore the molecular mechanisms of the action of kuguacin J and to determine its properties *in vivo*.

2.2. Anticancer *in vivo* studies

Kuguacin J has only been recently isolated [62], thus the chemopreventive effects of kuguacin J on cancer or the study of carcinogenesis *in vivo* have not been elucidated yet. An important limitation is that the yield of kuguacin J obtained after purification was not enough to perform *in vivo* experiments. On the other hand, bitter melon extract (BME), from which kuguacin J was purified, was reported to have anticancer effects in *in vivo* studies. The bitter melon seed or fruit extracts were shown to have anticancer activities in a rat colonic aberrant crypt foci model [96] and a mouse mammary tumor model [20]. Extracts of bitter melon fruits were reported to inhibit tumor formation of lymphoma cells (L1210 and P388) with intraperitoneal injections of BME inhibited tumor formation in CBA/H mice [8]. BME also inhibited aberrant crypt foci, which is known as preneoplastic lesion, in the rat colon [97]. In addition, seed oil from bitter melon was reported to inhibit aberrant crypt foci and carcinogenesis induced by azoxymethane in the rat colon through an elevation of peroxisome proliferator-activated receptor gamma expression and an alteration of lipid composition [98].

Other purified materials from BME were also reported to inhibit cancer and/or carcinogenesis. Momordica protein of 30 kDa (MAP30) from MC was reported to inhibit breast cancer in the tumor xenograft model. The treatment of human breast cancer-bearing SCID mice with MAP30 resulted in significant increases in survival, with 20–25% of the mice remaining tumor free for 96 days [99]. Administration of MCP30 decreased PC3 human prostate cancer cell growth by the induction of apoptosis in nude mice [71]. Recent studies further indicate that the chemical modification and reduction of ribosome-inactivating protein in BME, significantly reduced its *in vivo* immunogenicity, but retained its anti-proliferative activity as measured by DNA fragmentation and caspase-3 activation [100]. Cucurbitane-type triterpenoids, charantosides, from a methanol extract of the fruits of MC also inhibited mouse skin carcinogenesis induced by 7,12-dimethylbenz[a]anthracene (DMBA) or peroxynitrite plus 12-O-tetradecanoylphorbol-13-acetate (TPA) [45] α-ESA in bitter melon seed oil suppressing the growth of DLD-1 human colon cancer cells by apoptosis induction via lipid peroxidation [101]. α-ESA, which is converted to conjugated linoleic acid *in vivo*, had a stronger suppressive effect than the conjugated linoleic acid on tumor cell growth.

We also have reported the anti cancer abilities of BMLE *in vivo* [72,73]. Dietary BMLE treatment tended to reduce lung weight and the number of lung metastatic tumors in a model in which intravenous inoculation of androgen-independent rat prostate cancer cells was injected into nude mice, resulting in a 100% incidence of lung metastasis [72]. Treatment of BMLE significantly reduced the percentage of the tumor area in the lungs in a dose-response manner.

In another study, while kuguacin J inhibited the migration and invasion of PC3 cells *in vitro*, dietary BMLE did not reduce metastasis to the lymph node but significantly reduced the growth of PC3 xenografts [73]. One reason why the differences in the incidence of lymph node metastasis between the control and the BMLE-diet fed animals could not be determined is that the PC3 xenograph model had a very low incidence of metastasis. Taking all the mice together, PC3 cells metastasized to the lymph node with an incidence of only 3/20, 15%, while metastasis to other organs was not detected.

Our *in vitro* data presented that the mechanism of the anticancer effects of kuguacin J were similar to BMLE in androgen-dependent and -independent prostate cancer via cell cycle arrest, apoptosis and invasion [61,72,73], suggesting that the possibility of *in vivo* anticancer effects of kuguacin J might be similar to BMLE. Therefore, further work using suitable *in vivo* models will be necessary to fully understand the *in vivo* activity of kuguacin J.

With respect to *in vivo* toxicity, MC was shown to be safe with no signs of nephrotoxicity and hepatotoxicity without any adverse influence on food intake, growth organ weights and hematological parameters in experimental animals when ingested in low doses up to a period of 2 months [4,102]. The relatively low toxicity of all parts of this plant has also been reported when ingested, while toxicity and even death in laboratory animals has only been reported when the extracts were administered intravenously or by intraperitoneal injection in high doses [103]. MC has shown abortifacient activity traditionally, as well as experimentally [3,7]. The fruit and seeds demonstrated greater toxicity than the leaf or aerial parts of the plant. The documented adverse effects of MC are hypoglycemic coma and convulsions in children, reduced fertility in mice, a favism-like syndrome, increases in gamma-glutamyltransferase and alkaline phosphatase levels in animals, as well as headaches [3].

3. Conclusion

A current strategy for the evaluation of anticancer phytochemicals is based in part on: (1) cell cycle and apoptosis regulation; (2) anti-oxidative stress and anti-inflammatory activities;

(3) drug resistance of cancer cells, and (4) specific molecular targets targeting carcinogenesis and metastasis. In our studies, BMLE and one of the tritepenoids included in BMLE, kuguacin J, have shown that they possess potent anticancer capabilities to induce apoptosis/cell cycle arrest in pre-initiated/initiated tumor cells, while in more advanced tumors, these compounds could block resistance to anticancer drugs, tumor progression and metastasis (Figure 3). These findings provide evidence of the anticancer effects of BMLE and kuguacin J (as summarized in Figure 3) and suggest the strong possibility that these natural products can be developed for cancer chemoprevention and chemotherapy.

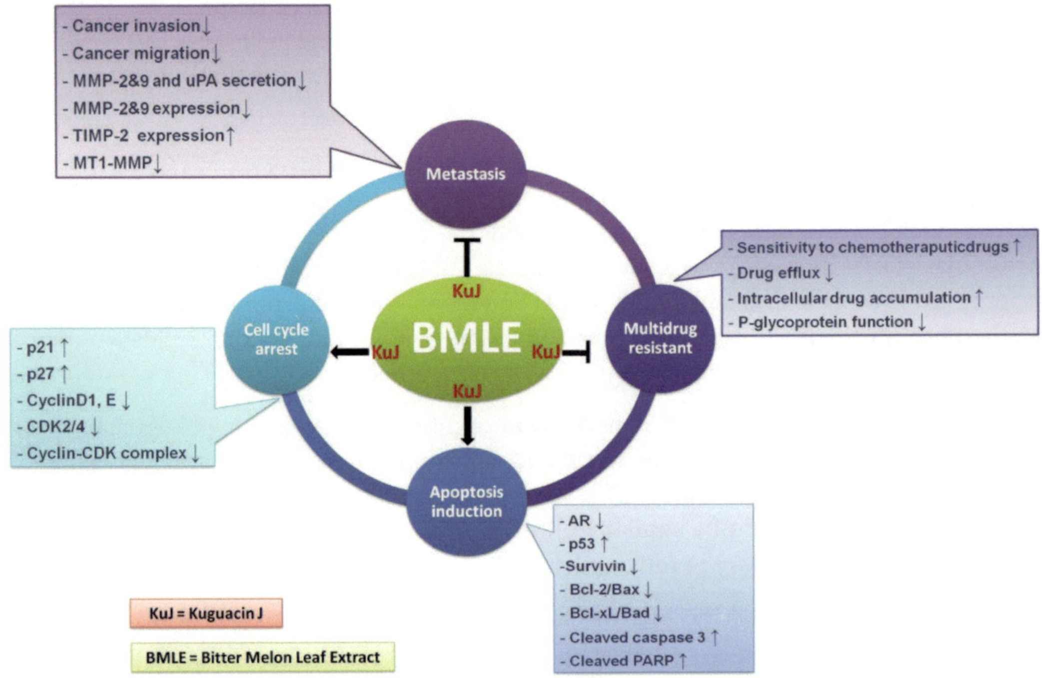

Figure 3. Summary of reported anticancer effects of bitter melon leaf extract and kuguacin J [59-61,72,73].

The critical points to be investigated in future experiments include the fact that Kuguacin J accounts for only approximately 1.6% of BMLE [61]. BMLE is known to include several triterpenoids and flavoniods. Recently various triterpenoids have shown promising effects when applied as anticancer agents [104,105]. Cucurbitacin B (cucB), a triterpenoid from Cucurbitaceae vegetables also found in bitter melon seeds, caused cell cycle arrest and apoptosis induction in human colon adenocarcinoma cancer cells [53]. Additionally, Rutin, a flavonoid present in bitter melon leaves, has been reported to display growth inhibition of leukemia and ovarian carcinoma cells, with anti-invasive effects on melanoma cells [35,56-58]. Therefore, BMLE may include other bioactive compounds apart from kuguacin J, which exert anti-tumor effects, although human studies have not yet been published. Thus, a characterization of other active components present in BMLE needs to be further elucidated.

In addition, the absorption and metabolism of the bioactive compounds after consumption remains to be investigated as to whether a test tube study can be applicable to people.

Author details

Pornngarm Limtrakul and Pornsiri Pitchakarn
Department of Biochemistry, Faculty of Medicine, Chiang Mai University, Chiang Mai, Thailand

Shugo Suzuki
Department of Experimental Pathology and Tumor Biology, Nagoya City University, Graduate School of Medical Sciences, Japan

Acknowledgement

We would like to gratefully acknowledge our research grants, including the National Research Council of Thailand and the Research Foundation for Oriental Medicine and the Society for Promotion of Pathology of Nagoya, Japan. Our research work would not have been a complete success without their financial support. The authors are also grateful for the English correction from Russell Kirk Hollis of the English Department, Faculty of Humanities, Chiang Mai University.

4. References

[1] Ahmed, I., Lakhani, M.S., Gillett, M., John, A. and Raza, H. (2001) Hypotriglyceridemic and hypocholesterolemic effects of anti-diabetic Momordica charantia (karela) fruit extract in streptozotocin-induced diabetic rats. Diabetes Res Clin Pract, 51, 155-61.

[2] Krawinkel, M.B. and Keding, G.B. (2006) Bitter gourd (Momordica Charantia): A dietary approach to hyperglycemia. Nutr Rev, 64, 331-7.

[3] Basch, E., Gabardi, S. and Ulbricht, C. (2003) Bitter melon (Momordica charantia): a review of efficacy and safety. Am J Health Syst Pharm, 60, 356-9.

[4] Virdi, J., Sivakami, S., Shahani, S., Suthar, A.C., Banavalikar, M.M. and Biyani, M.K. (2003) Antihyperglycemic effects of three extracts from Momordica charantia. J Ethnopharmacol, 88, 107-11.

[5] Cakici, I., Hurmoglu, C., Tunctan, B., Abacioglu, N., Kanzik, I. and Sener, B. (1994) Hypoglycaemic effect of Momordica charantia extracts in normoglycaemic or cyproheptadine-induced hyperglycaemic mice. J Ethnopharmacol, 44, 117-21.

[6] Clouatre, D.L., Rao, S.N. and Preuss, H.G. (2011) Bitter melon extracts in diabetic and normal rats favorably influence blood glucose and blood pressure regulation. J Med Food, 14, 1496-504.

[7] Grover, J.K. and Yadav, S.P. (2004) Pharmacological actions and potential uses of Momordica charantia: a review. J Ethnopharmacol, 93, 123-32.

[8] Jilka, C., Strifler, B., Fortner, G.W., Hays, E.F. and Takemoto, D.J. (1983) In vivo antitumor activity of the bitter melon (Momordica charantia). Cancer Res, 43, 5151-5.

[9] Lee-Huang, S., Huang, P.L., Chen, H.C., Bourinbaiar, A., Huang, H.I. and Kung, H.F. (1995) Anti-HIV and anti-tumor activities of recombinant MAP30 from bitter melon. Gene, 161, 151-6.

[10] (1980) WHO Expert Committee on Diabetes Mellitus: second report. World Health Organ Tech Rep Ser, 646, 1-80.

[11] Leung, L., Birtwhistle, R., Kotecha, J., Hannah, S. and Cuthbertson, S. (2009) Anti-diabetic and hypoglycaemic effects of Momordica charantia (bitter melon): a mini review. Br J Nutr, 102, 1703-8.

[12] Ross, I.A. (2003) Medicinal plants of the world. Chemical constituents, traditional and modern uses. Totowa NJ: Humana Press. 489 p.

[13] Kubola, J. and Siriamornpun, S. (2008) Phenolic contents and antioxidant activities of bitter gourd (Momordica charantia L.) leaf, stem and fruit fraction extracts in vitro. Food Chemistry, 110, 881-890.

[14] Mathew, S. and Abraham, T.E. (2006) In vitro antioxidant activity and scavenging effects of Cinnamomum verum leaf extract assayed by different methodologies. Food Chem Toxicol, 44, 198-206.

[15] Lotlikar, M.M. and Rajarama, R.M.R. (1996) Pharmacology of a hypoglycemic principle: Isolated from the fruits of *Momordica charantia* Linn. . Indian Journal of Pharmacy, 28, 129-133.

[16] Matsuda, H., Li, Y., Murakami, T., Matsumura, N., Yamahara, J. and Yoshikawa, M. (1998) Antidiabetic principles of natural medicines. III. Structure-related inhibitory activity and action mode of oleanolic acid glycosides on hypoglycemic activity. Chem Pharm Bull (Tokyo), 46, 1399-403.

[17] Yuan, X.-Q., Gu, X.-H., Tang, J. and Wasswa, J. (2008) Hypoglycemic effect of semipurified peptides from momordica charantia l. var. abbreviata ser. in alloxan-induced diabetic micE. Journal of food biochemistry, 32, 107-121.

[18] Zhang, S.Y., Yao, W. Z., Xue, Q. F., Wang, G. Y., Han, J. H., Lei, Q. J., et al. (1980) Isolation, purification and characterization of peptides with hypoglycemic effect in *Momordica Charantia* L. Acta Biochimica et Biophysica Sinica, 12, 391.

[19] Lee, S., Eom, S., Kim, Y., Park, N. and Park, S. (2009) Cucurbitane-type triterpenoids in *Momordica charantia* Linn. Medicinal Plants Res, 3, 1264-1269.

[20] Nagasawa, H., Watanabe, K. and Inatomi, H. (2002) Effects of bitter melon (Momordica charantia l.) or ginger rhizome (Zingiber offifinale rosc) on spontaneous mammary tumorigenesis in SHN mice. Am J Chin Med, 30, 195-205.

[21] Deep, G., Dasgupta, T., Rao, A.R. and Kale, R.K. (2004) Cancer preventive potential of Momordica charantia L. against benzo(a)pyrene induced fore-stomach tumourigenesis in murine model system. Indian J Exp Biol, 42, 319-22.

[22] Shi, H., Hiramatsu, M., Komatsu, M. and Kayama, T. (1996) Antioxidant property of Fructus Momordicae extract. Biochem Mol Biol Int, 40, 1111-21.

[23] Cunnick, J.E., Sakamoto, K., Chapes, S.K., Fortner, G.W. and Takemoto, D.J. (1990) Induction of tumor cytotoxic immune cells using a protein from the bitter melon (Momordica charantia). Cell Immunol, 126, 278-89.

[24] Kirtikar, K.R. (1918) Indian Medicinal Plants: By K.R. Kirtikar, B.D. Basu, and I.C.S: Sudhindra Nath Basu.

[25] Chopra, R.N., Chopra, I.C., Handa, K.L. and Kapoor, L.D. Indigenous Drugs Of India: Academic Publishers.

[26] Raza, H., Ahmed, I., Lakhani, M.S., Sharma, A.K., Pallot, D. and Montague, W. (1996) Effect of bitter melon (Momordica charantia) fruit juice on the hepatic cytochrome P450-dependent monooxygenases and glutathione S-transferases in streptozotocin-induced diabetic rats. Biochem Pharmacol, 52, 1639-42.

[27] Watt, J.M. (1962) The medicinal and poisonous plants of southern and eastern Africa; being an account of their medicinal and other uses, chemical composition, pharmacological effects and toxicology in man and animal by John Mitchell Watt and Maria Gerdina Breyer-Brandwijk. Edinburgh: E. & S. Livingstone.

[28] Chhabra, S.C., Mahunnah, R.L.A. and Mshiu, E.N. (1989) Plants used in traditional medicine in Eastern Tanzania. II. Angiosperms (capparidaceae to ebenaceae). Journal of Ethnopharmacology, 25, 339-359.

[29] Goldstein, S.W., Jenkins, G.L. and Thompson, M.R. (1937) A chemical and pharmacological study of phytolacca Americana, N. F. J. Pharm. Sci., 26, 306-312.

[30] Bryant, A.T. (1909) Zulu medicine and medicine men. In Annals of the Natal Museum. Adlard & Son, vol. 2, pp. 1-76.

[31] Rosales, R. and Fernando, R. (2001) An inquiry into the Hypoglycemic Action of Momordica Charantia among type-2 diabetic patients. Phil J Intern Med, 39, 213-16.

[32] Dans, A.M., Villarruz, M.V., Jimeno, C.A., Javelosa, M.A., Chua, J., Bautista, R., et al. (2007) The effect of Momordica charantia capsule preparation on glycemic control in type 2 diabetes mellitus needs further studies. J Clin Epidemiol, 60, 554-9.

[33] Xie, H., Huang, S., Deng, H., Wu, Z. and Ji, A. (1998) [Study on chemical components of Momordica charantia]. Zhong Yao Cai, 21, 458-9.

[34] Braca, A., Siciliano, T., D'Arrigo, M. and Germano, M.P. (2008) Chemical composition and antimicrobial activity of Momordica charantia seed essential oil. Fitoterapia, 79, 123-5.

[35] Zhang, M., Hettiarachchy, N.S., Horax, R., Chen, P. and Over, K.F. (2009) Effect of maturity stages and drying methods on the retention of selected nutrients and phytochemicals in bitter melon (Momordica charantia) leaf. J Food Sci, 74, C441-8.

[36] Mahato, S.B., Nandy, A.K. and Roy, G. (1992) Triterpenoids. Phytochemistry, 31, 2199-49.

[37] Connolly, J.D. and Hill, R.A. (2008) Triterpenoids. Nat Prod Rep, 25, 794-830.

[38] Chen, J.C., Chiu, M.H., Nie, R.L., Cordell, G.A. and Qiu, S.X. (2005) Cucurbitacins and cucurbitane glycosides: structures and biological activities. Nat Prod Rep, 22, 386-99.

[39] Beloin, N., Gbeassor, M., Akpagana, K., Hudson, J., de Soussa, K., Koumaglo, K., et al. (2005) Ethnomedicinal uses of Momordicacharantia (Cucurbitaceae) in Togo and relation to its phytochemistry and biological activity. J Ethnopharmacol, 96, 49-55.

[40] Mulholland, D.A., Sewram, V., Osborne, R., Pegel, K.H. and Connolly, J.D. (1997) Cucurbitane triterpenoids from the leaves of Momordica foetida. Phytochemistry, 45, 391-395.

[41] Murakami, T., Emoto, A., Matsuda, H. and Yoshikawa, M. (2001) Medicinal foodstuffs. XXI. Structures of new cucurbitane-type triterpene glycosides, goyaglycosides-a, -b, -c, -d, -e, -f, -g, and -h, and new oleanane-type triterpene saponins, goyasaponins I, II, and III, from the fresh fruit of Japanese Momordica charantia L. Chem Pharm Bull (Tokyo), 49, 54-63.

[42] Kimura, Y., Akihisa, T., Yuasa, N., Ukiya, M., Suzuki, T., Toriyama, M., et al. (2005) Cucurbitane-type triterpenoids from the fruit of Momordica charantia. J Nat Prod, 68, 807-9.

[43] Chang, C.I., Chen, C.R., Liao, Y.W., Cheng, H.L., Chen, Y.C. and Chou, C.H. (2006) Cucurbitane-type triterpenoids from Momordica charantia. J Nat Prod, 69, 1168-71.

[44] Nakamura, S., Murakami, T., Nakamura, J., Kobayashi, H., Matsuda, H. and Yoshikawa, M. (2006) Structures of new cucurbitane-type triterpenes and glycosides, karavilagenins and karavilosides, from the dried fruit of Momordica charantia L. in Sri Lanka. Chem Pharm Bull (Tokyo), 54, 1545-50.

[45] Akihisa, T., Higo, N., Tokuda, H., Ukiya, M., Akazawa, H., Tochigi, Y., et al. (2007) Cucurbitane-type triterpenoids from the fruits of Momordica charantia and their cancer chemopreventive effects. J Nat Prod, 70, 1233-9.

[46] Chang, C.I., Chen, C.R., Liao, Y.W., Cheng, H.L., Chen, Y.C. and Chou, C.H. (2008) Cucurbitane-type triterpenoids from the stems of momordica charantia. J Nat Prod, 71, 1327-30.

[47] Ma, J., Whittaker, P., Keller, A.C., Mazzola, E.P., Pawar, R.S., White, K.D., et al. (2010) Cucurbitane-type triterpenoids from Momordica charantia. Planta Med, 76, 1758-61.

[48] Liu, J.Q., Chen, J.C., Wang, C.F. and Qiu, M.H. (2009) New cucurbitane triterpenoids and steroidal glycoside from Momordica charantia. Molecules, 14, 4804-13.

[49] Chen, J., Tian, R., Qiu, M., Lu, L., Zheng, Y. and Zhang, Z. (2008) Trinorcucurbitane and cucurbitane triterpenoids from the roots of Momordica charantia. Phytochemistry, 69, 1043-1048.

[50] Chen, J.-C., Liu, W.-Q., Lu, L., Qiu, M.-H., Zheng, Y.-T., Yang, L.-M., et al. (2009) Kuguacins F–S, cucurbitane triterpenoids from Momordica charantia. Phytochemistry, 70, 133-140.

[51] Lavhale, M.S., Kumar, S., Mishra, S.H. and Sitasawad, S.L. (2009) A novel triterpenoid isolated from the root bark of Ailanthus excelsa Roxb (Tree of Heaven), AECHL-1 as a potential anti-cancer agent. PLoS ONE, 4, 53-65.

[52] Sun, C., Zhang, M., Shan, X., Zhou, X., Yang, J., Wang, Y., et al. (2009) Inhibitory effect of cucurbitacin E on pancreatic cancer cells growth via STAT3 signaling. J Cancer Res Clin Oncol.

[53] Yasuda, S., Yogosawa, S., Izutani, Y., Nakamura, Y., Watanabe, H. and Sakai, T. (2009) Cucurbitacin B induces G(2) arrest and apoptosis via a reactive oxygen species-dependent mechanism in human colon adenocarcinoma SW480 cells. Mol Nutr Food Res.

[54] Yanamandra, N., Berhow, M.A., Konduri, S., Dinh, D.H., Olivero, W.C., Nicolson, G.L., et al. (2003) Triterpenoids from Glycine max decrease invasiveness and induce caspase-mediated cell death in human SNB19 glioma cells. Clin Exp Metastasis, 20, 375-83.

[55] Weng, C.J., Chau, C.F., Chen, K.D., Chen, D.H. and Yen, G.C. (2007) The anti-invasive effect of lucidenic acids isolated from a new Ganoderma lucidum strain. Mol Nutr Food Res, 51, 1472-7.

[56] Lin, J.P., Yang, J.S., Lu, C.C., Chiang, J.H., Wu, C.L., Lin, J.J., et al. (2009) Rutin inhibits the proliferation of murine leukemia WEHI-3 cells in vivo and promotes immune response in vivo. Leuk Res, 33, 823-8.

[57] Luo, H., Jiang, B.H., King, S.M. and Chen, Y.C. (2008) Inhibition of cell growth and VEGF expression in ovarian cancer cells by flavonoids. Nutr Cancer, 60, 800-9.

[58] Martinez Conesa, C., Vicente Ortega, V., Yanez Gascon, M.J., Alcaraz Banos, M., Canteras Jordana, M., Benavente-Garcia, O., et al. (2005) Treatment of metastatic melanoma B16F10 by the flavonoids tangeretin, rutin, and diosmin. J Agric Food Chem, 53, 6791-7.

[59] Limtrakul, P., Khantamat, O. and Pintha, K. (2004) Inhibition of P-glycoprotein activity and reversal of cancer multidrug resistance by Momordica charantia extract. Cancer Chemother Pharmacol, 54, 525-30.

[60] Pitchakarn, P., Ohnuma, S., Pintha, K., Pompimon, W., Ambudkar, S.V. and Limtrakul, P. (2012) Kuguacin J isolated from Momordica charantia leaves inhibits P-glycoprotein (ABCB1)-mediated multidrug resistance. J Nutr Biochem, 23, 76-84.

[61] Pitchakarn, P., Suzuki, S., Ogawa, K., Pompimon, W., Takahashi, S., Asamoto, M., et al. (2011) Induction of G1 arrest and apoptosis in androgen-dependent human prostate cancer by Kuguacin J, a triterpenoid from Momordica charantia leaf. Cancer Lett, 306, 142-50.

[62] Chen, J.C., Liu, W.Q., Lu, L., Qiu, M.H., Zheng, Y.T., Yang, L.M., et al. (2009) Kuguacins F-S, cucurbitane triterpenoids from Momordica charantia. Phytochemistry, 70, 133-40.

[63] Hanahan, D. and Weinberg, R.A. (2000) The hallmarks of cancer. Cell, 100, 57-70.

[64] Ramos, S. (2008) Cancer chemoprevention and chemotherapy: dietary polyphenols and signalling pathways. Mol Nutr Food Res, 52, 507-26.

[65] Kaur, M., Agarwal, C. and Agarwal, R. (2009) Anticancer and cancer chemopreventive potential of grape seed extract and other grape-based products. J Nutr, 139, 1806S-12S.

[66] Neergheen, V.S., Bahorun, T., Taylor, E.W., Jen, L.S. and Aruoma, O.I. (2010) Targeting specific cell signaling transduction pathways by dietary and medicinal phytochemicals in cancer chemoprevention. Toxicology, 278, 229-41.

[67] Surh, Y.J. (2003) Cancer chemoprevention with dietary phytochemicals. Nat Rev Cancer, 3, 768-80.

[68] Ray, R.B., Raychoudhuri, A., Steele, R. and Nerurkar, P. (2010) Bitter melon (Momordica charantia) extract inhibits breast cancer cell proliferation by modulating cell cycle regulatory genes and promotes apoptosis. Cancer Res, 70, 1925-31.

[69] Brennan, V.C., Wang, C.M. and Yang, W.H. (2012) Bitter Melon (Momordica charantia) Extract Suppresses Adrenocortical Cancer Cell Proliferation Through Modulation of the Apoptotic Pathway, Steroidogenesis, and Insulin-Like Growth Factor Type 1 Receptor/RAC-alpha Serine/Threonine-Protein Kinase Signaling. J Med Food, 15, 325-34.

[70] Ru, P., Steele, R., Nerurkar, P.V., Phillips, N. and Ray, R.B. (2011) Bitter melon extract impairs prostate cancer cell-cycle progression and delays prostatic intraepithelial neoplasia in TRAMP model. Cancer Prev Res (Phila), 4, 2122-30.

[71] Xiong, S.D., Yu, K., Liu, X.H., Yin, L.H., Kirschenbaum, A., Yao, S., et al. (2009) Ribosome-inactivating proteins isolated from dietary bitter melon induce apoptosis and inhibit histone deacetylase-1 selectively in premalignant and malignant prostate cancer cells. Int J Cancer, 125, 774-82.

[72] Pitchakarn, P., Ogawa, K., Suzuki, S., Takahashi, S., Asamoto, M., Chewonarin, T., et al. (2010) Momordica charantia leaf extract suppresses rat prostate cancer progression in vitro and in vivo. Cancer Sci, 101, 2234-40.

[73] Pitchakarn, P., Suzuki, S., Ogawa, K., Pompimon, W., Takahashi, S., Asamoto, M., et al. (2012) Kuguacin J, a triterpeniod from Momordica charantia leaf, modulates the progression of androgen-independent human prostate cancer cell line, PC3. Food Chem Toxicol, 50, 840-7.

[74] Syed, D.N., Khan, N., Afaq, F. and Mukhtar, H. (2007) Chemoprevention of prostate cancer through dietary agents: progress and promise. Cancer Epidemiol Biomarkers Prev, 16, 2193-203.

[75] Moldovan, G.L., Pfander, B. and Jentsch, S. (2007) PCNA, the maestro of the replication fork. Cell, 129, 665-79.

[76] Pilat, M.J., Kamradt, J.M. and Pienta, K.J. (1998) Hormone resistance in prostate cancer. Cancer Metastasis Rev, 17, 373-81.

[77] Zhu, M.L. and Kyprianou, N. (2008) Androgen receptor and growth factor signaling cross-talk in prostate cancer cells. Endocr Relat Cancer, 15, 841-9.

[78] Rozan, L.M. and El-Deiry, W.S. (2007) p53 downstream target genes and tumor suppression: a classical view in evolution. Cell Death Differ, 14, 3-9.

[79] Polyak, K., Xia, Y., Zweier, J.L., Kinzler, K.W. and Vogelstein, B. (1997) A model for p53-induced apoptosis. Nature, 389, 300-5.

[80] Tan, B., Piwnica-Worms, D. and Ratner, L. (2000) Multidrug resistance transporters and modulation. Curr Opin Oncol, 12, 450-8.

[81] Aimes, R.T. and Quigley, J.P. (1995) Matrix Metalloproteinase-2 Is an Interstitial Collagenase. J. Biol. Chem., 270, 5872-5876.

[82] Lehnert, M. (1998) Chemotherapy resistance in breast cancer. Anticancer Res, 18.

[83] Ambudkar, S.V., Dey, S., Hrycyna, C.A., Ramachandra, M., Pastan, I. and Gottesman, M.M. (1999) Biochemical, cellular, and pharmacological aspects of the multidrug transporter. Annu Rev Pharmacol Toxicol, 39, 361-98.

[84] Larsen, A.K., Escargueil, A.E. and Skladanowski, A. (2000) Resistance mechanisms associated with altered intracellular distribution of anticancer agents. Pharmacol Ther, 85, 217-29.

[85] Ambudkar, S.V., Sauna, Z.E., Gottesman, M.M. and Szakacs, G. (2005) A novel way to spread drug resistance in tumor cells: functional intercellular transfer of P-glycoprotein (ABCB1). Trends Pharmacol Sci, 26, 385-7.

[86] Maki, N., Hafkemeyer, P. and Dey, S. (2003) Allosteric modulation of human P-glycoprotein. Inhibition of transport by preventing substrate translocation and dissociation. J Biol Chem, 278, 18132-9.

[87] Sauna, Z.E. and Ambudkar, S.V. (2000) Evidence for a requirement for ATP hydrolysis at two distinct steps during a single turnover of the catalytic cycle of human P-glycoprotein. Proc Natl Acad Sci U S A, 97, 2515-20.

[88] Ambudkar, S.V. (1998) Drug-stimulatable ATPase activity in crude membranes of human MDR1-transfected mammalian cells. Methods Enzymol, 292, 504-14.

[89] Braun-Falco, M., Holtmann, C., Lordick, F. and Ring, J. (2006) Follicular drug reaction from cetuximab: a common side effect in the treatment of metastatic colon carcinoma. Hautarzt, 57, 701-4.

[90] Yodkeeree, S., Garbisa, S. and Limtrakul, P. (2008) Tetrahydrocurcumin inhibits HT1080 cell migration and invasion via downregulation of MMPs and uPA. Acta Pharmacol Sin, 29, 853-60.

[91] Lin, S.S., Lai, K.C., Hsu, S.C., Yang, J.S., Kuo, C.L., Lin, J.P., et al. (2009) Curcumin inhibits the migration and invasion of human A549 lung cancer cells through the inhibition of matrix metalloproteinase-2 and -9 and Vascular Endothelial Growth Factor (VEGF). Cancer Lett, 285, 127-33.

[92] Li, Y. and Cozzi, P.J. (2007) Targeting uPA/uPAR in prostate cancer. Cancer Treat Rev, 33, 521-7.

[93] Pulukuri, S.M., Gondi, C.S., Lakka, S.S., Jutla, A., Estes, N., Gujrati, M., et al. (2005) RNA interference-directed knockdown of urokinase plasminogen activator and urokinase plasminogen activator receptor inhibits prostate cancer cell invasion, survival, and tumorigenicity in vivo. J Biol Chem, 280, 36529-40.

[94] Nagase, H., Visse, R. and Murphy, G. (2006) Structure and function of matrix metalloproteinases and TIMPs. Cardiovasc Res, 69, 562-73.

[95] Fisher, J.F. and Mobashery, S. (2006) Recent advances in MMP inhibitor design. Cancer Metastasis Rev, 25, 115-36.

[96] Kohno, H., Suzuki, R., Noguchi, R., Hosokawa, M., Miyashita, K. and Tanaka, T. (2002) Dietary conjugated linolenic acid inhibits azoxymethane-induced colonic aberrant crypt foci in rats. Jpn J Cancer Res, 93, 133-42.

[97] Chiampanichayakul, S., Kataoka, K., Arimochi, H., Thumvijit, S., Kuwahara, T., Nakayama, H., et al. (2001) Inhibitory effects of bitter melon (Momordica charantia Linn.) on bacterial mutagenesis and aberrant crypt focus formation in the rat colon. J Med Invest, 48, 88-96.

[98] Kohno, H., Yasui, Y., Suzuki, R., Hosokawa, M., Miyashita, K. and Tanaka, T. (2004) Dietary seed oil rich in conjugated linolenic acid from bitter melon inhibits azoxymethane-induced rat colon carcinogenesis through elevation of colonic PPARgamma expression and alteration of lipid composition. Int J Cancer, 110, 896-901.

[99] Lee-Huang, S., Huang, P.L., Sun, Y., Chen, H.C., Kung, H.F. and Murphy, W.J. (2000) Inhibition of MDA-MB-231 human breast tumor xenografts and HER2 expression by anti-tumor agents GAP31 and MAP30. Anticancer Res, 20, 653-9.

[100] Li, M., Chen, Y., Liu, Z., Shen, F., Bian, X. and Meng, Y. (2009) Anti-tumor activity and immunological modification of ribosome-inactivating protein (RIP) from Momordica charantia by covalent attachment of polyethylene glycol. Acta Biochim Biophys Sin (Shanghai), 41, 792-9.

[101] Tsuzuki, T., Tokuyama, Y., Igarashi, M. and Miyazawa, T. (2004) Tumor growth suppression by alpha-eleostearic acid, a linolenic acid isomer with a conjugated triene system, via lipid peroxidation. Carcinogenesis, 25, 1417-25.

[102] Platel, K., Shurpalekar, K.S. and Srinivasan, K. (1993) Influence of bitter gourd (Momordica charantia) on growth and blood constituents in albino rats. Nahrung, 37, 156-60.

[103] Kusamran, W.R., Ratanavila, A. and Tepsuwan, A. (1998) Effects of neem flowers, Thai and Chinese bitter gourd fruits and sweet basil leaves on hepatic monooxygenases and glutathione S-transferase activities, and in vitro metabolic activation of chemical carcinogens in rats. Food Chem Toxicol, 36, 475-84.

[104] Sung, B., Park, B., Yadav, V.R. and Aggarwal, B.B. (2010) Celastrol, a triterpene, enhances TRAIL-induced apoptosis through the down-regulation of cell survival proteins and up-regulation of death receptors. J Biol Chem, 285, 11498-507.

[105] Yeh, C.T., Wu, C.H. and Yen, G.C. (2010) Ursolic acid, a naturally occurring triterpenoid, suppresses migration and invasion of human breast cancer cells by modulating c-Jun N-terminal kinase, Akt and mammalian target of rapamycin signaling. Mol Nutr Food Res, 54, 1285-95.

Chapter 14

Regulation of Apoptosis, Invasion and Angiogenesis of Tumor Cells by Caffeic Acid Phenethyl Ester

Mohamed F. El-Refaei and Essam A. Mady

Additional information is available at the end of the chapter

http://dx.doi.org/10.5772/55275

1. Introduction

Cancer is a multistage disease involving a series of events and generally occurs over an extended period. During this period, accumulation of genetic and epigenetic alterations leads to the progressive transformation of a normal cell into a malignant cell. Cancer cells acquire several abilities that most healthy cells do not possess: they become resistant to growth inhibition, proliferate without dependence on growth factors, replicate without limit, evade apoptosis, and invade, metastasize and support angiogenesis [1]. Unlike heart disease, death rates for cancer remained approximately the same in the United States from 1975 through 2002. Indeed, it is predicted that by 2020 approximately 15 million new cancer cases will be diagnosed worldwide and 12 million cancer patients will die [2].

Cancer is a disease characterized by uncontrolled growth and division of genetically altered cells and its emergence requires several elements, including self-sufficiency in growth signals, insensitivity to growth-inhibitory signals, evasion of apoptosis, limitless replicative potential, tissue invasion and metastasis, and sustained angiogenesis [1, 3]. Cancer is thought to evolve along a multi-step process. Cancer cells are the descendants of a normal cell in which some kind of internal or external stress causes a change in its genetic code. This event is said to initiate the cell to a precancerous state. In a second stage, this precancerous cell divides in response to a promoting agent to produce daughter cells, and these daughter cells divide to produce more daughter cells, and so on. The genetic instabilities passed down through the generations finally result in one cell that no longer requires the promoting agent to stimulate its proliferation. A cancer cell is thus born with the ability to make proteins such as growth factors that stimulate proliferation. Finally in the third stage of carcinogenesis, progression, this cancer cell divides to produce daughter cells, which also divide, and soon there is a population of cancer cells with the ability to invade and metastasize [4].

It is now clear that cancer phenotypes result from the dysregulation of more than 500 genes at multiple steps in cell signaling pathways. This indicates that inhibition of a single gene product or cell signaling pathway is unlikely to prevent or treat cancer. However, most current anticancer therapies are based on the modulation of a single target [5, 6].

One of the most important findings to have emerged during the past three decades is that cancer is a largely preventable disease. Thus, people need to be educated about the risk factors for cancer and those that prevent the disease. As many as 90% of all cancers have been shown to be due to environmental/acquired factors such as tobacco, diet, radiation and infectious organisms, etc., and only the remaining 5–10% of cases are caused by internal factors such as inherited mutations, hormones, and immune conditions [7].

The ineffective, unsafe, and expensive monotargeted therapies have led to a lack of faith in these approaches. Therefore, the current paradigm for cancer treatment is either to combine several monotargeted drugs or to design drugs that modulate multiple targets. As a result, pharmaceutical companies have been increasingly interested in developing multitargeted therapies. Many plant-derived dietary agents, called nutraceuticals, have multitargeting properties. In addition, these products are less expensive, safer, and more readily available than are synthetic agents [5].

Prevention is better than cure and this is very true in case of cancer. Chemoprevention was defined as the administration of agents to prevent induction, to inhibit or to delay the progression of cancer [8], or as the inhibition or reversal of carcinogenesis at a premalignant stage [9]. Chemoprevention involves the use of synthetic or natural compounds to inhibit, slow, or reverse carcinogenesis. It is based on the hypothesis that the disruption of biological events involved in carcinogenesis will inhibit this process and can be applied to any stage of carcinogenesis. Chemoprevention utilizes appropriate pharmacological agents [10,11] or dietary agents, consumed in diverse forms like macronutrients, micronutrients, or nonnutritive phytochemicals [12–14]. It is estimated that from 10 to 80 percent of cancer patients use some form of natural compounds as a part of complementary medicine as part of their overall therapy without any real guidance. This explains the growing interest in using the natural compounds properly in the treatment of cancer.

Phytochemicals are one wide class of nutraceuticals found in plants, which are extensively researched by scientists for their health-promoting potential. Honey has a wide range of phytochemicals including polyphenols which act as antioxidants. Polyphenols and phenolic acids found in the honey vary according to the geographical and climatic conditions. Some of them were reported as a specific marker for the botanical origin of the honey. Considerable differences in both composition and content of phenolic compounds have been found in different unifloral honeys [15]. Terpenes, benzyl alcohol, 3, 5-dimethoxy-4-hydroxybenzoic acid (syringic acid), methyl 3, 5-dimethoxy-4-hydroxybenzoate (methyl syringate), 3, 4, 5-trimethoxybenzoic acid, 2-hydroxy-3- phenylpropionic acid, 2-hydroxybenzoic acid and 1, 4- dihydroxybenzene are some of the phytochemicals a ascribed for the antimicrobial activity of honey [16]. Among these phytochemicals, polyphenols were reported to have antiproliferative potential.

2. Active compounds in propolis

Polyphenolic compounds are widely distributed in the plant kingdom and display a variety of biological activities, including chemoprevention and tumor growth inhibition. Propolis and honey have been known to mankind from the remotest of ancient times and have been widely used by many cultures for different purposes. Propolis is a complex resinous mixture gathered from plants and used by honeybees in their hives as a general-purpose sealer and antibiotic. It is made up of a variety of polyphenolic compounds. Some of the isolated compounds have shown anti-inflammatory activity, carcinostatic, anti-carcinogenic activity and induction of apoptosis. Caffeic acid (CA) and caffeic acid phenethyl ester (CAPE) are members of the polyphenolic compounds and present in high concentrations in medicinal plants and propolis. CAPE showed a wide variety of biological activities at non-toxic concentrations. It has shown antibacterial, anti-inflammatory, antioxidant, antitumor and anti-proliferative activities [17].

CAPE [2-propenoic acid, 3-(3,4-dihydroxy phenyl)-,2-phenethyl ester] (Fig.1) is an active component of propolis with a variety of biological activities. CAPE has been used in folk medicine as a potent antibacterial, anti-inflammatory, antioxidant, antitumor and antiproliferative with a wide variety of biological and pharmacological activities at non-toxic concentrations in a mammal's organs [18].

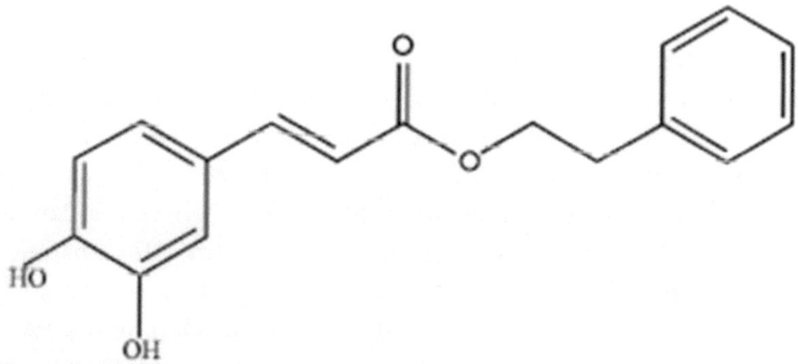

Figure 1. Structure of caffeic acid phenethyl ester (CAPE)

CAPE is chemopreventive against intestinal, colon and skin cancer, and also has been shown to decreases the formation of preneoplastic hepatic lesions when is administrated in a rat model of liver carcinogenesis [19-21], but the mechanism of these properties is not completely understood. Recently, CAPE, in a concentration dependent fashion, was shown to inhibit MCF-7 (hormone receptor positive, HR+) and MDA-MB-231 (a model of triple negative BC (TNBC)) tumor growth, either *in vitro* or *in vivo* without much effect on normal mammary cells [22]. At the same time, CAPE was found to cause pronounced changes in bCSC characteristics manifested by inhibition of self renewal, progenitor formation, clonal growth in soft agar, and concurrent significant decrease in CD44 content, all signs of decreased malignancy potential [23]. Besides CAPE, other caffeic acid esters in propolis may have biological effects.

Here we will focus on CAPE and its biological effects against cancer *in vitro* and *in vivo*. Specifically, we will discuss how CAPE can modulate inflammatory pathways and thus affect the survival, proliferation, invasion, angiogenesis, and metastasis of the tumor.

2.1. Regulation of inflammatory pathways by CAPE

Inflammation is a localized reaction of tissue to infection, irritation, or other injury. Inflammation is a necessary response to clear bacterial and viral infections, repair tissue insults, and suppress tumor initiation/progression. However, when inflammation persists or control mechanisms are dysregulated, diseases such as cancer can develop. Interestingly, inflammation functions at all stages of tumor development: initiation, promotion and progression including metastasis. During the initiation phase, inflammation induces the release of a variety of cytokines and chemokines that promote the activation of inflammatory cells and associated factors. This causes further oxidative damage, DNA mutations, and other changes in the tissue microenvironment, making it more conducive to cell transformation, increased survival, and proliferation [24]. At the molecular level, inflammation, transformation, survival and proliferation are regulated by the proinflammatory transcription factor Nuclear Factor-κB (NF-κB), a family of ubiquitously expressed transcription factors. NF-κB regulates the expression of genes involved in the transformation, survival, proliferation, invasion, angiogenesis and metastasis of tumor cells [25].

TNF-α is also one of the prime signals that induces apoptosis in many different types of cells. Whereas acute activation of NF-κB may be therapeutic, chronic activation may lead to the development of chronic inflammation, cancer and other chronic diseases. There is a strong association between chronic inflammatory conditions and cancer specific to the organ. Epidemiological evidence points to a connection between inflammation and a predisposition for the development of cancer, i.e., long-term inflammation leads to the development of dysplasia. Various factors are known to induce chronic inflammatory responses that further cause cancer. These include bacterial, viral, and parasitic infections (e.g., Helicobacter pylori, Epstein-Barr virus, human immunodeficiency virus, flukes, schistosomes) and chemical irritants (i.e., tumor promoters). Active NF-κB has now been identified in tissues of most cancer patients, including those with leukemia and lymphoma and cancers of the prostate, breast, oral cavity, liver, pancreas, colon and ovary [26].

In the resting stage, NF-κB resides in the cytoplasm as a heterotrimer consisting of p50, p65, and the inhibitory subunit IκBα. On activation, the IκBα protein undergoes phosphorylation, ubiquitination, and degradation. p50 and p65 are then released, are translocated to the nucleus, bind specific DNA sequences present in the promoters of various genes, and initiate their transcription. A number of proteins are involved in the NF-κB signaling pathway. Because of the relevance of the NF-κB signaling pathway in cancer, this pathway has been proven to be an attractive target for therapeutic development. Active NF-κB complexes can contribute to tumorigenesis by regulating genes that promote the growth and survival of cancer cells, during the cell cycle. NF-κB has ability to regulate the G1-phase expression of key proto-oncogenes is subject to regulation by the integrated activity of IkappaB kinase (IKK)alpha, IKKbeta, Akt and Chk1. The coordinated binding of NF-κB subunits to the Cyclin D1, c-Myc and Skp2 promoters is dynamic with distinct changes in promoter occupancy and RelA(p65) phosphorylation occurring through G1, S and G2 phases, concomitant with a switch from coactivator to corepressor recruitment. Akt activity is required for IKK-dependent phosphorylation of NF-κB subunits in G1 and G2 phases, where Chk1 is inactive. However, in S-phase, Akt is inactivated, while Chk1 phosphorylates RelA and associates with IKKalpha, inhibiting the processing of the p100 (NF-κB2) subunit, which also plays a critical role in the regulation of these genes. This reveals a complex regulatory network integrating NF- κB with the DNA-replication checkpoint and the expression of critical regulators of cell proliferation [27]. Thus, its inhibition could be a novel approach to breaking the vicious cycle of tumor cell proliferation [28-30] More than 700 inhibitors of the NF-κB activation pathway have been reported, including antioxidants, peptides, small RNA/DNA, microbial and viral proteins, small molecules, and engineered dominant-negative or constitutively active polypeptides [31,32].

Caffeic acid phenethyl ester has been shown to suppress NF-κB activation by suppressing the binding of the p50–p65 complex directly to DNA [33-35]. The molecular basis of CAPE action was elucidated by Natarajan et al. [36]. Since NF-κB has a role in these activities, they examined the effect of CAPE on this transcription factor in an exhaustive manner. They preincubated the U-937 cells with CAPE at various concentrations for 2 hours before treating with TNF (0.1 nM) for 15 minutes. CAPE inhibited the TNF-dependent activation of NF-κB in a dose-dependent manner with maximum effect occurring at 25 μg/mL. NF- κB activation induced by the phorbol ester, phorbol-12- myristate 13-acetate (PMA), ceramide, okadaic acid and hydrogen peroxide was also inhibited by CAPE. It prevented the translocation of the p65 subunit of NF-κB to the nucleus without affecting the TNF-induced IκBα degradation. It did not show any inhibitory effects on the other transcription factors like AP-1, TFIID and oct-1. With these findings they concluded that CAPE is a potent and a specific inhibitor of NF-κB activation and this may provide the molecular basis for its multiple immunomodulatory and antiinflammatory activities of CAPE.

Abdel-Latif et al.[37] have demonstrated for the first time that CAPE is a major component of propolis, modulates H. pylori-induced NF-κB, AP-1 DNA binding activity and COX-2 expression in gastric epithelial cells. In addition, CAPE reduced TNF-α and IL-8 levels and suppressed the proliferative response of AGS cells to H. pylori. They found also that pretreatment of gastric epithelial cells with CAPE upregulated IkB-a levels and prevented nuclear translocation of NF-κB/ p65 in H. pylori-treated AGS cells. NF-κB is present in the cytosol in an inactive state bound to the inhibitory IkB protein. H. pylori infection of gastric epithelial cells results in phosphorylation and degradation of the IkB, thus allowing nuclear translocation of NF-κB.

It is mechanistically proven that inflammation produces reactive oxygen species (ROS) and reactive nitrogen species (RNS). In particular, ROS and RNS lead to oxidative damage and nitration of DNA bases, which increases the risk of DNA mutations and further leads to cancer. Nitric oxide (NO) is associated with inflammatory reaction and is produced by inducible nitric oxide synthase (iNOS) in certain cells activated by various proinflammatory agents. NO acts as a host defense by damaging membranes of pathogenic bacteria and as a regulatory molecule with homeostatic activities. However, excessive production of NO is pathogenic for host tissue itself because NO, as a reactive radical directly damages functions of normal tissue. Thus, effective inhibition of NO accumulation by inflammatory stimuli represents a beneficial therapeutic strategy [38,39].

Nagaoka et al. [40] reported that CAPE possesses potent NO inhibitory activities and suggested that the NO inhibitory effect can directly correlate with anti-inflammatory properties of the Netherlands propolis. They suggested that the active principles of the Netherlands propolis, i.e., CAPE and its analogues, should block the activation of iNOS through the suppression of NF-kB activation and resulted in potent NO inhibition.

We investigated the anti-inflammatory and antioxidant potential of CAPE on a tumor cell line (ZR-75-1). We found that CAPE at the concentration of 15μM inhibited NO production by ($>$ 47%) compared to NO level of untreated tumor cells ($P < 0.05$). In addition, superoxide dismutase (SOD) was at the highest level in the maintained basal tumor culture cell supernatant (231.9± 4.2 μU/L). This level reduced intensively to (169.3 ± 3.7 μU/L), in the CAPE-treated culture cells, which was significantly less than the level in untreated cells ($P < 0.001$). On the other hand, malonaldehyde (MDA) level, which is considered to be an important parameter for the oxidative damage determination, was inhibited to (17.3 ± 2.3 μmol/L) in the CAPE-treated cells when compared with untreated tumor cells (23.8 ± 2.5 μmol/L), but was not statistically significant (Table 1).

Group Parameters	NO· (μ mol/L)	SOD (μ U/ L)	MDA (μ mol/L)
I	19.6 ± 1.9	231.9 ± 4.2	23.8 ± 2.5
II	10.2 ± 1.3	169.3 ± 3.7	17.3 ± 2.3
P	$<$ 0.05	$<$ 0.001	N.S

(I). Untreated tumor cells , (II). Treated tumor cells at 15μM CAPE.

Table 1. Nitric oxide (NO·), Superoxide dismutase (SOD) and Malondialdehyde (MDA) values in culture supernatant.

2.2. Regulation of tumor cell development by CAPE

Under normal physiological conditions, the human body maintains homeostasis by eliminating unwanted, damaged, aged, and misplaced cells. Homeostasis is carried out in a genetically programmed manner by a process referred to as apoptosis (programmed cell death). Cancer cells are able to evade apoptosis and grow in a rapid and uncontrolled manner. One of the most important ways by which cancer cells have gained this ability is through mutation in the p53 tumor suppressor gene. Without a functional p53 gene, cells lack the DNA-damage-sensing capability that would normally induce the apoptotic cascade [41-43].

A complex set of proteins, including caspases, proapoptotic and antiapoptotic B cell lymphoma (Bcl)-2 family proteins, cytochrome c, and apoptotic protease activating factor (Apaf)-1, execute apoptosis either by an intrinsic or extrinsic pathway. The intrinsic pathway is mitochondria dependent, whereas the extrinsic pathway is triggered by death receptors (DRs). Some antiapoptotic proteins such as Bcl-2 and B cell lymphoma extra large (Bcl-xL) and survivin are overexpressed in a wide variety of cancers. Therefore, selective downregulation of antiapoptotic proteins and upregulation of proapoptotic proteins and p53 in cancer cells offer promising therapeutic interventions for cancer treatment [44,45].

We tested the effect of CAPE on the viability of human breast cancer ZR-75-1 cells derived from a malignant ascitic effusion in a 63 year-old, white female with infiltrating ductal carcinoma [46]. CAPE induced a significant inhibitory effect on the growth and viability of tumor cells in vitro. We observed that this inhibitory action was highly dosage and time-dependent. The maximum inhibitory action was obtained at 15μM (Figure 2A) on culture media.

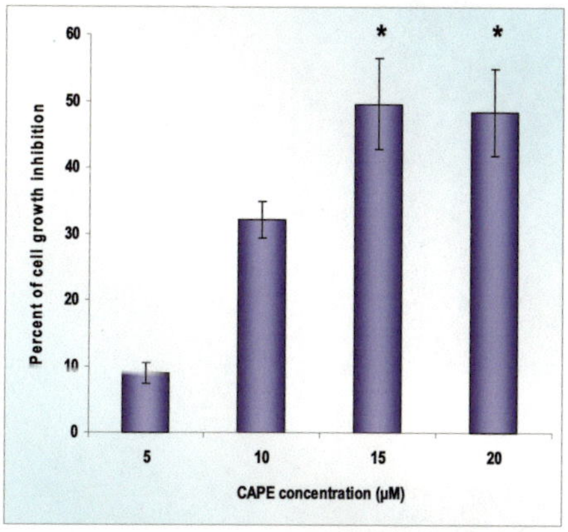

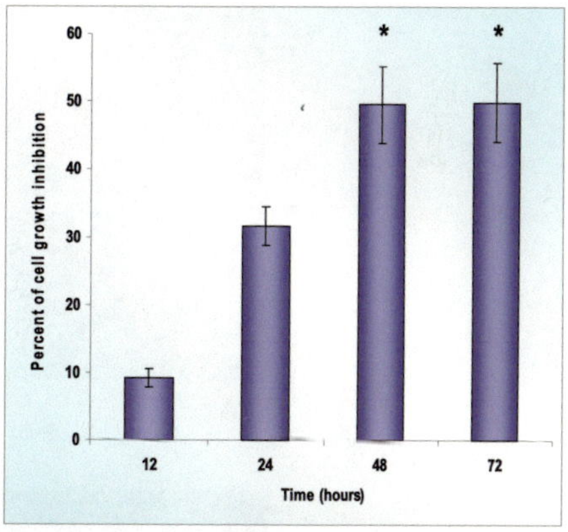

Figure 2. CAPE induced ZR-75-1 cell death (A); cell viability was observed in tumor cells treated with different CAPE concentrations (5, 10, 15 and 20μM), while (B) cells showed maximum alteration of viability at 48 hrs. of incubation, indicating that CAPE induced cell death in a dose and time dependent manner. The results shown in the histogram were the mean ± S.D. Assay was performed in 12 – well plate (2 x 10^6) cells/well, using trypan blue dye for viability detection.

On the other hand, after 48 hours of administration, the percentage of cell death increased significantly to 49.6±6.9 (Figure 1B). No further changes were observed after 72 hours of treatment. To investigate the induced effect of apoptosis on cell viability, we analyzed the DNA fragmentation using DAPI. The nuclear structure exhibited condensation and fragmentation of some nuclei that were caused by 15μM CAPE at 48 hours. Apoptotic cells count significantly increased by 27% as compared to control tumor cells ($P < 0.01$) (Figure 3B) [47].

Additionally, the microscopic examination did not reveal any signs of morphological changes after 12 hours of administration. However, a scattered retraction of the monolayer, vacuoles, and the granulation of the cytoplasm were observed after 24 hours. The alterations were further aggravated after 48 hours. The cells were rounded up. Later, they became phase-dense and formed floating aggregates, which gradually increased in size and most of the cells were detached from the flasks. The cell membranes burst, which was followed by a gradual decrease of the cell count. These changes were not reversible. Transferring the cells into a fresh medium did not alter their state (Figure 4) [47].

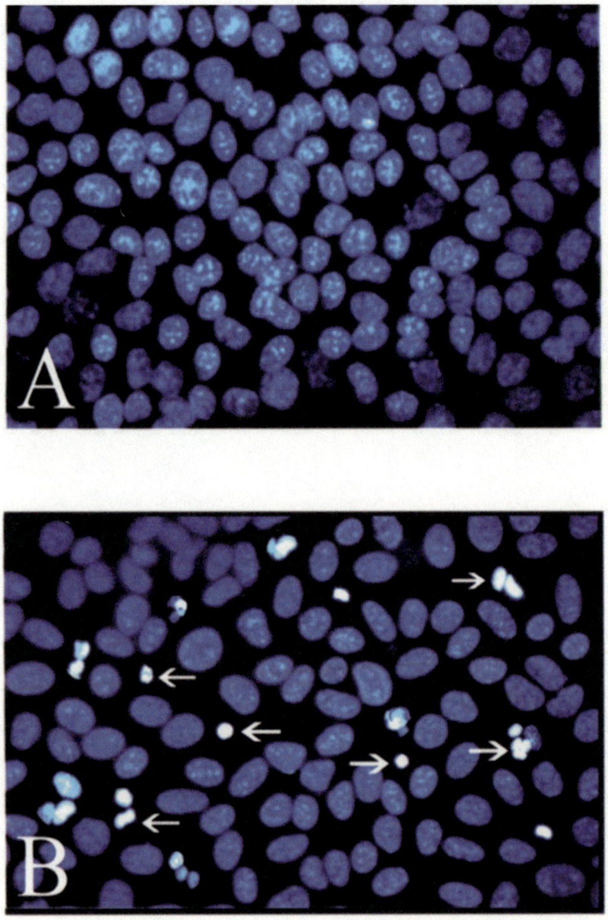

Figure 3. Effect of CAPE on expression of apoptotic cells. (A) ZR-75-1 cells without treatment. (B) Cells were treated with 15μM CAPE for the indicated time of 48 hrs. Condensation and apoptotic bodies were examined by immunofluorescence microscopy. Magnification, X20.

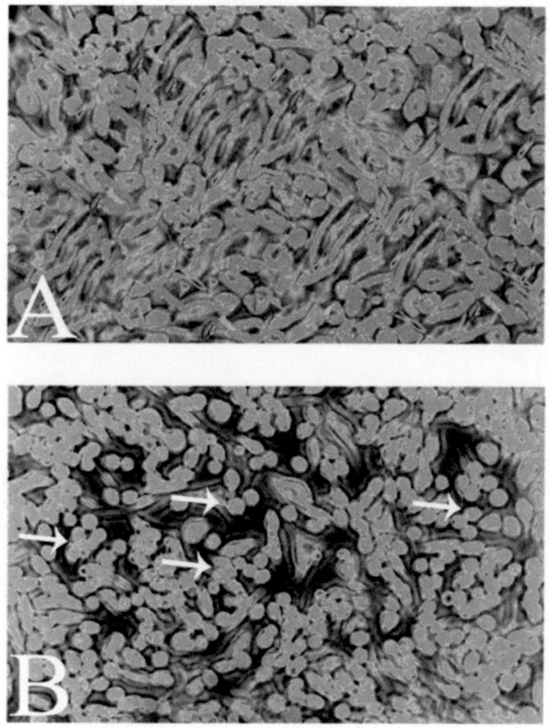

Figure 4. CAPE induced cell detaching (A) ZR-75-1 cells kept without treatment during experiments. (B) 15μM CAPE treatment after 48 hrs. Morphology changes in cells were examined by phase-contrast microscopy. Magnification, X40

2.3. Tumor growth inhibition *in vivo* by CAPE

The effects of CAPE on the survival of mice bearing tumor are shown in figure 5. The median survival time for the untreated group of mice was 21 days. On the other hand, the group of mice bearing tumor and treated with 10mg/kg S.C/ every 5 days had a median survival time of 29 days. Two mice were completely cured. The median survival time of the group treated with 15mg/kg S.C/ every 5 days was found to be 43 days and 3 mice were completely cured. However, those mice treated with 5mg /kg S.C/ every 5 days did not show any remarkable changes in their survival percentage. It has also been observed that giving treatment more than once a week caused sores and increased irritability in the mice, vehicle (1:1/DMSO: NaCl).

We studied the effect of CAPE (15mg/kg S.C/ every 5 days) on the growth of transplanted Ehrlich carcinoma into Swiss mice. The solid tumor volume showed a reduced rate in CAPE-treated mice and appreciably smaller volume (1.9 ± 0.46) mm^3, with respect to the untreated group (3.7 ± 0.82) mm^3. This value was significant ($P < 0.01$). The difference was observed from the beginning of tumor measurement i.e. since the 6th day after tumor implantation to the host, and was maintained until the end of observation (Figure 6). This finding is one of the characteristic effects of anti-tumor drugs. It is also in accordance with the other findings, which suggest that subcutaneous administration of an aqueous crude water-soluble propolis (CWSP) resulted in marked regression of transplanted tumors [48].

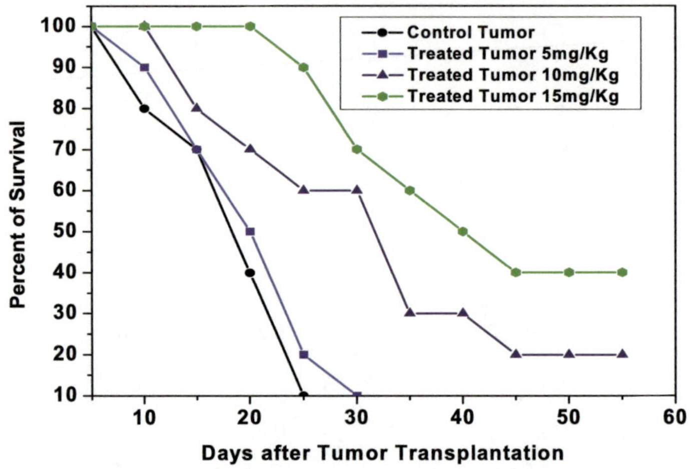

Figure 5. Effect of CAPE treatment on the time of survival for mice bearing solid tumor at different doses compared with untreated group.

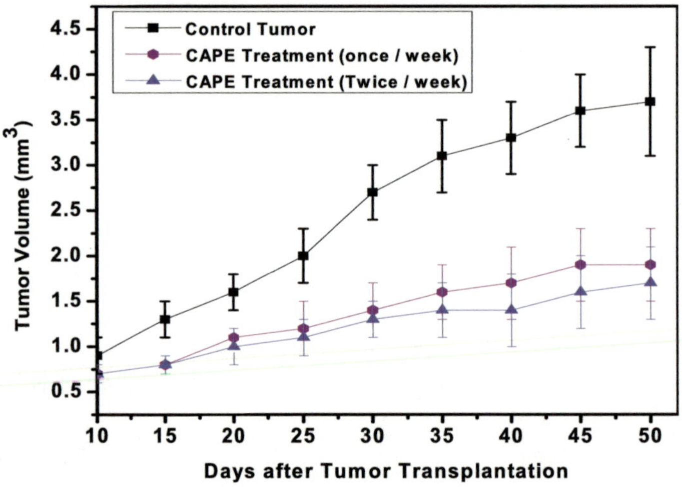

Figure 6. Effect of CAPE (15mg/kg S.C), once/week and twice/week treatment on tumor volume against untreated group of mice. Data represented as mean ± S.D.

The percentage of apoptotic cells with hypodiploid DNA content was determined from DNA histograms. Untreated tumor-bearing mice showed a peak pattern which represented proliferative and high metastatic tumor activity (Figure 7A). However the mice which had their tumor treated at 15mg/kg S.C did not alter the relative size of the peak, but induced a significant parallel shift to less-intense fluorescence (D- area). This decrease in the intensity and shift may be termed as nuclear apoptosis and fragmentation (Figure 7B).

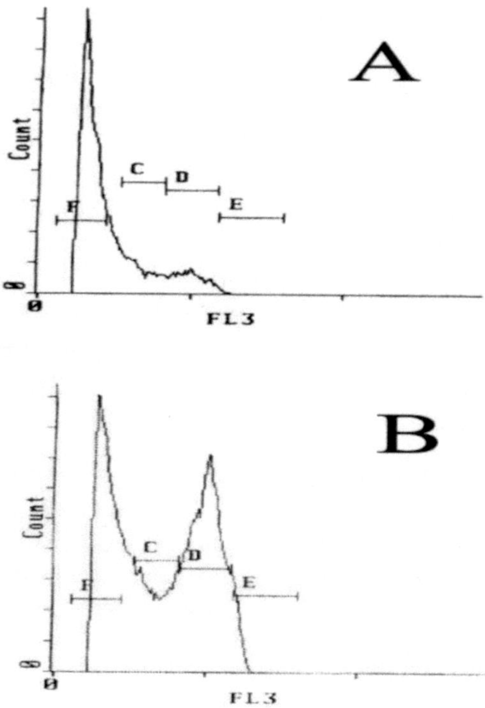

Figure 7. The value in the tumor apoptosis histogram was higher in mice-bearing tumors, which were treated with CAPE (15mg/kg/S.C). (B) as compared to mice-bearing tumors untreated with CAPE (A). The apoptosis was identified by PI staining (D-area) with increased DNA fragmentation [47].

Chung et al., [49] showed that both CA and CAPE selectively inhibit matrix metalloproteinases (MMP) 2 and 9. CAPE inhibited strongly MMPs 2 and 9 with IC_{50} of 2–5μM, while CA required 10–20 μM for such inhibition. In contrast, MMPs 1, 3, 7 and Cathepsin-K were not completely inhibited by either of them. CA and CAPE had a dose-dependent inhibitory effect on the proliferation of HEPG2 cells. In HepG2 cells, CA at the concentration of 200 μg/mL reduced the viability to 61% , while CAPE, at 10 times lower concentration, inhibited the viability to 72% as compared to the respective controls. CAPE and CA suppressed the MMP 9 expression in HepG cells exposed to phorbol 12-myristate 13-acetate (PMA). They also confirmed that CA (20 mg/kg) and CAPE (5mg/kg) repressed the growth of HepG2 tumor xenografts in nude mice as well as liver metastasis when administered subcutaneous or orally. Finally they concluded their observation that CA and its derivative CAPE: (1) inhibited the enzymatic activity of MMP-9 that plays an important role in cancer invasion and metastasis, (2) blocked the invasive potential through the suppression of MMP-9 gene transcription by inhibiting NF-κB function in PMA-stimulated HepG2 cells and (3) suppressed the growth of HepG2 cell xenografts in nude mice. Therefore, these two drugs were reported as strong candidates for treatment of cancer and metastasis via dual mechanisms (dual inhibition of metastasis-specific enzyme activity and gene transcription) [50].

2.4. Regulation of tumor cell proliferation by CAPE

Dysregulated proliferation is one of the major characteristics of tumorigenesis. In normal cells, proliferation is regulated by a delicate balance between growth signals and antigrowth signals. Cancer cells, however, acquire the ability to generate their own growth signals and become insensitive to antigrowth signals [51]. Their growth is controlled by cell cycle regulators at the G1/S-phase boundary, in the S phase, and during the G2/M phases of the cell cycle. A precise set of proteins called cyclins and cyclin-dependent kinases (CDKs) control the progression of cell cycle events. Whereas cyclin binding is required for CDK activity, CDK inhibitors (CKIs) such as p21 and p27 prevent CDK activity and prevent cell cycle progression. The G1-to-S-phase transition also requires cellular v-myc myelocytomatosis viral oncogene homolog (c-Myc), and inhibition of c-Myc expression leads to growth arrest [52,53].

The expression of c-Myc in turn is regulated by cdc25, a phosphatase that activates CDKs. The well-characterized tumor suppressor p53 has been implicated in controlling the G1-to-S-phase transition and in blocking cell cycle progression at the G1 phase in response to DNA damage [54]. A number of genes controlling cell cycle progression, including the CKI p21, are transcribed in a p53-dependent manner [55,56].

Rb is a tumor suppressor retinoblastoma protein that, like p53, functions as a negative regulator of cell growth [57]. Rb inactivation or deletion has been found in many cancers, including retinoblastomas and carcinomas of the lung, breast, bladder, and prostate. By binding to and inhibiting transcription factors such as elongation 2 factor (E2F), which are necessary for S-phase entry, Rb is believed to inhibit cell cycle progression [58]. On the other hand, phosphorylation of Rb (pRb) by CDK/cyclin complexes results in the release of active E2F species to stimulate the transcription of genes involved in DNA synthesis and S-phase progression [59,60].

Currently, a number of inhibitors based on cell cycle regulators, including nutraceuticals, are being developed as therapeutic intervention for cancer prevention. Nutraceuticals have been shown to have potential in cancer prevention for halting cell cycle progression by targeting one or more steps in the cell cycle. Most nutraceuticals prevent the transition of cancer cells from the G1 to S phase. Some of these nutraceuticals act through p53 and some through Rb. Acetyl-keto-beta-boswellic acid was shown to arrest colon cancer cells at the G1 phase, which was associated with decreases in cyclin-D1, cyclin-E, CDK-2, CDK-4, and pRb and an increase in p21[61].

In Ehrlich ascites tumor cells, acetoxychavicol acetate was shown to stimulate the accumulation of tumor cells in the G1 phase of the cell cycle, which was accompanied by a decrease in pRb and an increase in Rb [62]. β-Escin, a triterpene saponin, induced cell cycle arrest at the G1/S phase by inducing p21 and reducing pRb in a p53-independent manner in HT-29 human colon cancer cells [63]. In gastric cancer cells, curcumin was shown to suppress the transition of cells from the G1 to S phase, which was accompanied by a decrease in cyclin-D1 and p21-activated kinase 1 activity [64].

The therapeutic goal of cancer treatment is to induce apoptotic death of cancer cells rather than necrosis due to the deleterious consequences of the latter, which include leakage of lysosomal enzymes to the extracellular media and spawning a substantial inflammatory reaction. Several investigators have demonstrated that CAPE has an anti-proliferative effect and an apoptosis inducing effect against various tumor cell lines. Cavaliere et al., showed that CAPE treatment increased the percentage of cells in G0/G1 and decreased the percentage of cells in S and G2/M phase in addition to its ability to inhibit DNA, RNA, and protein synthesis , thus delaying cell cycle progression to G2/M phase. CAPE also caused high levels of apoptotic cell death of 77.1%, with no signs of significant necrosis in PL104 cells [65]. Also, Wang et al., demonstrated that CAPE treatment was associated with a strong inhibition of proliferation in a dose- and time-dependent manner, along with induction of G0/G1 arrest and apoptosis in HCT116 cells [66].

2.5. Regulation of tumor cell invasion by CAPE

Tumor cell invasion and metastasis are interrelated processes involving cell growth, cell adhesion, cell migration, and proteolytic degradation of tissue barriers such as the extracellular matrix and basement membrane. Several proteolytic enzymes, including MMPs (chiefly MMP-2 and MMP-9) [67,68] and intercellular adhesion molecule (ICAM; chiefly ICAM-1), participate in the degradation of these barriers [69,70]. A number of studies in lung, colon, breast, and pancreatic carcinomas have demonstrated overexpression of MMPs in malignant tissues compared with adjacent normal tissues [71-78]. Apart from MMPs, cysteine proteases [79] and serine proteases [80] such as urokinase-type plasminogen activator (u-PA) have also been involved in the invasion and metastasis of cancer cells. Since both u-PA and u-PA receptor (u-PAR) contain binding sites for NF-κB and activator protein (AP)-1 in their promoter regions [81-83], inhibition of these transcription factors will eventually result in the inhibition of u-PA–u-PAR complex and subsequent suppression of invasive behavior.

Furthermore, Hwang et al. [84] investigated the effect of CAPE on tumor invasion and metastasis in HT 1080 fibrosarcoma cells by determining the regulation of matrix metalloproteinases (MMPs). HT 1080 cells were treated with increasing concentration of CAPE and the m-RNA transcripts of MMP-2 and MMP-9 were analyzed using semi-quantitative RT-PCR. Both MMP- 2 and 9 proteins levels were significantly suppressed in a dose dependent manner. Gelatin zymography also indicated constitutively expressed MMP-2 and 9 proteins in HT 1080 cells, which gradually reduced after treating with CAPE. To further corroborate the down regulation of MMP-2, activation studies of pro-MMP2 were performed using organomercuric compound, 4-aminophenylmercuric acetate (APMA), and the result indicated the down regulation of MMP-2 by CAPE. It has been shown that mRNA levels of tissue inhibitor of matrix metalloproteinases (TIMPs) and membrane type-matrix metalloproteinases (MT-1 MMPs) were also reduced significantly. CAPE also inhibited the cell invasion, cell migration and colony formation of tumor cells. Thus CAPE acts as a vital antimetastatic agent, by inhibiting the metastatic and invasive potential of malignant cells.

2.6. Regulation of tumor cell angiogenesis by CAPE

Angiogenesis, the process during which new blood vessels are formed from preexisting ones, can be classified as either physiological or pathological. Physiological angiogenesis provides a driving force for organ development in ontogeny, is necessary for ovulation, and is a prerequisite for wound healing; pathological angiogenesis occurs during tumor growth at primary and metastatic sites [85]. The angiogenic cascade during tumor development consists of the release of angiogenic factors, binding of angiogenic factors to receptors on endothelial cells (ECs), EC activation, degradation of the basement membrane by proteases, and migration and proliferation of ECs. Adhesion molecules then help to pull the sprouting blood vessels forward, and ECs are finally organized into a network of new blood vessels [86].

The signaling pathway governing tumor angiogenesis is exceedingly complex, involving various angiogenic mediators. The major signaling mediators include VEGF, platelet-derived growth factor, fibroblast growth factors (FGFs), epidermal growth factor, ephrins, angiopoietins, endothelins, integrins, cadherins, and notch [87].

Group Parameters	Normal Group n = 10	Tumor Group n = 10	Treated Group n = 10	P_1	P_2
MMP-9 (ng/ml)	130.9	181.9	142.1	$P < 0.001$	$P < 0.01$
Median Range	79.6 – 166.4	88.2 – 216.1	84.5 – 196.3		
Endostatin (ng/ml)	2.2	1.4	1.9	$P = 0.01$	$P < 0.01$
Median Range	1.1 – 6.3	1.0 – 5.4	1.3 – 9.3		

P1 Tumor group Vs Normal group
P2 Treated group Vs Tumor group

Table 2. Levels of MMP-9 and Endostatin serum in normal mice group, tumor bearing group and treated tumor group.

We found that the untreated mice bearing Ehrlich tumor elicited a highly significant increase of serum MMP-9 level (181.9 ng/ml), which was reduced (142.1 ng/ml) in mice treated with CAPE at a dose of 15mg/kg ($P < 0.01$) close to the normal mice serum level. However, in the untreated mice bearing tumor serum endostatin (sE) was significantly lowered (1.4 ng/ml) compared with the normal mice. In CAPE-treated mice serum endostatin level was significantly higher (1.9 ng/ml) than the serum level in the untreated group (Table 2)[47]. On the other hand, there was a negative correlation between (sMMP-9 and sE) and the total white blood cells (WBCs), hemoglobin (HB) and the platelet count of mice (Table 3)[47]. Based on these findings, we concluded that; the endogenous inhibitor of the angiogenic serum (endostatin) has been shown to be overexpressed, significantly higher in treated mice compared to untreated mice (1.9 ng/ml), and nearly to the value of normal serum mice (Table 2). These findings may help to utilize endostatin itself in the therapy. It also indicates that

CAPE has the potential of an anti-metastatic agent. It may mediate CAPE effects by inhibiting the cell proliferation. The findings of this study are in accordance with Schuch et al. [88] who, claimed that endostatin microbeads significantly inhibit the growth of subcutaneous choloromas in SCID mice as compared to control mice. On the other hand, MMP-9 and endostatin did not correlate with the white blood cells (WBCs), hemoglobin (HB) and platelet count (Table 3). It may be concluded that MMP-9 and endostatin are independent factors.

	HB	WBCs Count	Platelets Count
MMP-9	R= 0.11, ›0.05	R= 0.19, ›0.05	R= 0.24, ›0.05
Endostatin	R= 0.09, ›0.05	R= 0.1, ›0.05	R= 0.04, ›0.05

Table 3. Correlation between investigated angiogenic factors and, hemoglobin (HB), white blood cells count (WBCs) and platelets count in tumor treated mice.

3. Conclusion

These findings obtained suggest that CAPE is a potent agent, which has antioxidant properties. *In vitro* findings support that CAPE could be potentially useful in the control of tumor cell proliferation as well as, an apoptotic-inducing agent. Furthermore, CAPE exhibits anti-metastatic and anti-angiogenic properties. CAPE could be potentially useful in the control of tumor growth in experimental models. Its action is accompanied by the shifting and elevating of the angiostatic and inhibiting angiogenic factors. Finally, it has been demonstrated that CAPE has many biological and pharmacological properties with predictive future applications in human clinical trials.

Author details

Mohamed F. El-Refaei*

Engineering and Biotechnology Institute, Menoufiya University, Sadat City, Egypt
Dept. of Molecular Biology, Institute of Genetic, Menoufia University, Egypt
Faculty of Medicine, Al-Baha University, Al-Baha Province, KSA

Essam A. Mady

Dept. of Biochemistry, Faculty of Science, Ain Shams University, Egypt
Faculty of Medicine, Al-Baha University, Al-Baha Province, KSA

Acknowledgement

The authors wish to express gratitude for Al-Baha University for their support. Deepest gratitude is also due to the Dean and the staff members, faculty of Medicine, Al-Baha University, KSA.

* Corresponding Author

4. References

[1] Hanahan D, Weinberg RA (2000) The hallmarks of cancer. Cell. J.100(1) :57–70.
[2] Bray F, Moller B (2006) Predicting the future burden of cancer. Nat Rev Can.J.6: 63–74.
[3] Hanahan D, Weinberg RA (2011) The hallmarks of cancer: the next generation.. Cell. J . 4;144(5):646-674.
[4] Vincent TL, Gatenby RA (2008) An evolutionary model for initiation, promotion, and progression in carcinogenesis. Int J Oncol 32(4): 729-737.
[5] Anand P, Sundaram C, Jhurani S, Kunnumakkara AB, Aggarwal BB(2008) Curcumin and cancer: An "old-age" disease with an "age-old" solution. CanLet J. 267:133–164.
[6] Vogelstein B, Kinzler KW (2004) Cancer genes and the pathways they control. Nat Med. J .10:789–799.
[7] Aggarwal BB, Vijayalekshmi RV, Sung B (2009) Targeting inflammatory pathways for prevention and therapy of cancer: short-term friend, longterm foe. Clin Can Res. J .15: 425–430.
[8] Sporn MB, Newton DL (1979) "Chemoprevention of cancer with retinoids," *Feder Proce.* J . 38(11) 2528–2534.
[9] Kelloff GJ (1999) "Perspectives on cancer chemoprevention research and drug development" *Adva in CanRes.*J.78:320–334.
[10] Kelloff, GJ, Boone CW (1994) Eds., "Cancer chemopreventive agents: drug development status and future prospects *Cell Biochem.* J . 20:1–303.
[11] Kelloff GJ, Hawk ET, Sigman CC (2004) Eds., *Cancer Chemoprevention: Prom Can Chemop Ag* vol. 1, Humana Press, Totowa, NJ, USA.
[12] Ferguson LR (1994) "Antimutagens as cancer chemopreventive agents in the diet," *Mut Res.*j. 307(1) 395–410.
[13] Ferguson LR, Philpott M, Karunasinghe N (2004) "Dietary cancer and prevention using antimutagens," *Toxico.* J .198(1–3):147–159.
[14] Surh YJ, (2003) "Cancer chemoprevention with dietary phytochemicals,"*Nat Rev Can.* J .3(10):768–780.
[15] Amiot MJ, Aubert S, Gonnet M, Tacchini M, (1989) "Les compos´es ph´enoliques des miels: ´etude pr´eliminaire sur l'identifi cation et la quantifi cation par familles," *Apidologie.* J .20:115–125.
[16] World Wide Wounds, (2002) "Honey as a topical antibacterial agent for treatment of infected wounds,"http://www.worldwidewounds.com/2001/november/Molan/ honey-as-topical agent.html.
[17] Orsolic N, Terzic S, Mihaljevic Z, Sver L, basic I (2005) Effects of local administration of propolis and its polyphenolic compounds on tumor formation and growth. Biol Pharm Bull. J . 28:1928-1933.
[18] Carrasco-Legleu CE, Márquez-Rosado L, Fattel-Fazenda S, Arce-Popoca E et al., (2004) Chemoprotective effect of caffeic acid phenethyl ester on promotion in a medium-term rat hepatocarcinogenesis assay. Int J Can.. 10;108(4):488-92.
[19] Mahmoud NN, Carothers AM, Grunberger D, Bilinski RT, Churchill MR, Martucci C, et al.,(2000) Plant phenolics decrease intestinal tumors in an animal model of familial adenomatous polyposis.Carcinog. 21(5):921-927.

[20] Huang MT, Ma W, Yen P, Xie JG, Han J, Frenkel K, Grunberger D, Conney AH (1996) Inhibitory effects of caffeic acid phenethyl ester (CAPE) on 12-O-tetradecanoylphorbol-13-acetate-induced tumor promotion in mouse skin and the synthesis of DNA, RNA and protein in HeLa cells. Carcinog .17(4):761-765.

[21] Carrasco-Legleu CE, Sánchez-Pérez Y, Márquez-Rosado L et al., (2006) A single dose of caffeic acid phenethyl ester prevents initiation in a medium-term rat hepatocarcinogenesis model. W Gastroen . J .14;12(42):6779-85.

[22] Wu J, Omene C, Karkoszka J, Bosland M, Eckard J, Klein CB, Frenkel K (2011) Caffeic acid phenethyl ester (CAPE), derived from a honeybee product propolis, exhibits a diversity of anti-tumor effects in pre-clinical models of human breast cancer.Cancer Lett. 1;308(1):43-53.

[23] Omene CO, Wu J, Frenkel K (2012) Caffeic Acid Phenethyl Ester (CAPE) derived from propolis, a honeybee product, inhibits growth of breast cancer stem cells. Invest. New D. J.30(4):1279-1288.

[24] Subash C,Gupta Ji, Hye Kim, Sahdeo Prasad, Bharat B, Aggarwal BB (2010) Regulation of survival, proliferation, invasion, angiogenesis, and metastasis of tumor cells through modulation of inflammatory pathways by nutraceuticals. Can. Meta. J .29(3): 405–434.

[25] Aggarwal BB, Gehlot P (2009) Inflammation and cancer: How friendly is the relationship for cancer patients? Current Opin. in Pharm.. J . 9:351–369.

[26] Coussens LM, Werb Z (2002) Inflammation and cancer. Nat.. J . 420: 860–867.

[27] Dey A, Tergaonkar V, Lane DP. (2008) Double-edged swords as cancer therapeutics: simultaneously targeting p53 and NF-kappaB pathways. *Nat. Rev. D. Disc. 7, 1031-1040.*

[28] Kabrun N, Enrietto PJ (1994) The Rel family of proteins in oncogenesis and differentiation. Seminars in Can. Biol. 5:103–112.

[29] Ghosh S, Karin M (2002) Missing pieces in the NF-kappaB puzzle. Cell. J . 109(Suppl):S81–S96.

[30] Hussain SP, Hofseth LJ, Harris CC (2003) Radical causes of cancer. Nat. Rev. J .3: 276–285

[31] Gupta SC, Sundaram C, Reuter S, Aggarwal BB (2010) . Inhibiting NF- kappaB activation by small molecules as a therapeutic strategy. Bioch. et Bioph. Act.. J .1799(10-12):775-787.

[32] de Visser KE, Eichten A, Coussens LM (2006) Paradoxical roles of the immune system during cancer development. Nat. Rev Can.. J .6: 24–37.

[33] Chaturvedi MM, Kumar A, Darnay BG, Chainy GB, Agarwal S, Aggarwal BB(1997) Sanguinarine (pseudochelerythrine) is a potent inhibitor of NF-kappaB activation, IkappaBalpha phosphorylation, and degradation. Biol. Chem.. J .272:30129–30134.

[34] Kumar A, Dhawan S, Aggarwal BB. (1998) Emodin (3-methyl-1,6,8-trihydroxyanthraquinone) inhibits TNF-induced NF-kappaB activation, IkappaB degradation, and expression of cell surface adhesion proteins in human vascular endothelial cells. Onco. ;17:913–918.

[35] Jing Y, Yang J, Wang Y, Li H, Chen Y, Hu Q, et al. (2006) Alteration of subcellular redox equilibrium and the consequent oxidative modification of nuclear factor kappaB are critical for anticancer cytotoxicity by emodin, a reactive oxygen species-producing agent. Free Radic. Biol. & Med.. J .40:2183–2197.

[36] Natarajan K, Singh S, Burke T Jr TR, Grunberger D Aggarwal BB (1996) "Caffeic acid phenethyl ester is a potent and specific inhibitor of activation of nuclear transcription factor NF-κB," *Proce. of the Nati.Acad. of Sci.of theUSA.* 93(17)9090–9095.
[37] Abdel-Latif MM, Windle HJ, El Homasany BS, Sabra K, Kelleher D (2005). Caffeic acid phenethyl ester modulates Helicobacter pylori-induced nuclear factor-kappa B and activator protein-1 expression in gastric epithelial cells. B J. of Pharm .146: 1139–1147.
[38] Moncada S, Palmer RMJ, Higgs EA (1991) Nitric oxide: physiology, pathophysiology, and pharmacology. Pharm. Rev J . 43:109—142.
[39] Kou PC, Schroeder RA (1995) The emerging multifacated roles of nitric oxide.Annal. Sur. J .221:220—235.
[40] Nagaoka T, Banskota AH, Tezuka Y, Midorikawa K, Matsushige K, Kadota S (2003) Caffeic acid phenethyl ester (CAPE) analogues: potent nitric oxide inhibitors from the Netherlands propolis. *Biol. Pharm. Bull.* J . 26: (4) 487—491.
[41] Steller H (1995) Mechanisms and genes of cellular suicide. Sci.. J . 267:1445–1449.
[42] Green DR (2000) Apoptotic pathways: Paper wraps stone blunts scissors. Cell. J.102:1–4.
[43] Meier P, Finch A, Evan G (2000) Apoptosis in development. Nat.. J . 407:796–801.
[44] Wang S, Yang D, Lippman ME (2003) Targeting Bcl-2 and Bcl-XL with nonpeptidic small-molecule antagonists. Seminars in Onco.. 30:133–142.
[45] Ambrosini G, Adida C, Altieri DC (1997) A novel anti-apoptosis gene, survivin, expressed in cancer and lymphoma. Nat. Med..J. .3:917–921.
[46] Engel L, Young N (1978) Human breast carcinoma cells in continuous culture: a review. Can. Res. 38: 4327-4339.
[47] El-Refaei M, El-Naa M (2010) Inhibitory effect of caffeic acid phenethyl ester on mice bearing tumor involving angiostatic and apoptotic activities. Chemi Biologi Interact 186:152-156. [48] Suzuki I, Hayashi I, Takaki T, Groveman D, Fujimiya Y (2002) Antitumor and Anticytopenic Effects of Aqueous Extracts of Propolis in Combination with Chemotherapeutic Agents. Can. Bioth.y & Radiopharmac., 17:553-562.
[48] Chung TW, Moon SK, Chang YC et al., (2004) "Novel and therapeutic effect of caffeic acid and caffeic acid phenyl ester on hepatocarcinoma cells: complete regression of hepatoma growth and metastasis by dual mechanism," *The FASEB.* J .18(14):1670–1681.
[49] Ryan KM, Birnie GD (1987) Deregulated expression of c-Myc has been implicated in a number of human malignancies. Myc oncogenes: The enigmatic family. Nat.. J . 328:445–449.
[50] Hanahan D, Weinberg RA (2000) The hallmarks of cancer. Cell J;100:57–70.
[51] Heikkila R, Schwab G, Wickstrom E, Loke SL, Pluznik DH et al., (1987) A c-myc antisense oligodeoxynucleotide inhibits entry into S phase but not progress from G0 to G1 Nat. J.. 5;328(6129):445-449.
[52] Evan GI, Littlewood TD (1993) The role of c-myc in cell growth. Curr. Opin. in Gen. & Dev..3:44–49.
[53] Kuerbitz SJ, Plunkett BS, Walsh WV, Kastan MB (1992) Wild-type p53 is a cell cycle checkpoint determinant following irradiation. Proc. of the Nat. Acad. of Sci. of the USA. 89:7491–7495.
[54] Dulic V, Kaufmann WK, Wilson SJ, Tlsty TD, Lees E, Harper JW, et al.(1994) p53-dependent inhibition of cyclin-dependent kinase activities in human fibroblasts during radiation-induced G1 arrest. Cell. J . 76:1013–1023.

[55] El-Deiry WS, Tokino T, Velculescu VE, Levy DB, Parsons R, Trent JM (1993) WAF1, a potential mediator of p53 tumor suppression. Cell. J . 75:817–825.

[56] Weinberg RA (1995) The retinoblastoma protein and cell cycle control. Cell .J. 81:323–330.

[57] King KL, Cidlowski JA (1998) Cell cycle regulation and apoptosis. Ann. Rev. of Phys. 60:601–617.

[58] Hiebert SW (1993) Regions of the retinoblastoma gene product required for its interaction with the E2F transcription factor are necessary for E2 promoter repression and pRb-mediated growth suppression. Mol.and Cell. Biol. 13:3384–3391.

[59] Qian Y, Luckey C, Horton L, Esser M, Templeton DJ (1992) Biological function of the retinoblastoma protein requires distinct domains for hyperphosphorylation and transcription factor binding. Mol. Cell Biol. J. 12(12): 5363–5372.

[60] Liu JJ, Huang B, Hooi SC (2006) Acetyl-keto-beta-boswellic acid inhibits cellular proliferation through a p21-dependent pathway in colon cancer cells. B. J. of Pharm.. J. 148:1099– 1107.

[61] Xu S, Kojima-Yuasa A, Azuma H, Huang X, Norikura T, Kennedy DO, et al.(2008) (1′S)-Acetoxychavicol acetate and its enantiomer inhibit tumor cells proliferation via different mechanisms. Chem. Biol. Interact.172:216–223.

[62] Patlolla JM, Raju J, Swamy MV, Rao CV (2006) Beta-escin inhibits colonic aberrant crypt foci formation in rats and regulates the cell cycle growth by inducing p21(waf1/cip1) in colon cancer cells Mol. Can. Therapeu.. 5:1459–1466.

[63] Cai XZ, Wang J, Li XD, Wang GL, Liu FN, Cheng MS, et al.(2009) Curcumin suppresses proliferation and invasion in human gastric cancer cells by downregulation of PAK1 activity and cyclin D1 expression. Can. Biol. & Ther 8:1360–1368.

[64] Cavaliere V, Papademetrio DL, Lorenzetti M, Valva P, Preciado MV, Gargallo P, Larripa I, Monreal MB, et al. (2009) Caffeic Acid Phenylethyl Ester and MG-132 Have Apoptotic and Antiproliferative Effects on Leukemic Cells But Not on Normal Mononuclear Cells. Transl Oncol. ;2(1):46-58.

[65] Wang D, Xiang DB, He YJ, Li ZP, Wu XH, Mou JH, Xiao HL, Zhang QH (2005) Effect of caffeic acid phenethyl ester on proliferation and apoptosis of colorectal cancer cells in vitro. Wor. J Gastro. 14;11(26):4008-4012

[66] Sternlicht MD, Werb Z (2001) How matrix metalloproteinases regulate cell behavior. Annual Review of Cell and Dev. Biol.. 17:463–516.

[67] Jiang MC, Liao CF, Lee PH (2001) Aspirin inhibits matrix metalloproteinase-2 activity, increases Ecadherin production, and inhibits in vitro invasion of tumor cells. Bioch. and Bioph. Res. Commu.. 282:671–677.

[68] Aimes RT, Quigley JP (1995) Matrix metalloproteinase-2 is an interstitial collagenase. Inhibitor-free enzyme catalyzes the cleavage of collagen fibrils and soluble native type I collagen generating the specific 3/4- and 1/4-length fragments. Biol.Chem. J . 270:5872– 5876.

[69] Kleiner DE Jr, Stetler-Stevenson WG (1993) Structural biochemistry and activation of matrix metalloproteases. Current Opinion in Cell Bio. ;5:891–897.

[70] Lochter A, Bissell MJ (1999) An odyssey from breast to bone: Multi-step control of mammary metastases and osteolysis by matrix metalloproteinases. APMIS 107:128–136.

[71] Davidson B, Goldberg I, Liokumovich P, Kopolovic J, Gotlieb WH et al., (1998) Expression of metalloproteinases and their inhibitors in adenocarcinoma of the uterine cervix.Intern. J. of Gyn. Path..17:295–301.

[72] Kugler A, Hemmerlein B, Thelen P, Kallerhoff M, Radzun HJ, Ringert RH(1998) Expression of metalloproteinase 2 and 9 and their inhibitors in renal cell carcinoma. J d'Urologie.160:1914–1918.

[73] Hashimoto K, Kihira Y, Matuo Y, Usui T (1998) Expression of matrix metalloproteinase-7 and tissue inhibitor of metalloproteinase-1 in human prostate. J d'Urologie. 160:1872–1876.

[74] Sutinen M, Kainulainen T, Hurskainen T, Vesterlund E, Alexander JP, Overall CM, et al.(1998) Expression of matrix metalloproteinases (MMP-1 and -2) and their inhibitors (TIMP-1, -2 and -3) in oral lichen planus, dysplasia, squamous cell carcinoma and lymph node metastasis. B. J. of Can.. 77:2239–2245.

[75] Gonzalez-Avila G, Iturria C, Vadillo F, Teran L, Selman M, Perez-Tamayo R (1998) 72-kD (MMP-2) and 92-kD (MMP-9) type IV collagenase production and activity in different histologic types of lung cancer cells. Pathob. J. . 66:5–16.

[76] Nawrocki B, Polette M, Marchand V, Monteau M, Gillery P, Tournier JM, et al. (1997) Expression of matrix metalloproteinases and their inhibitors in human bronchopulmonary carcinomas: Quantificative and morphological analyses. Intern. J.of Can.. 72:556–564.

[77] Bramhall SR (1997) The matrix metalloproteinases and their inhibitors in pancreatic cancer. From molecular science to a clinical application. International Journal of Pancreatology 21:1–12.

[78] Chapman HA, Riese RJ, Shi GP (1997) Emerging roles for cysteine proteases in human biology. Ann. Rev. of Phys.. 59:63–88.

[79] Andreasen PA, Kjoller L, Christensen L, Duffy MJ (1997) The urokinase-type plasminogen activator system in cancer metastasis: A review. Intern.J. of Can.. 72:1–22.

[80] Nerlov C, Rorth P, Blasi F, Johnsen M (1991) Essential AP-1 and PEA3 binding elements in the human urokinase enhancer display cell type-specific activity. Onco.6:1583–1592.

[81] Lengyel E, Gum R, Stepp E, Juarez J, Wang H, Boyd D (1996) Regulation of urokinase-type plasminogen activator expression by an ERK1-dependent signaling pathway in a squamous cell carcinoma cell line. J. of Cell.Bio. 61:430–443.

[82] Wang Y (2001) The role and regulation of urokinase-type plasminogen activator receptor gene expression in cancer invasion and metastasis. Medi. Res. Rev.. 21:146–170.

[83] Hwang HJ, Park HJ, Chung HJ, et al. (2006) "Inhibitory effects of caffeic acid phenethyl ester on cancer cell metastasis mediated by the down-regulation of matrix metalloproteinase expression in human HT1080 fibrosarcoma cells," J. of Nut. Bio..17(5): 356–362.

[84] Folkman J (2007) Angiogenesis: An organizing principle for drug discovery? Nature Reviews. Drug Disc. 6:273–286.

[85] Fan TP, Yeh JC, Leung KW, Yue PY, Wong RN (2006) Angiogenesis: From plants to blood vessels. Trends in Pharma. Sci.. 27:297–309.

[86] Gordon MS, Mendelson DS, Kato G (2010) Tumor angiogenesis and novel antiangiogenic strategies. Intern. J. of Can.. 126:1777–1787.

[87] Schuch G, Oliveira-Ferrer L, Loges S, Laack E, Bokemeyer C, Hossfeld DK, Fiedler W, Ergun S. (2005) Antiangiogenic treatment with endostatin inhibits progression of AML in vivo.Leuk.;19(8):1312-1317.